Dealing with Drugs

New Histories of Risk and Benefit

Edited by
Nils Kessel, Joseph M. Gabriel, and
David Herzberg

UNIVERSITY OF ROCHESTER PRESS

First published 2026

University of Rochester Press
www.urpress.com
and Boydell & Brewer Limited
www.boydellandbrewer.com

Our Authorised Representative for product safety in the EU is Easy Access System Europe – Mustamäe tee 50, 10621 Tallinn, Estonia, gpsr.requests@easproject.com

ISBN-13: 978-1-64825-169-6
ISSN: 1526-2715

Library of Congress Cataloging-in-Publication Data
CIP data is available from the Library of Congress.

Dealing with Drugs

Rochester Studies in Medical History

Senior Editor: Christopher Crenner
Professor and Chair, History and Philosophy of Medicine
University of Kansas Medical Center

ISSN 1526-2715

Recent Titles in the Series

Children's Health and Urban Ecology in England, 1885–1919
Jim Harris

Putting Plastic Surgery on Paper: How Art and Archives Defined Second World War Reconstructive Surgery in Britain
Christine Slobogin

Rethinking the Public Fetus: Historical Perspectives on the Visual Culture of Pregnancy
Edited by Elisabet Björklund and Solveig Jülich

Benjamin Rush, Civic Health, and Human Illness in the Early American Republic
Sarah E. Naramore

Reimagining Psychiatric Epidemiology in a Global Frame: Toward a Social and Conceptual History
Edited by Anne M. Lovell and Gerald M. Oppenheimer

Cancer, Research, and Educational Film at Midcentury: The Making of the Movie Challenge: Science Against Cancer
David Cantor

The Filth Disease: Typhoid Fever and the Practices of Epidemiology in Victorian England
Jacob Steere-Williams

Sickness in the Workhouse: Poor Law Medical Care in Provincial England, 1834–1914
Alistair Ritch

A complete list of titles in the Rochester Studies in Medical History Series may be found on our website, www.urpress.com.

Contents

Introduction[1]

Nils Kessel, Joseph M. Gabriel, and David Herzberg

Dealing with Drugs: New Histories of Risk and Benefit brings together an interdisciplinary group of scholars to explore two framing concepts in the history of these powerful substances: risk and benefit. This approach enables us to tell new stories about a set of objects that has often been defined in European and North American historiography through categorizations of similarity and difference: medicines (or "pharmaceuticals") assumed to share a set of conditions and dynamics separate from intoxicants (or "drugs") that follow a different shared logic – with both seemingly disconnected from other products such as tobacco, alcohol, and caffeine. Such categorizations have, of course, been persuasively critiqued by many scholars (some of whom are represented in this collection). This volume is an effort to take a next step: we seek to move beyond both critique and exposé of internal contradictions and instead build new stories about medicines and drugs that reckon with, but are not defined or constrained by, this inherited architecture of categorization. "Risk" and "benefit" already factor in the history and historiography of all these substances. Yet foregrounding these two concepts, and how they have changed over time, allows us to tell new stories that cut across inherited categories, revealing similarities and continuities without ignoring the material and discursive significance of differences and ruptures.

Historicizing Risk and Benefit

Risk and benefit are, of course, themselves historically contingent categories that shape the world in which we currently live. We cannot apply them as if

1 We are particularly grateful to the following institutions for their support: Laboratoire SAGE (UMR 7363), Université de Strasbourg; Université de Strasbourg Scientific excellence program (IDEX) "Attractivité" (Project CONSENS, 2019–2021); ERC Advanced Grant "Body Capital" (2016–2022, ID: 694817); ANR Research Project "MEDICI. Les conflits d'intérêts dans le domaine du médicament"(2016–2019, ANR 16-CE26-0007), Florida State University College of Medicine; College of Arts and Sciences, University at Buffalo, State University of New York.

they do not carry their own inherited meanings. On the one hand, narratives about risk and benefit have been historically mobilized to create, reinforce, reshape, and occasionally challenge or even transcend the medicine/drug divide by a diverse range of people pursuing many different goals. On the other hand, risk and benefit are also concepts that remain analytically useful for both drug scholars and policymakers searching for alternative frameworks for governing such useful and dangerous products. Employing these concepts means carefully attending to these past and present uses.

Contemporary ideas about risk and benefit grow, as Ian Hacking put it, out of the "taming of chance" since the eighteenth century through the development of quantitative and statistical scientific methods and forms of reasoning.[2] Over the past several decades, the conceptual and practical utility of efforts to calculate risk have led to sustained scholarly attention, including a wealth of sociological, philosophical, historical, and anthropological research. This scholarly creativity has resulted in a series of now-canonical works and a large amount of scholarship on topics such as disasters and accidents, safety and security, and the social and technological production of knowledge, ignorance, and uncertainty. The transformation of risk from a possibility of danger to a calculable probability of a specific danger has been directly linked to scientific, epistemic, and political practices directed toward a wide variety of goals, including efforts to predict and mitigate the harms of disasters and other large-scale events; efforts to regulate the supply of food, pesticides, and other goods; and both industry profitability and the mitigation of legal and financial exposure within business organizations.[3] By show-

2 Ian Hacking, *The Taming of Chance* (Cambridge University Press, 1990).

3 Classic accounts include Thomas Schlich and Ulrich Tröhler, eds., *The Risks of Medical Innovation: Risk Perception and Assessment in Historical Context* (Routledge, 2004); Anthony Giddens, "Risk and responsibility," *The Modern Law Review* 62 (1999): 1–10; Ulrich Beck, *Risk Society: Towards a New Modernity* (SAGE Publications, 1992), 1–10; Mary Douglas and Aaron Wildavsky, *Risk and Culture: An Essay on the Selection of Technological and Environmental Dangers* (University of California Press, 1983). Studies of risk and disasters include but are not limited to Soraya Boudia and Nathalie Jas, eds., *Risk and Risk Society in Historical Perspective*, special issue of *History and Technology* 23, no. 4 (2007); Soraya Boudia and Emmanuel Henry, eds., *La mondialisation des risques: Une histoire politique et transnationale des risques sanitaires et environnementaux* (Presses universitaires de Rennes, 2015); Scott Gabriel Knowles, *The Disaster Experts: Mastering Risk in Modern America* (University of Pennsylvania Press, 2012); Kim Fortun, *Advocacy after Bhopal: Environmentalism, Disaster, New Global Orders* (University of Chicago Press, 2009). Studies of safety and security preparedness include Nicolas Sternsdorff-Cisterna, *Food Safety after Fukushima: Scientific Citizenship and the Politics of Risk* (University of Hawaii Press, 2018); Andrew Lakoff, *Unprepared:*

ing that "risk" evaluation by elite experts is not politically neutral but rather a messy way of integrating and omitting dimensions of technological realities, these studies have challenged older frameworks that essentialized risk as a naturally existing truth lying beneath conflicting human perceptions.[4]

Considerations of risk are also ubiquitous in the historiography of medicines and drugs, including work on the history of controlled clinical trials, histories of public health disasters caused by pharmaceuticals such as elixir sulfanilamide and thalidomide, and studies that link shifting ideas about risk to notions of individual and collective health.[5] Much of this rich literature

---

Global Health in a Time of Emergency (University of California Press, 2017). On the production of ignorance and uncertainty, see Janet Kourany and Martin Carrier, eds., *Science and the Production of Ignorance: When the Quest for Knowledge is Thwarted* (MIT Press, 2020); Naomi Oreskes and Erik M. Conway, *Merchants of Doubt: How a Handful of Scientists Obscured the Truth on Issues from Tobacco Smoke to Global Warming* (Bloomsbury Publishing USA, 2011); Robert Proctor and Londa L. Schiebinger, *Agnotology: The Making and Unmaking of Ignorance* (Stanford University Press, 2008); Stefan Böschen, Karen Kastenhofer, Luitgard Marschall, Ina Rust, Jens Soentgen, and Peter Wehling, "Scientific cultures of non-knowledge in the controversy over genetically modified organisms (GMO): the cases of molecular biology and ecology," *GAIA-Ecological Perspectives for Science and Society* 15, no. 4 (2006): 294–301. On the history of risk management in business, see Phil Kelly, "The evolution of risk management thinking in organizations," in *The Routledge Companion to Risk, Crisis and Security in Business*, ed. Kurt J. Engemann (Routledge, 2018), 20–46; G. Neil Crockford, "The bibliography and history of risk management: Some preliminary observations," *Geneva Papers on Risk and Insurance* 7, no. 23 (1982): 169–79.

4 For examples, see Douglas and Wildavsky, *Risk and Culture*, 9. Thomas Schlich, "Risk and Medical Innovation: A Historical Perspective" in *Risks of Medical Innovation*, ed. Schlich and Tröhler, 16.

5 On the history of randomized controlled trials, see Peter Keating and Alberto Cambrosio, *Cancer on Trial: Oncology as a New Style of Practice* (University of Chicago Press, 2019); Scott H. Podolsky, *The Antibiotic Era: Reform, Resistance, and the Pursuit of a Rational Therapeutics* (Johns Hopkins University Press, 2015); Linda Bryder, "The Medical Research Council and treatments for tuberculosis before streptomycin," *Journal of the Royal Society of Medicine* 107, no. 10 (2014): 409–15; Joseph M. Gabriel, "The testing of sanocrysin: science, profit, and innovation in clinical trial design, 1926–31," *Journal of the History of Medicine and Allied Sciences* 69, no. 4 (2014): 604–632; Ted J. Kaptchuk, "Intentional ignorance: a history of blind assessment and placebo controls in medicine," *Bulletin of the History of Medicine* 72, no. 3 (1998): 389–433; Harry M. Marks, *The Progress of Experiment: Science and Therapeutic Reform in the United States, 1900–1990* (Cambridge University Press, 1997). Studies of risk and notions of individual and public health

is based on the relatively narrow conception of risk developed by biomedical experts and other actors with scientific and technical expertise. As Thomas Schlich notes in the influential 2006 anthology *The Risks of Medical Innovation*, "using the notion of 'risk' implies a specific strategy for dealing with uncertainty, based on calculation of probabilities."[6] This concept of risk as a calculated uncertainty that is open to human intervention has deep historical roots, but it also differs from other ways of understanding danger and mitigating its effects that have their own deep histories. We cannot use risk as if it were a timeless, universal analytical tool. In this volume we therefore understand "risk" as a geographically and temporally situated experience of potential danger, one that has developed distinctive forms in the regional context of Europe and North America. This potential is sometimes – but not always – formally calculated by different groups of actors occupying different social, institutional, and epistemic positions.

We take the same approach to "benefit," a much less historiographically or theoretically developed concept. The concept of benefit, in the sense of an expected positive result from the consumption of a substance, has appeared in both "pharmaceutical" and "drug" contexts – although in somewhat different ways. For pharmaceuticals, "benefit" is often embedded in contexts of evaluation, promotion, and therapeutic utility with respect to diagnosis. As the history and sociology of the valuation and evaluation of medicines have shown, processes for determining and defining this specific type of benefit have evolved over time.[7] Indeed, there is a growing body of scholarship on pharmaceutical evaluation in a wide variety of fields. Much of the literature

---

include Nike Ayo, "Understanding health promotion in a neoliberal climate and the making of health conscious citizens," *Critical Public Health* 22, no. 1 (2012): 99–105; Jeremy A. Greene, *Prescribing By Numbers: Drugs and the Definition of Disease* (Johns Hopkins University Press, 2007); Alan Petersen and Deborah Lupton, *The New Public Health: Health and Self in the Age of Risk* (Sage Publications, 2000).

6 Schlich, "Risk and Medical Innovation," 1.

7 In French economic sociologist François Vatin's work, a linguistic distinction is made between valorization (*valorisation*) and evaluation (*évaluation*), in order to show how evaluation practices participate all over the valuation process: "All along the chain of production, valorization is present in acts of evaluation, in that they are provisional modalities for establishing a value that is under construction." This is particularly true for medicines for which the value is not merely based on commercial success but also on scientific "value," therapeutic comparative benefit of efficacy or, in the contrary, comparative benefit of accumulated knowledge about risks. François Vatin, "Valuation as Evaluating and Valorizing," *Valuation Studies* 1, no. 1 (2013): 31–50.

on pharmaceutical risk cited previously either implicitly or explicitly pairs sciences of risk with sciences of (therapeutic) benefit. A central area of focus is the mechanisms of evaluation and how those who propose or implement them – often elite figures in medicine, industry, or policymaking – recognize these as dynamic arenas of epistemological and political struggle. Key strands in this focus include the development and institutionalization of evaluative technological settings (e.g., clinical trials) to ascertain therapeutic efficacy; the development of marketing and promotional systems that expand and promote efficacy; and disputes about the reliability, veracity, and intent of these technologies.[8]

Notably absent from the literature on the mechanisms of evaluation are a wide swath of benefits that people have sometimes derived from the use of medicines outside the context of the formal, medically sanctioned pursuit of efficacy in treatment of a diagnosed illness. Such benefits have ranged from physical and psychological betterment, including performance enhancement

8 On the complexity of stabilizing "benefit," see Magaly Tornay, *Zugriffe auf das Ich. Psychoaktive Stoffe und Personenkonzepte in der Schweiz, 1945 bis 1980* (Mohr Siebeck, 2018); Viola Balz, *Zwischen Wirkung und Erfahrung – eine Geschichte der Psychopharmaka. Neuroleptika in der Bundesrepublik Deutschland, 1950–1980* (Transcript, 2010). Examples of work on evaluation include Jonathan Simon and Christoph Gradmann, eds., *Evaluating and Standardizing Therapeutic Agents, 1890–1950* (Palgrave Macmillan, 2010); Jean-Paul Gaudillière and Volker Hess, eds., *Ways of Regulating Drugs in the 19th and 20th Centuries* (Palgrave Macmillan UK, 2013); Maurice Cassier, *Il y a des alternatives. Une autre histoire des medicaments, XIX–XXIe siècles* (Éditions du Seuil, 2023). For examples of work on the relationship between pharmaceutical marketing and clinical trials, among other aspects of drug research and development, see Sergio Sismondo, *Ghost-Managed Medicine: Big Pharma's Invisible Hands* (Mattering Press, 2018); Laurence Monnais, *Médecine(s) et Santé: Une Petite Histoire Globale – 19e et 20e Siècles* (Presses de l'Université de Montréal, 2016); Joanne Collin and Marcelo Otero, "De l'ère du Valium à celle du Prozac: publicité sur les médicaments psychotropes et pharmaceuticalisation," In *Vers une pharmaceuticalisation de la société? Le Médicament comme objet social*, ed. Joanne Collin and Pierre Marie David (Presses de L'Université du Québec, 2016), 32–55; Jean-Paul Gaudillière and Ulrike Thoms, eds., *The Development of Scientific Marketing in the Twentieth Century* (Pickering and Chatto, 2015); Greene, *Prescribing by Numbers*; David Healy, *The Antidepressant Era* (Harvard University Press, 1997). There is now an extensive literature critiquing the role of the pharmaceutical marketing and promotion in drug evaluation; for examples, see Jacob Stegenga, *Medical Nihilism* (Oxford University Press, 2018); David Healy, *Pharmageddon* (University of California Press, 2012); Ben Goldacre *Bad Pharma: How Drug Companies Mislead Doctors and Harm Patients* (Macmillan, 2014).

and self-treatment for psychological and physical ailments, to potential benefits such as pleasure, human connection, community formation, and spiritual and religious transcendence. The same, of course, can be said of the literature on "drugs": although ethnographic accounts and scholarly work in cultural history, literary studies, and related fields sometimes examine these themes in relation to drug use, most scholarship on the history, use, and regulation of intoxicating goods silently assumes, rather than explicitly engages with, the potential for these commodities to bring a variety of benefits to their users outside the narrow scope of therapeutic efficacy or "self-treatment."[9] We have tried to avoid this presupposition: authors in this volume do not begin with the assumption that benefit from medically sanctioned products is limited to narrowly calculable forms of therapeutic utility; nor do we assume that the medically unsanctioned use of intoxicating goods or other products automatically means the absence of benefit. Indeed, authors in this volume seek to complicate notions of benefit by situating the scientific and political practices of elite experts in relation to other actors, including drug consumers and their communities, who, often in tension with authorities, arrived at their own notions of benefit and implemented their own mechanisms for pursuing it.

Risk and benefit, in other words, are real but situational. Scholars and scientists in the social and behavioral sciences, including historians, have long noted that the meanings, effects, and contexts of drug use cannot be

9 Kane Race, *Pleasure Consuming Medicine: The Queer Politics of Drugs* (Duke University Press, 2020); David Moore, "Erasing pleasure from public discourse on illicit drugs: On the creation and reproduction of an absence," *The International Journal of Drug Policy* 19, no. 5 (2008): 353–58. For exceptions that prove the rule, see, Natasha Du Rose, "Marginalised drug-using women's pleasure and agency," *The Social History of Alcohol and Drugs* 31, no. 1 (2017): 42–64; Caroline Jean Acker, *Creating the American Junkie: Addiction Research in the Classic Era of Narcotic Control* (Johns Hopkins University Press, 2003); John Christopher Feudtner, *Bittersweet: Diabetes, Insulin, and the Transformation of Illness* (University of North Carolina Press, 2003). Examples of literary, cultural history, and other approaches that take pleasure, transcendence, community, and related experiences of drug use seriously include Martin Torgoff, *Bop Apocalypse: Jazz, Race, the Beats, and Drugs* (Hachette+ORM, 2025); Neil Carrier and Lisa L. Gezon, *The Anthropology of Drugs* (Routledge, 2023); Mafalda Pardal, ed., *The Cannabis Social Club* (Taylor & Francis, 2022); Mike Jay, *Mescaline: A Global History of the First Psychedelic* (Yale University Press, 2019); Ingrid Walker, *High: Drugs, Desire, and a Nation of Users* (University of Washington Press, 2017); Geoffrey Hunt, Molly Moloney, and Kristin Evans, *Youth, Drugs, and Nightlife* (Routledge, 2010); Marcus Boon, *The Road of Excess: A History of Writers on Drugs* (Harvard University Press, 2005).

reduced to a type of pharmacological determinism; they are shaped by the complex interplay between pharmacological, social, and psychological factors.[10] These factors include, but are not limited to, social hierarchies of race, class, and gender which simultaneously structure unequal exposure to harm and care and unequal power to determine how risk and benefit are defined and managed. This volume therefore aims to move away from the assumption that risk and benefit are objectively inscribed in objects that reinforce a medicine/drug divide, and to instead recognize, and reckon with, the wide diversity of people who characterize risk and benefit in different ways, including not just scientific and medical "experts" but also political actors, drug consumers, and other parties – always bearing in mind that risk and benefit, in addition to being conceptual and regulatory categories, are also real, embodied experiences that matter in peoples' lives and are therefore linked to hope, uncertainty, and fear.[11]

10 Examples of work that make this point from historical and sociological perspectives include Howard I. Kushner, "Taking biology seriously: The next task for historians of addiction?," *Bulletin of the History of Medicine* 80, no. 1 (2006): 115–43; Sarah W. Tracy and Caroline Jean Acker, *Altering American Consciousness: The History of Alcohol and Drug Use in the United States, 1800–2000* (University of Massachusetts Press, 2004); Craig Reinarman and Harry G. Levine, eds., *Crack in America: Demon Drugs and Social Justice* (University of California Press, 1997); Howard S. Becker, "Becoming a marihuana user," *American Journal of Sociology* 59, no. 3 (1953): 235–42. There is a vast literature on drug use in the behavioral sciences; see for example, Judith S. Brook, David W. Brook, Mario De La Rosa, Martin Whiteman, Erica Johnson, and Ivan Montoya, "Adolescent illegal drug use: The impact of personality, family, and environmental factors," *Journal of Behavioral Medicine* 24, no. 2 (2001): 183–203; Maury Nation and Craig Anne Heflinger, "Risk factors for serious alcohol and drug use: the role of psychosocial variables in predicting the frequency of substance use among adolescents," *The American Journal of Drug and Alcohol Abuse* 32, no. 3 (2006): 415–33. For an influential effort to integrate perspectives, see Norman Earl Zinberg *Drug, Set, and Setting: The Basis for Controlled Intoxicant Use* (Yale University Press, 1984).

11 Hope is a recurring theme in the historiography of drugs and medicines. Examples include Bharat Jayram Venkat, *At the Limits of Cure* (Duke University Press, 2021); Toine Pieters and Stephen Snelders, "Managing double binds in the pharmaceutical prescription market: the case of Halcion," in *Ways of Regulating Drugs in the 19th and 20th Centuries*, ed. Gaudillière and Hess, 270–86; Christer Nordlund, *Hormones of Life: Endocrinology, the Pharmaceutical Industry, and the Dream of a Remedy for Sterility, 1930–1970* (Science History Publications, 2011); David Cantor, "Cancer, Quackery and the Vernacular Meanings of Hope in 1950s America," *Journal of the History of Medicine and Allied Sciences* 61, no. 3 (2006): 324–68; Toine Pieters, *Interferon: The Science and Selling of a Miracle Drug* (Routledge, 2005).

Chapters in this volume provide different, and sometimes contradictory, histories of risk and benefit in Europe and North America. Instead of providing one overarching narrative we instead show how historically diverse these categories and their implementations have been. As Joseph M. Gabriel's chapter shows, therapeutic benefit tends to be attributed to scientific and technological innovation by expert authorities, while risk tends to be understood as either an iatrogenic danger properly managed by medical expertise at the level of the individual patient or, on the other hand, as the result of supposedly deviant behavior among individuals and communities of users that require other forms of control. Alex Mold's chapter argues that this individualization of risk introduces new forms of responsibility among users while also serving other ends such as managing health care budgets. The risks and benefits seemingly inscribed in pharmaceutical objects thus change over time, as demonstrated by Solène Lellinger's analysis of the French drug Mediator, which lost its official status as beneficial for diabetes between 1976 and 1999. Indeed, the definition of objects themselves are historically contingent as shown in Jeremey Greene and Avery Gulino's chapter tracking experts' shifting determinations of whether the anti-diarrhea drug loperamide should be classified as an opioid or not.

Of course, scientific experts and regulators do not act alone in defining and calculating risk and benefit; drug manufacturers also use their brands and specific products to reorganize markets and increase sales. In Joséphine Eberhart's chapter, for example, pharmaceutical companies successfully positioned the opioid Tramadol as "weak" and posing little risk, in part by persuading physicians to prescribe risk management behaviors along with the medicine. Professional organizations also wield real power to shape risk and benefit, as Dan Malleck shows in his chapter. The professional agenda of physicians (to know exactly what they were prescribing) and pharmacists (to protect their professional interests) intersected to shape risk/benefit calculations into a binary framework dividing proprietary and "ethical" medicines. Beyond the immediate context of medical markets, the legal system also acts to define risk and benefit. Jay Sosa shows how gay men, and boutique pharmaceutical companies, created their own contested system of risk and benefit in a relatively free market for nitrite "poppers" opened by the absence of legal or regulatory certainty, while David Herzberg's chapter tracks how federal US narcotics authorities re-narrated Demerol consumers' stories of benefiting from the drug as the "typical lying of addicts."

Contesting Risk and Benefit

This volume thus takes seriously longstanding debates among health professionals about the evolving character of efforts to balance risk and benefit. Historically, therapeutic authorities in Europe and North America have weighed the potential benefits and harms of medicines by either clinical experience, statistical calculation, or some combination of the two.[12] Over the course of the late nineteenth and twentieth centuries their efforts were complicated by a growing number of other actors, from marketing departments, to crusading politicians, to insurance companies, to pharmacists, and, not least of all, to drug consumers themselves, who sometimes embraced and sometimes resisted – and sometimes benefited from, and sometimes paid the price for – authorities' judgements. Therapeutic authorities, of course, often saw these manifold actors as interlopers interfering in the proper evaluation of risk and benefit, and could be particularly judgmental of patients either resisting their encouragements to take a drug or appropriating a drug for unsanctioned ("non-medical") purposes. At the same time, and perhaps ironically, authorities were aware that they had to integrate behavior itself as structuring a drug's risk and benefit.[13]

12 On the role of statistical reasoning in medicine, in addition to Keating and Cambrosio, *Cancer on Trial*, and Greene, *Prescribing by Numbers*, see William G. Rothstein, *Public Health and the Risk Factor: A History of An Uneven Medical Revolution*, vol. 3 (Boydell & Brewer, 2003); James H. Cassedy, *American Medicine and Statistical Thinking, 1800–1860* (Harvard University Press, 1984). As far as we know, no comprehensive history of clinical pharmacology has yet been written, but see also Lawrence J. Lesko and Piet H. van der Graaf, "History and evolution of innovations in clinical pharmacology," *Clinical Pharmacology & Therapeutics* 118, no. 6 (2025): 1313–28; Robert M. Elenbbaas and Dennis B. Worthen, *Clinical Pharmacy in the United States: Transformation of a Profession* (American College of Clinical Pharmacy, 2009).

13 Martin D. Moore, *Managing Diabetes, Managing Medicine: Chronic Disease and Clinical Bureaucracy in Post-War Britain* (Manchester University Press, 2019); Nancy Tomes, *Remaking the American Patient: How Madison Avenue and Modern Medicine Turned Patients into Consumers* (UNC Press Books, 2016); Rothstein, *Public health and the risk factor*; David Herzberg, "Blockbusters and controlled substances: Miltown, Quaalude, and consumer demand for drugs in postwar America," *Studies in History and Philosophy of Science Part C: Studies in History and Philosophy of Biological and Biomedical Sciences* 42, no. 4 (2011): 415–26; David Armstrong, "Origins of the problem of health-related behaviours: a genealogical study," *Social Studies of Science* 39, no. 6 (2009): 909–26; James A. Trostle, "The history and meaning of patient compliance as an ideology," in *Handbook of Health Behavior Research II: Provider Determinants*, ed. David S. Gochman (Springer US, 1997), 109–24.

Therapeutic authorities have often attempted to build standardized systems of drug risks and benefits, often characterized as an effort to definitively establish the "value" of drugs or to list drugs of true "value." The long history of pharmacopeias, dating back to the early modern period, is an important example of this.[14] Despite their aspirations to objective scientific processes, however, their determinations, like those of the drug-consuming interlopers they so often complain about, are structured by social context and emerge dialogically through interactions with others. The "value" of a drug thus changes over time and space. As early as 1930, Heidelberg chair of pharmacology Wolfgang Heubner pointed out that physicians, academics, patients, consumers, manufacturers, and health insurance each value a drug differently, for different reasons.[15] A drug's market value, for example, could differ considerably from its therapeutic value. Heubner held up cardiac drug Strophantin, insulin, malaria drug quinine, and the syphilis drug Neosalvarsan as truly life-saving medications, i.e., medicines of incontrovertible worth or value, whose benefits definitively outweighed their risks. Fifty years after Heubner, WHO's list of essential medicines updated such efforts to determine a universal list of definitively valuable drugs, even if – or especially if – they no longer carried enough commercial value to sustain market availability.[16]

The historicity of value attributions reminds us that scientific and/or therapeutic authority never stands alone but rather emerges through contest and collaboration with other actors and interests. Therapeutic authorities, police, and daily consumers bring very different assessments of opioid risks and benefits, for example. Or, too, a general practitioner might prescribe a combination drug with several active principles despite – and based on very different calculations than – a pharmacologist's skepticism. Often such contestations have played out in a specific arena of risk characterized as "side effects," i.e., unwanted drug effects. But this simple definition hides enormous complexity: unwanted by whom; in what circumstances; and weighed against which

14 Stuart Anderson, *Pharmacopoeias, Drug Regulation, and Empires: Making Medicines Official in Britain's Imperial World, 1618–1968* (McGill-Queen's University Press, 2024); Matthew James Crawford and Joseph M. Gabriel, eds., *Drugs on the Page: Pharmacopoeias and Healing Knowledge in the Early Modern Atlantic World* (University of Pittsburgh Press, 2019). Lee Anderson and Gregory Higby, *The Spirit of Voluntarism: A Legacy of Commitment and Contribution; The United States Pharmacopeia 1820–1995* (American Institute of the History of Pharmacy, 1995).

15 Wolfgang Heubner, *Arznei als Wert. Antrittsvorlesung gehalten zu Heidelberg am 29. November 1930* (Springer, 1931).

16 Jeremy A. Greene, "Making medicines essential: The emergent centrality of pharmaceuticals in global health," *BioSocieties* 6, no. 1 (2011): 10–33.

benefits? In this sense, "side effects," like risks more broadly, are not static qualities but evolve over time through interaction between medical, legal, and political authorities and the social contexts in which the drugs are used. There is no universal expert view on drug risks, as shown by Nils Kessel's chapter on tensions in the 1950s and 1960s between clinical experts, who measured risk and benefit at an individual level, and public health experts, who calculated risk and benefit epidemiologically. Even severe "side effects" may be considered tolerable for a lifesaving drug, but not for a headache pill. In other words, changing social and therapeutic contexts result in changing valuations of risk and benefit over time, and even "scientifically" established calculations of risk and benefit can change dynamically. Indeed, as Greene and Gulino's chapter on the anti-diarrhea drug loperamide shows, a side effect may be transformed into a therapeutic benefit based on shifting evaluations of a drug's utility.

The early-twenty-first-century form of European and North American therapeutic authorities' style of benefit-risk calculation must therefore be understood not as a final truth to be retroactively applied to the past, but instead as one form of knowledge that is useful for a variety of purposes, including both state-building and regulatory decision-making, and that has emerged contextually over the course of the nineteenth and twentieth centuries. Social hierarchies of gender, class, and race have been central factors influencing the historical development and application of this type of calculation, as have exclusionary and stigmatizing practices based on physical and mental ability, aesthetic criteria such as beauty, sexual and gender identity, and other complex markers. Therapeutic authority has long been linked to professional legitimacy and credentialing, which are of course themselves structured by these social hierarchies and practices; positions of authority have been overwhelmingly occupied by white European or US men with a high degree of social legitimacy in their roles as medical experts, chemists and pharmacists, regulators, politicians, journalists, lawyers, businessmen, and so on. The French media authorities censoring educational films in Christian Bonah's chapter, for example, or the British experts championing the birth control hormone Depo-Provera in Caroline Rusterholz's chapter, were exclusively middle-aged white men able to maintain and deploy social legitimacy toward their own goals. This matters, in part, because, as a result, disputes between therapeutic authorities and marginalized groups over questions of risk and benefit often play out along lines structured by these hierarchies and exclusionary practices; Nancy D. Campbell's chapter, for example, shows how therapeutic authorities did not just ignore but actively resisted the production of legitimized knowledge from socially marginalized and highly stigmatized people ("addicts") about the life-saving benefits of naloxone.

Campbell's naloxone activists were not unusual among socially marginalized people in their refusal to remain silent in evaluating drug risks and benefits. Rather, racialized minorities, women, economically disadvantaged people, youths, gender and sexual minorities, and many others with less access to the levers of power have practiced their own evaluations and advocated for them. Samuel Kelton Roberts Jr.'s chapter on African American resistance to methadone maintenance and harm reduction programs in New York, for example, shows the significance of "lay" communities in determining a drug's risks and benefits. As Roberts (and others) make clear, this resistance to expert guidance should not be derided as "irrational." Rather, in the case of methadone, African Americans' long history of oppression equipped them to accurately assess not just pharmacological risks but the risks produced by the racist social and political context in which the drug was provided – and which could not be ameliorated by any drug alone, or indeed any other form of individualized therapy alone. Early twentieth-century US consumers of the stigmatized substance cannabis, as discussed in Robert Beach's chapter, made the opposite move, rejecting increasingly negative assessments by experts in order to pursue what they understood as the health, social, and economic benefits of the drug. And people who used Demerol in the 1940s, David Herzberg argues, unsuccessfully sought to make use of the medicine's ambiguous legal status to reap the benefits of opioid use without the social harms created by criminalization of heroin.

This volume suggests that those methadone-skeptical African Americans, cannabis smokers, Demerol consumers, and naloxone champions were correct in believing that drug risks and benefits are both real *and* profoundly shaped by social context. We do not, however, simply invert the hierarchy of knowledge and place marginalized knowers on the pedestal previously occupied by scientific and medical experts with high degrees of social, institutional, and political authority; rather, we recognize the practical significance of how different actors shape the various contexts in which they operate and how different actors' positioning gives them access to distinct insights into the social production and experience of risk and benefit. This volume thus tracks political contestations over expertise as, themselves, factors that have influenced not just the calculation of risk and benefit, but the subjective experience of it. Risk and benefit is an analytical framing, not an analytical straitjacket: rather than defining and applying our own system of risk and benefit, we explore how these powerful concepts have been constructed and experienced by a wide diversity of actors.

Separating "Pharmaceuticals" from "Drugs"

Calculations of risk and benefit are deeply intertwined with the process of storytelling and, in particular, narratives about what it means to be cured and what it means to be harmed. Too-neat categories of "wonder drugs" versus "intoxicants" are, of course, only one way to narrate risks and benefits, which in many historical contexts have been seen as always operating together in every potentially medicinal substance.[17] In Europe and North America, however, the binary between cure and harm has often been narrated in precisely this way, with pleasure serving as the *de facto* dividing line between the rational pursuit of health and the irrational pursuit of intoxication. Indeed, as Benjamin Breen and others have shown, a particularly intense investment dividing "medicines" and "drugs" was one important strategy by which Europeans and later scientific authorities in North and South America imposed a hierarchy of therapeutic knowledges and practices by extracting, or "isolating" medicines from the supposedly messy, dangerous forms of healing and harm practiced by nonwhite and often women healers in colonized places.[18] This cultural trope long outlasted the era of formal empire, as Beat Bächi shows in his chapter's analysis of Swiss LSD discoverer Albert Hoffman's argument that the inward-looking "Eastern" effects of cannabis rendered it riskier than the "active attention" inspired by psychedelic medicines.

The salience of pleasure as an unspoken dividing line between drug and medicine places particular importance on pain and pain relief in broader efforts to systematize and operationalize risk and benefit. Like other such evaluations, risk and benefit in pain relief cannot be reduced to pharmacological categories or even relatively narrow social phenomena such as prescription and dispensing errors. Instead, risk and benefit emerge from historically constituted structural determinants, unequal encounters between many kinds of social authorities and patients and other drug users, and consumers and illicit commercial actors operating without a "legitimate" basis on which to effectuate their views. Like all such encounters, perhaps more vividly than in other medicinal contexts, these have been deeply structured

17 For example, Yan Liu, *Healing With Poisons: Potent Medicines in Medieval China* (University of Washington Press, 2021).

18 Benjamin Breen, *The Age of Intoxication: Origins of the Global Drug Trade* (University of Pennsylvania Press, 2019). For other examples of this argument, see Seth Garfield, "Guaraná's forgotten history: The rise and fall of an Indigenous Brazilian phytotherapy in Anglo-American medicine," *History of Science* 63, no. 2 (2025); Joseph M. Gabriel, "Indian Secrets, Indian Cures, and the Pharmacopoeia of the United States of America," in *Drugs on the Page*, ed. Crawford and Gabriel, 240–62.

by social hierarchies of race, class, and gender. Because pain and pain relief have played such an outsized role in building the inherited architecture of similarity and difference – with the medicine/drug divide as its most serious manifestation – explorations of this topic play an important role in this volume as well, in chapters by Jeremy A. Greene, Nancy D. Campbell, David Herzberg, Alex Mold, and Joséphine Eberhart.

Pain and pain relief is just one particularly important element of a more general historical and historiographical divide between psychoactive substances and other medicines. This is not a perfect binary, of course, and it does not always fit neatly with the binary architecture of licit/illicit – indeed, "psychoactive" is itself a category embedded within a rich history of debate about drug classification and taxonomy; it is therefore not surprising that numerous drugs are sometimes considered "psychoactive" and/or "psychotropic" and sometimes not – including antidepressants, anticonvulsants, and mood stabilizers – and that such drugs tend to fall squarely in the "licit" category. Still, historians of psychoactive substances – or, at least, historians of psychoactive substances that are frequently used for pleasure or other non-medically sanctioned use – must reckon with the licit/illicit divide in ways that historians of pharmaceuticals more broadly can avoid. Indeed, pharmaceutical historians often take a supposed lack of criminality among their research subjects as an obvious and *a priori* condition rather than as an end product to be analyzed and explained.

Linking histories of psychoactive and non-psychoactive substances – and exploring the messy and contested boundaries between such categories – through the concepts of risk and benefit therefore raises complex questions about the presumed divide between regulation and criminalization. As historians and other scholars of drugs such as heroin, cocaine, cannabis, and LSD have persuasively shown, divisions between legal and illegal products have not followed naturally from pharmacological distinctions but have rather emerged at the intersection of science, commerce, and social hierarchies and stigmatizing practices of exclusion in the context of conflict over urban governance, border policing, regulatory procedures, and other sociopolitical flashpoints.[19] Yet the analytic centrality of the licit/illicit divide tends to

19 Recent examples include David Farber, *The War on Drugs: A History* (New York University Press, 2021); Stephen Snelders, *Drug Smuggler Nation: Narcotics and the Netherlands, 1920–1995* (Manchester University Press, 2021); David A. Guba Jr., *Taming Cannabis: Drugs and Empire in Nineteenth-Century France* (McGill-Queen's University Press, 2020); David Herzberg, *White Market Drugs: Big Pharma and the Hidden History of Addiction in America* (University of Chicago Press, 2020); Diana S. Kim, *Empires of Vice: The Rise of Opium Prohibition Across Southeast Asia* (Princeton University Press, 2020); Lucas Richert, *Strange Trips: Science, Culture, and the*

vastly oversimplify the many and varied meanings of both "licit" and "illicit." There is an extensive literature on the regulation of medicines in Europe and North America that explores it as a complex, multifaceted affair, undertaken by many different actors in quite different ways in the pursuit of a wide range of goals.[20] This sophistication tends to disappear, however, in analyses of criminalized drugs due to the way that the category "illegal" homogenizes a similarly rich complexity of the ways prohibition can be conceived, defined, enforced, and resisted.[21] At the same time, the category of "criminal" tends to focus attention on products and peoples that are subject to the violence of the state, thus obscuring the regulatory complexity that underpins the production of counterfeit products, adulterated goods, and other illicit substances that may or may not be psychoactive in nature – whatever we mean by that fraught term.

There are other significant challenges to the licit/illicit divide – and to the binary between "medicines" and "drugs" that we engage with in this volume. The rich and complex histories and historiographies of alcohol and

---

Regulation of Drugs (McGill-Queen's Associated Media, 2018); Dan Malleck, *When Good Drugs Go Bad: Opium, Medicine, and the Origins of Canada's Drug Laws* (University of British Columbia Press, 2015); Alex Mold, *Heroin: The Treatment of Addiction in Twentieth-Century Britain* (Northern Illinois University Press, 2008). Older examples include Acker, *Creating the American Junkie*; and David T. Courtwright, *Forces of Habit: Drugs and the Making of the Modern World* (Harvard University Press, 2002).

20 Sabrina Röttger-Wirtz, *The Interplay of Global Standards and EU Pharmaceutical Regulation: The International Council for Harmonisation* (Bloomsbury Publishing, 2021); Matthew Oram, *The Trials of Psychedelic Therapy* (Johns Hopkins University Press, 2018); Gaudillière and Hess, eds., *Ways of Regulating Drugs in the 19th and 20th Centuries*; Dominique Tobbell, *Pills, Power, and Policy: The Struggle for Drug Reform in Cold War America and Its Consequences* (University of California Press, 2012); Daniel Carpenter, *Reputation and Power: Organizational Image and Pharmaceutical Regulation at the FDA* (Princeton University Press, 2010); John Abraham and Graham Lewis, *Regulating Medicines in Europe: Competition, Expertise and Public Health* (Routledge, 2014); Joseph M. Gabriel, "Restricting the Sale of 'Deadly Poisons': Pharmacists, Drug Regulation, and Narratives of Suffering in the Gilded Age," *The Journal of the Gilded Age and Progressive Era* 9, no. 3 (2010): 313–36; Arthur A. Daemmrich, *Pharmacopolitics: Drug Regulation in the United States and Germany* (University of North Carolina Press, 2004).

21 One recent exception is Matthew Lassiter, *The Suburban Crisis: White America and the War on Drugs* (Princeton University Press, 2023), which explores how US "drug war" policy was designed to protect white youths from drugs (by punishing "drug dealers") while also protecting white youths from drug laws by making cannabis laws flexible.

tobacco products, for example, challenge both the licit/illicit and medicine/drug divides, with both sets of substances having multifaceted and varied meanings over time that defy easy categorization. The same can be said of food and spices. Whether or not these histories and historiographies can, or should, be integrated with discussions about "medicines" and "drugs" is very much an open question; adopting an analytic focus on risk and benefit may be one way of doing so. Another even more fundamental challenge can be found in the rich literature on early modern *materia medica*, where categories that historians who work on more recent periods often take for granted are instead destabilized or even non-existent. Other pairings – and their origins – instead come to the fore, such as the binary between poisons and medicines, simple and compound, pure and adulterated, secret and revealed. Indeed, even categories such as "intoxication" and "healing" look different from an early modern perspective. Yet even here stories of risk and benefit abound – although, of course, such stories may not mean what they mean today.[22]

There are, in other words, many questions left to explore in the rich territory cracked open by thinking past the binary categorizations of goods into licit "pharmaceuticals" and illicit psychoactive "drugs."

Structure of the Book

This volume is drawn from a series of workshops exploring risk and benefit in medicines and drugs within the transnational context of Europe and North America. Calculations of risk and benefit in this context were part of global – imperial – systems of drug governance that were adopted, adapted, resisted, challenged, and ignored by people across the world with their own complex and evolving ways governing risk and benefit in relation to the

22 Chelsea Berry, *Poisoned Relations: Healing, Power, and Contested Knowledge in the Atlantic World* (University of Pennsylvania Press, 2025); Alisha Rankin, *The Poison Trials: Wonder Drugs, Experiment, and the Battle for Authority in Renaissance Science* (University of Chicago Press, 2021); Zachary Dorner, *Merchants of Medicines: The Commerce and Coercion of Health in Britain's Long Eighteenth Century* (University of Chicago Press, 2020); Paula S. De Vos, *Compound Remedies: Galenic Pharmacy from the Ancient Mediterranean to New Spain* (University of Pittsburgh Press, 2020); Pablo F. Gómez, *The Experiential Caribbean: Creating Knowledge and Healing in the Early Modern Atlantic* (UNC Press Books, 2017); William Eamon, *Science and the Secrets of Nature: Books of Secrets in Medieval and Early Modern Culture* (Princeton University Press, 1994).

substances they consumed.[23] Since the early modern era a long series of scientists, explorers, imperialists, merchants, and other groups from the northern Atlantic region have tried to "order" the ambiguous world of substances through constant boundary work and purification practices. Best known in this context is the history of natural substances such as coca, opium, and cannabis that faced criminalization after industrially manufactured substitutes with supposedly higher benefits or fewer risks became available. Such moves depended on a colonial imagining of a hierarchically structured globe, with Europe and eventually the US as "modern" and scientifically advanced societies with the technological capacity to extract benefit from supposedly unstable and dangerous "backwards" remedies. This dynamic intensified during the late nineteenth and twentieth centuries as an ever more sophisticated and explicitly global pharmaceutical industry centered in Europe and North America has come to dominate the global supply of medicines despite increasing challenges from countries such as Brazil, China, India, and Japan.

Given this context, a largely inward-focused exploration of risk and benefit in the North Atlantic is itself a risky endeavor – it elides dimensions that stretch beyond, or are centered outside, the North Atlantic and runs the danger of reproducing the imperial structures so deeply embedded in its histories. We therefore feel it is important to recognize and embrace that this volume is a regional history, with a clear sense of its own limitations. It

23 Examples include Nandini Bhattacharya, *Disparate Remedies: Making Medicines in Modern India* (McGill-Queen's University Press, 2023); Maziyar Ghiabi, *Drug Politics: Managing Disorder in the Islamic Republic of Iran* (Cambridge University Press, 2019); Laurence Monnais, *The Colonial Life of Pharmaceuticals: Medicines and Modernity in Vietnam*, trans. Noémi Tousignant (Cambridge University Press, 2019); Eirik Saethre and Jonathan Stadler, *Negotiating Pharmaceutical Uncertainty: Women's Agency in a South African HIV Prevention Trial* (Vanderbilt University Press, 2017); Paul Gootenberg and Isaac Campos, "Toward a new drug history of Latin America: A research frontier at the center of debates," *Hispanic American Historical Review* 95, no. 1 (2015): 1–35; Melissa Graboyes, *The Experiment Must Continue: Medical Research and Ethics in East Africa, 1940–2014* (Ohio University Press, 2015); Miriam Kingsberg, *Moral Nation: Modern Japan and Narcotics in Global History* (University of California Press, 2014); Kristin Peterson, *Speculative Markets: Drug Circuits and Derivative Life in Nigeria* (Duke University Press, 2014); Isaac Campos, *Home Grown: Marijuana and the Origins of Mexico's War on Drugs* (University of North Carolina Press, 2012); Laurent Pordié and Jean-Paul Gaudillière, "The reformulation regime in drug discovery: Revisiting polyherbals and property rights in the Ayurvedic industry," *East Asian Science, Technology and Society: An International Journal* 8, no. 1 (2014): 57–79; Andrew Lakoff, *Pharmaceutical Reason: Knowledge and Value in Global Psychiatry* (Cambridge University Press, 2006).

does not present an origin story of risk and benefit that then spreads to other regions; nor does it offer a universal or universalizing story about the nature of risk and benefit itself. Instead, the volume approaches the North Atlantic as one of many sites where different communities of actors have used these concepts to shape the circulation, use, experience, and definition of one set of goods – the boundaries of which are themselves contested and change over time. It is, in short, a practical context for an effort to reframe the binary between licit and illicit substances through a new analytic approach. It is not intended to be the final word on risk and benefit in medicines and drugs and we very much hope it will not be – rather, we hope that it will prove useful for scholars pursuing similar goals in other contexts both within and outside Europe and North America. We recognize that that these categories may themselves need to be modified, may not apply, or may be highly problematic in other contexts. Yet we hope that by broaching such questions we will provoke new conversations and reformulations across a variety of intellectual networks and communities; interrogating whether or not this analytic framework makes sense in other contexts, and if so how, seems to us to be a valuable direction for future work.

The book is organized into five overlapping thematic sections. The first section, "Systematizing Risk and Benefit," analyzes authorities' efforts to systematize the identification and evaluation of benefits and risks, and identifies fundamental problems they faced in doing so. Malleck explores how physicians, pharmacists, and government regulators sought to impose order on early twentieth-century Canadian medical markets by grouping risks into proprietary and "ethical" drugs. In Gabriel's chapter, early twentieth-century therapeutic authorities obscured social and racial logic through their increasing investment in drug specificity during the era of the "magic bullet." Kessel analyzes how therapeutic reformers redefined drug risks in the 1960s through technocratic parsing of undesired drug effects from the broad category of "side effects" to the more restrictive "adverse drug reaction."

The second section, "Narrating Risk and Benefit," looks at the cultural underpinnings of systems of risk and benefit by exploring the stories circulated about medicines and drugs by a diverse set of authorities. Bächi investigates a variety of attempts by Albert Hofmann and other Swiss experts to define and "disenchant" the seemingly magical traces left on psychedelics by their exotic (to Europeans) origins – in essence, to reassert European authority over stories of psychedelic risk and benefit. As Bonah shows through a case study of French censorship of psychedelic medical films as "inciting illegal drug abuse," state authorities were well aware of the power of stories in this context and actively sought to control their circulation. Finally, Mold's analysis of British public health campaigns in the 1980s shows that they relied on narrative tropes (such as tragedy) to popularize their categorizations of "good" and "bad" modes of consumption in a medically paternalistic but commercial market.

The third section, "Crises of Risk and Benefit," looks at dynamic political struggles over – and public health consequences of – flaws or loopholes in formal systems of evaluating risk and benefit. Rusterholz's chapter on resistance to the injectable contraceptive Depo Provera in 1970s and 1980s Britain argues that race and gender structured experts' ideas of the drug's benefits – just as the experience of racism and sexism structured activists' battle to highlight risks such as coercion. Eberhart argues that the manufacturer of the analgesic Tramadol outwitted the usual obstacles to "blockbuster" opioid sales in late-twentieth-century France by successfully downplaying the risks of what they pitched as a "weak," aspirin-like remedy whose safety could be ensured by properly training consumers. In Lellinger's chapter on the French appetite suppressant Mediator, competing claims of risk and benefit from regulatory, therapeutic, and industry authorities created enough uncertainty to shield the drug from regulatory constraints, resulting in the worst drug scandal in that nation's recent history.

The fourth section, "Resisting Systems of Risk and Benefit," examines moments when alternative or insurgent ways to understand, characterize, and respond to risk and benefit emerged to challenge or at least bedevil authoritative paradigms. These were not always deliberate or even fully coherent, as Herzberg shows in his study of people who used the synthetic opioid Demerol in the 1940s before it was fully categorized as a "narcotic" under US law. Relatively free of the social risks of criminalization, these consumers generated their own individual ways of managing opioids' pharmacological risks and benefits before they were shut down by federal authorities. Roberts, on the other hand, finds and analyzes the revealing coherence of Black communities' resistance to methadone maintenance and other forms of harm reduction. These, he argues, should be understood as an insistence on incorporating the political – in this case, Black communities' experiences of and political adaption to America's long history of medical racism – in any assessment of risk and benefit. Finally, in her account of harm reductionists' long struggle to get regulatory approval for over-the-counter availability of the overdose reversing drug naloxone, Campbell identifies a partially successful effort to radically reinterpret risk to incorporate the social circumstances of drug use, revealing *abstinence* from opioid use as a real risk for people who use drugs.

The final section, "Consumer Paradigms of Risk and Benefit," takes a deeper look at how communities of consumers developed and implemented their own approaches to risk and benefit – often in the interstices opened by rudimentary, incomplete, or conflicting formal regulations. Beach's chapter shows that even during the era of cannabis criminalization after 1937, consumers' alternate understandings of risk and benefit persisted, complicating the meaning of "recreational" use and its implicit limiting of real benefit to medically sanctioned use. In Greene and Gulino's chapter, consumers' unexpected uses of the antidiarrheal drug loperamide in the 1970s and 1980s provoked experts to reevaluate the risk and benefit profile of not just that drug, but the broader class "opioid" to which it belonged. And finally, Sosa's chapter explores how, in the relative absence of federal regulation, gay men built their own niche industry for nitrite "poppers" in the 1970s and 1980s, complete with their own coded language of risk and benefit.

Part One

Systematizing Risk and Benefit

Chapter One

Such Immoral Pharmacy: Pharmacists, Physicians, and Addressing the Harms and Benefits of Secret Remedies in Canada

Dan Malleck

This chapter examines how Canadian pharmacists attempted to influence understandings of the risks and benefits of patent and proprietary medicines at the beginning of the twentieth century. It argues that when addressing the proliferation of secret remedies, pharmacy leadership balanced the potential risks of such products against the benefits of supporting a marketplace in medicines that might help the public. Pharmacists balanced their role as vendors and sometimes producers of medicine who sought provide useful and safe medicine to the public against their status as learned professionals whose work in compounding medicine supported the work of physicians. Presenting themselves as respectable and responsible experts in pharmaceutical chemistry, they asserted their role as central to maintaining and assuring a safe supply of prefabricated medicines. Simultaneously, as entrepreneurs, they also saw their role as vendors and potentially manufacturers of such medicines as a noble cause that needed to be protected.

The chapter is divided into three sections. It begins with an overview of the main challenges presented by what I will refer to generally as prefabricated medicines, many of which had secret or proprietary ingredients, to both the profession of pharmacy and physicians. It was a complex issue because both pharmacists and physicians saw some usefulness in such remedies, but for different reasons, related to their central professional mandates. Seeing the potential value of prefabricated remedies, and their usefulness for physicians and for their own confreres, pharmacists sought to address the proliferation of proprietary remedies by advocating for a national standardized formulary that would ensure that physicians' prescriptions and pharmacists' compounding practices would adhere to agreed-upon standards. This strategy, focused internally upon the activities of pharmacists and physicians, was joined to an outward facing effort to influence national proprietary or patent medicine legislation. As the Dominion government contemplated restrictive legislation to limit the potential dangers of these products, pharmacists lobbied for changes that would protect the public but not damage their businesses. They emphasized their capability as highly educated pharmaceutical experts whose perspective was essential in shaping this legislation. Facing considerable hurdles in these efforts, pharmacists united to form the Canadian Pharmaceutical Association, which they felt would allow the profession to lobby with one more convincing voice and press the government to pass legislation that, while protecting the public, would not unduly burden the nation's pharmacists. Central to both of these efforts was the pharmacists' self-perception as educated and responsible protectors of the public's health who had a unique understanding of the pressures of market economics because they were embedded within it. Just as the risks and benefits of patent and proprietary medicines needed to be balanced and negotiated, so too pharmacists had to consider the risks and benefits of such regulations on their profession and their livelihoods. Overly restrictive legislation could affect their ability to do their job and earn a living, whereas advocating for legislation that was not sufficiently restrictive could undermine their own authority when discussing the increasingly complicated field of pharmaceuticals.

The creation and standardization of pharmaceuticals, and how they affected and were affected by the pharmacy profession, have seen increased attention recently. Stuart Anderson's *Pharmacopoeias* (2024) provides a comprehensive examination of the creation of and attempts to standardize a diverse and complicated medical industry across the British Empire.[1] He shows that no matter how standardized the format, the production of medical remedies was dependent upon an accommodating medical and pharmaceutical profession, and often sympathetic legislators to support the need for such standardized medical systems. Looking at the way the growing pharmaceutical industry developed and protected their drugs as products,

1 Stuart Anderson, *Pharmacopoeias, Drug Regulation and Empires: Making Medicines Official in Britain's Imperial World 1618–1968* (McGill-Queen's University Press, 2024).

in *Medical Monopoly* (2014) Joseph M. Gabriel examines the complexity of patent laws and the precedents created and then expanded as the pharmaceutical industry grew and expanded.[2] Connecting the complicated pharmaceutical market with the ebb and flow of medical professional power, in *Disorder* (2021) Peter Swenson discusses how a broad and complicated pharmaceutical market, notably the growth and concern over secret and proprietary medicines, affected and influenced reform of America's medical profession.[3] In these works, the pharmacist's traditional practice of compounding raw drugs in to a doctor's prescription, was replaced by prefabricated remedies manufactured, marketed, and distributed by increasingly large companies using innovative and sometimes deceptive marketing tactics. The expansion of the chemical industry, and global exploration for new compounds, increased pharmaceutical diversity and complicated the way that new products were viewed, whether their commercialization was considered "ethical" and whether physicians chose to incorporate them into their practices.

The range of prefabricated products of this diverse industry was vast. Traditionally, the most respectable manufacturers of medicines who sought to have innovative products appeal to and thus be prescribed by physicians, would publish their recipes and encourage physicians to use them and report on the results. Such an approach deemed such products "ethical remedies" because these manufacturers were not hiding knowledge that could be beneficial to the health of the people. Yet not all manufacturers were inclined to be so transparent. Many patented their remedies, thereby protecting the formulation in the expectation that only the manufacturer would profit from his or her innovation. Such secrecy was derided by the regular medical profession because patenting remedies that could help people would put profit ahead of human benefit. To be in the best interest of the public, they argued, such knowledge should be disseminated widely, not "hidden" by a patent. To be sure, not all products referred to as "patent medicines" were actually protected by a patent, but the vast majority – if not all – of the manufacturers of such products kept their ingredients secret, and were generally denounced by the medical leadership (if not by all physicians). To these two types of prefabricated products we must add a third, equally slippery in its definition: "proprietary" medicines. For these, a manufacturer would not degrade his product by protecting it with a patent, but he or she would trademark

2 Joseph M. Gabriel, *Medical Monopoly: Intellectual Property Rights and the Origins of the Modern Pharmaceutical Industry* (University of Chicago Press, 2014)

3 Peter A Swenson, *Disorder: A History of Reform, Reaction, and Money in American Medicine* (Yale University Press, 2021).

the name, and thus seek to profit from the reputation built on their formulation. Not all proprietary remedies were necessarily of dubious recipes or made excessive promises. Many manufacturers used a trademark in order to protect their investment, be it in chemical innovation such as the products of Bayer, or in the costs of pharmaceutical exploration into exotic locations to extract medicinal products from indigenous plants. Many observers contended that neither patenting nor trademarking proprietary medicines was considered entirely "ethical," but by the end of the nineteenth century, skepticism towards proprietary remedies had begun to ease as new discoveries – be they from chemical innovation or the results of exploration – were found to have genuinely beneficial therapeutic properties. Compared to the shameful practice of patenting a remedy, trademarking products was a less unethical way of ensuring that the costs of innovation could be recouped, along with a nice profit.[4]

The Growing Concern over Secret Remedies

The secrecy of patent and proprietary remedies was a key sticking point for physicians and pharmacists, two professional groups with a stake in protecting the health of the public, but for different reasons. For physicians, if they did not know the ingredients of a product, they could not in good conscience prescribe them to their patients. Not only were they potentially dangerous, but patent and proprietary remedies that claimed to treat specific conditions might encourage a sick person to avoid consulting a doctor (and paying a doctor's fee) by self-medicating. For pharmacists the challenge was similar, but also more rooted in the exigencies of the market. Pharmacists' professional status rested on their role as educated and capable compounders of medicines. Prefabricated remedies could thus undermine this key aspect of pharmacists' professional identity. At the same time, pharmacists who supported physicians by storing, maintaining, and assessing the potency of raw drugs, saw themselves and their skill in undertaking these tasks as essential to ensuring effective and properly assembled prescriptions. Prefabricated remedies with unknown ingredients undermined that key professional capability.

Despite these distinctions, by the turn of the twentieth century, such a complex pharmocopoeial wonderland meant that not all secret remedies were considered useless; a competent physician could distinguish good from bad. As the editor of the *Dominion Medical Monthly* noted in

4 Gabriel, *Medical Monopoly*, esp. Chapter 4, "Therapeutic Reform and the Reinterpretation of Monopoly."

1907: "It would be nothing more than foolish and nonsensical to say that all patent medicines and proprietary preparations in drugs were no good. Some of them are no doubt good prescriptions, accurately compounded." Nevertheless, he argued, "we consider [physicians] are the best qualified and fitted to diagnose disease ... and to prescribe best for its treatment." In this work, the physicians were assisted by loyal pharmacists: "The good druggist is he who follows out faithfully the doctor's prescription." The editorial concluded with a reminder that the main problem of secret remedies lie in "the harmful drugs incorporated in patents, for there can be no defence of such immoral pharmacy."[5] The editorial captured a key aspect of the relationship between doctors and druggists: physicians are the experts in healing, pharmacists are the experts in compounding, and a free medical market dominated by commercial tactics is an immediate "immoral" danger to be avoided. This argument was not new, but as the nineteenth century came to an end, it had gained increased urgency for the medical and pharmaceutical profession, as well as for the public.

By the beginning of the twentieth century, commentators inside and outside the medical and pharmaceutical professions were calling for something to be done to control the proliferation of this "immoral pharmacy." Journalists investigating the industry and publishing in periodicals as diverse as the *Ladies Home Journal*, *Collier's Weekly*, or *The Vancouver World* (in articles often reproduced elsewhere) manifested a stereotype of proprietary remedies that viewed any mass-marketed medicine as dangerous.[6] They lumped these products together, since, as Samuel Hopkins Adams noted in his introduction to his pivotal *Great American Fraud*, "the honest attempt to separate the sheep from the goats develops a lamentable lack of qualified candidates for the sheepfold."[7] Hopkins took a dim view of the rapacious and dodgy patent medical market, seeing secrecy and dubious marketing techniques as dangerous to the lives of the people and he saw physicians as complicit in the expansion of the market in dubious medicines.[8] Yet, as the *Dominion Medical Monthly* editorial illustrates, physician leadership tried to maintain their status as experts who could delineate good from bad remedies.

5 "The Federal Proprietary and Patent Medicine Act," *Dominion Medical Monthly and Ontario Medical Journal* 28 (March 1907): 138–39.

6 The *Vancouver World* undertook an extensive investigation in advance of a provincial patent medicine law (that was never passed). This may be found in articles in February 1905 with such excellent titles as "Often Obscene or Disgusting" (February 27, 1906); "1,000,000 Infants Die" (February 7, 1906); and my favourite, "Veritable Goblin Realm of Fakery" (February 20, 1906).

7 Samuel Hopkins Adams, *The Great American Fraud* (American Medical Association Press, 1905), 3.

8 Swenson, *Disorder*, 81.

Pharmacists found themselves in a tricky dilemma. Canadian pharmacists argued that they were respectable, responsible, and knowledgeable protectors of the public's health. They rested this status upon their knowledge of the medicinal properties of remedies; their skill in compounding prescriptions; their understanding of the problems of incorrect combinations; their dual role as responsible and respectable gatekeepers to powerful but potentially poisonous drugs like opium, strychnine, and arsenic; and their place as "faithful" assistants to physicians. These arguments appear to have been accepted by legislators who, starting in 1870, began to pass professional closure legislation granting pharmacy bodies the right to issues licenses, evaluate qualifications, discipline recalcitrant members, and define which drugs should be available only through a pharmacist if not always via a physician's prescription. By 1906, all provinces had enacted such legislation, and to all these laws was appended a list of remedies over which pharmacists would have unique control.[9]

The professionalization of pharmacy created a unique type of professional, however, and this is where the pharmacist was more threatened by the new medical innovations but also saw new benefits. In contrast to the incomes of lawyers and physicians, which were derived from being paid for their knowledge of law or medicine and skill in practicing their callings, a large proportion of pharmacists' income came from selling things.[10] Few if any pharmacists could make a living exclusively compounding and charging for physicians' prescriptions. So they carried perfume and soap, dispensed soda from fountains, developed photographs, and even sold spectacles. Many pharmacists also stocked prefabricated remedies. Some of these came from large ethical manufacturing businesses where common remedies, such as the ubiquitous tincture of opium were compounded in large volumes and distributed in reliable measured bottles. Others came from commercial travelers working for the new and expanding pharmaceutical companies that were selling new chemical formulations. Some of these were German corporations with familiar names such as Bayer or Merck producing new chemical compounds such as aspirin, phenacetin, and heroin, while others had less reliable although often more popular origins, such as Mrs. Winslow's Soothing Syrup and Dr. Williams' Pink Pills for Pale People. Many pharmacists also made up their own remedies and sold them in prefabricated forms. These were "proprietary" in that the medicine was a pharmacist's own formulation

9 Dan Malleck, *When Good Drugs Go Bad: Opium, Medicine, and the Origin of Canada's Drug Laws* (UBC Press, 2015), esp. Chapter 3, "Canada's First Drug Laws."

10 Stuart Anderson articulates this unique place of pharmacy inside and outside the market in *Pharmacy and Professionalization in the British Empire, 1780–1970* (Palgrave MacMillan, 2021).

and intended for customers to treat common conditions without a physician's intervention. Each of these types of remedies held their own benefits and harms, but as a profession whose feet were firmly in the marketplace, pharmacists saw the debates over the morality, danger, and need to restrict patent and proprietary remedies as threats both to their livelihoods and to their professional status.

Pharmacists, then, paid close attention as the muckraking investigations of Samuel Adams, and Norman Hapgood in *Colliers* (1905) joined Edward Bok's "The 'Patent-Medicine' Curse" (1904) in *The Ladies Home Journal* in raising attention and building concern about the unregulated patent medicine market, while the *Vancouver World* picked up on these reports and launched campaigns to restrict such products in their home province. William Dyas, editor of the Ontario-based *Canadian Druggist* railed against the perception of pharmacist in many of these articles, as a "mere shopkeeper... rather than a member of a profession whose primary object and office is the compounding and dispensing of medicine, in pursuance of a thorough and tested knowledge of his ability to do so" through appropriate education. Although Dyas admitted that "the sale of patent medicines, contribute[s] in some drug stores to a very large proportion of the sales" and that "the patent medicine is a legitimate factor in the business of the retail druggist," he characterized the pharmacist's trade in such products as "a minor portion of the business." Such undue attention to the role of the druggist in distributing such medicines seemed out of place, and Dyas called upon the pharmaceutical press to decry such characterizations.[11] Joseph Emery, editor of the *British Columbia Pharmaceutical Review*, published by the BC Pharmaceutical Association (BCPA), concurred. Commenting that *Colliers*' "diatribe on fraudulent patent medicine advertising" was motivated by a summertime need of "extra sensational" reading for its subscribers, Emery contended that the article entirely misunderstood the exigencies of the market.[12] The customers wanted these products, and limiting their access would take much more education and intervention than merely removing advertisements. Here the pharmacist played a pivotal role as a mediator between public needs and the unrestricted medical market. When faced with a request for a patent or proprietary remedy, Emery advised, it was improper for the druggist to substitute it for something else (substitution was itself an ethical problem). Instead, the druggist should "give what is asked for without question; but, if there follows a conversation – as there often does – on the merits

11 William Dyas, "The retail druggist and patent medicine," *Canadian Druggist* (July 1905): 298.

12 Joseph Emery, "Criminal Newspaper Alliance," *British Columbia Pharmaceutical Review* (September 1905): 37.

of the particular medicine – now is the retailer's opportunity to speak of his own preparation."[13] Here the pharmacist was not just a compounder, but an expert advisor to the health seeking general public. Although Emery's characterization may make pharmacists appear to be merely opportunistic, he was really articulating a core function of the pharmacy profession: a pharmacist provided good advice and more reliable products than some dubious and distant patent medicine manufacturer.

Emery's solution was a clever way to deal with the fact that prefabricated medicines could challenge the pharmacists' skill and knowledge of drugs by reiterating the pharmacist's authority, and in this strategy he was not alone. BCPA President John Cochrane laid out the problem to his colleagues at an address at the association's annual general meeting in June 1905. Faced with customers' demands for patent or proprietary remedies, Cochrane suggested a slightly different approach to undermining the popularity of such medicines. "In offering any of your own preparations ... do not state that it is 'just as good' as this or that patent medicine," which would "pay the patent medicine the compliment of setting it up as a standard by which to judge your preparations." Cochrane argued that it was "reasonable to suppose that a qualified pharmacist ... is able to produce better preparations than the majority of the patent medicines which flood the market to-day." Consequently, "let the public know that you make your preparations from the best obtainable ingredients and according to the latest scientific methods." Most cleverly, though, Cochrane offered a devious way to undermine the prefabricated medicine without actually saying anything bad: "When your opinion is asked as to the medicinal value of this or that patent medicine of secret formula, frankly admit your ignorance of its composition, but state that you do know what goes into your own preparations and that you believe it is all you represent it to be."[14] Again, the pharmacist's skill and familiarity, along with his place as respected expert dedicated to protecting the public by providing reliable medicine, could undermine the secret proprietary trade.

The picture of patent and proprietary remedies painted by these commentators placed the risk and benefit of such products in stark relief, as pharmacists sought to temper their need for revenue against their professional acumen and skill, simultaneously protecting the customer and boosting the pharmacists' own sales. This was a persistent feature of the debates, rhetoric, and actions of the pharmacists. Although they were a profession that drew their revenues from selling things, their professional status was based upon

13 Emery, "Criminal Newspaper Alliance," 37.

14 John Cochrane, "Provincial Pharmaceutical Associations: British Columbia," *Canadian Druggist* (July 1905): 367.

their knowledge, skill, and respectability, most essentially as noted above, to control access to dangerous drugs labelled "poisons" in most pharmacy laws. Yet the secrecy of patent and proprietary medicines meant they could contain any number of these "poisons" and be sold without a prescription or even by retailers who were not pharmacists. Hence for pharmacists the patent medicine debates that arose in the first decade of the twentieth century were especially poignant, problematic, and professionally threatening. Pharmacists took several approaches to addressing the issue. They sought to strengthen their authority in the area of drug composition, reinforce their place as the arbiters of risky and beneficial drugs, confirm their sometimes collegial, sometimes confrontational relationship with the medical fraternity and, ultimately, assert their professional rights at a national level.

The main challenge pharmacists faced came, probably not surprisingly, from a more active, established, and arguably more respected profession: physicians. The relationship between physicians and pharmacists is a topic that cannot be addressed in this short chapter, but it was complicated indeed.[15] Pharmacists positioned themselves as the doctors' helpers, and the doctors accepted this help. At the same time pharmacists had to defend themselves against what they saw as physician overreach into the professional realm of pharmacy. Canadian physicians already benefitted from being generally exempt from the restrictions of pharmacy acts. They could compound and dispense remedies to their patients if they chose to, an exemption that was based upon the tradition of doctors bringing remedies when on house calls, saving a patient a trip to the pharmacy, and the doctor the trouble of writing out a recipe, by putting together the prescription themselves. In some towns, physicians would open their own drugstores, a practice that was normally not illegal, although some provinces required the physician to pay a fee to the provincial pharmacy licensing body (but not sit exams) to legitimate the business. While physicians tread upon the pharmacists' turf, they decried the common and historically rooted practice of druggists recommending

15 The relationship between physicians and pharmacists with respect to drug use is complex. See, for examples, Swenson, *Disorder*; Joseph M. Gabriel, "Restricting the Sale of 'Deadly Poisons': Pharmacists, Drug Regulation, and Narratives of Suffering in the Gilded Age," *Journal of the Gilded Age and Progressive Era* 9, no. 3 (2010): 313–36; for Canada, see Dan Malleck, "'Its Baneful Influences Are Too Well Known': Debates over Drug Use in Canada, 1867–1908," *Canadian Bulletin of Medical History* 14, no. 2 (1997): 263–88; for the UK, see S. W. F. Holloway, "The Apothecaries' Act 1815: A Reinterpretation – Part 1," *Medical History* 10, no. 2 (1966): 107–29; "The Apothecaries' Act 1815: A Reinterpretation – Part 2," *Medical History* 10, no. 3 (1966): 221–36; and Anderson, *Pharmacy and Professionalization*.

remedies to customers without a physician's input, a practice known as "counter prescribing" (because it took place at the druggist's counter).[16]

Arguably, nowhere was the relationship between pharmacists and physicians more complicated than in the issue of patent and proprietary medicines. By many accounts, physicians were advocates for a broad class of proprietaries, and for the pharmacists who sold them. Many of these were ethical proprietaries. The vendors did not advertise to the general public (the "laity"), did not make excessive claims of miraculous cures, and many would indicate their active ingredients. These were the types of proprietaries that both pharmacists and physicians advocated, alluded to by the *Dominion Medical Monthly* in the passage quoted earlier. The *Canadian Practitioner and Review* presented a summary from an article by Wm. J. Robinson published in the *Journal of the American Medical Association*. Robinson divided physicians into three classes when it came to patent medicines: those who "prescribe everything and anything which may be brought to their notice, utterly regardless of composition"; those who "have gone to the other extreme, and object to every patented preparation"; and those who "investigate before they prescribe, adopting a scientific attitude which every physician should emulate."[17] Robinson had little time for the first two, and argued that properly-assessed proprietaries were essential to medical treatment. "The physician who refuses to use a thoroughly established remedy of known composition, merely because it is proprietary, is guilty of narrow-minded fanaticism, and he is not doing the best for his patients."[18] He did not argue that the ingredients of useful proprietaries needed to be revealed, just that the product needed to be known to be effective.

His was not a lone voice. As discussions over proprietaries expanded, physicians continued to support a broad range of patent or proprietary remedies in their practice, so long as the doctors be cautious in their use. Several Canadian medical journals reproduced an argument by Frederick Hadra of San Antonio, who, like Robinson, advised physicians not "to banish all or most of these drugs from his practice without investigating their merits." Hadra was advocating for a product called Antiphlogistine, a topical remedy that he argued was far superior to the traditional flax seed poultice. Given how frequently this article was reproduced, it is likely that, although originally presented at a medical society meeting, it amounted to sponsored content by the manufacturers of antiphlogistine itself, the Denver Chemical Company. Nevertheless, this article reiterates the ideas advocated by many in

16 Swenson, *Disorder*, 77.

17 "The relation of the Physician to Proprietary Remedies," *Canadian Practitioner and Review* (January 1905): 21.

18 "The relation of the Physician to Proprietary Remedies," 21.

the medical press, that proprietaries, properly vetted, were valuable adjuncts to medical practice. The *Dominion Medical Monthly* editorialized that proprietary remedies were useful, in fact, because they addressed a problem in medical practice: the apparent inability for many physicians to write a decent prescription: "We have seen many times prescriptions which when compounded would floor their master to tell what form the combination took when it had entered the stomach of his patient and what its therapeutic effect would be."[19] The *Maritime Medical News* agreed, and, after a proprietary medicine bill was defeated in the Nova Scotia legislature, waxed eloquent about the integral relationship between physicians and proprietary remedies: "There is a goodly list of proprietary medicines of undoubted merit, which we could not well do without, and which, in the future, will no doubt be developed by the chemists and pharmacologists parallel with the development of such general utilitarian products as the anilin dyes."[20] As proprietary medicine legislation began to be discussed at the federal level, the *Dominion Medical Monthly* reiterated its support for proprietaries, but with one caveat: "We are thoroughly of the belief ... like all physicians, we consider we are the best qualified and fitted to diagnose disease in all its forms and to prescribe best for its treatment. Therefore, always have doctors opposed the indiscriminate use of drugs by people who with swell headed wiseness diagnose their own ailments and so prescribe."[21] John Hunter, a leading figure in the Ontario Medical Association, saw doctors' enthusiasm for proprietaries as ethically problematic: "The ethical obligation of the medical citizen [the physician] in regard to this evil is somewhat unique, for he himself may be a contributing factor to it. Does he not err in the importance he attaches to the use of drugs?" Hunter concluded that to be ethical medical citizens, doctors were responsible for teaching "to the patient and to the laity" the best practices in drug-taking.[22]

Unfortunately for physicians and their professional reputation, not every doctor followed the advice to prescribe only the most ethical of proprietary remedies. In 1906 a committee of the Toronto retail druggists association reported to the Ontario College of Pharmacy, at its annual meeting, that it regretted to note "the increasing habit among physicians of prescribing trade marked and fancy named preparations." This characterization alluded to the secret nostrum trade even though, as Gabriel notes, by the turn of

19 Untitled editorial, *Dominion Medical Monthly* (June 1906): 304–5.

20 "Proprietary Medicines," *Maritime Medical News* (July 1906): 249.

21 "The Federal Proprietary and Patent Medicine Act," *Dominion Medical Monthly* (March 1907): 138.

22 John Hunter, "Ethics and deportment of the physician as a citizen," *Canadian Practitioner and Review* (April 1908): 217–19.

the century many remedies that would otherwise be considered ethical were trademarked (and might even have fancy names).[23] Emery of the *BC Pharmaceutical Review* expressed his concern with physicians indiscriminately prescribing such remedies. Instead of doing their own investigations or relying upon authoritative information from reputable medical and pharmaceutical sources, many a physician, he claimed, simply took the manufacturers' promotional literature at face value.[24] It was a significant problem, Emery noted, since, owing to "the desire for 'something new' the physician has allowed himself to be drawn into the vortex of the stream of proprietary preparations to the unfortunate exclusion of the known remedies which after years of world-wide trial find a place in the *Pharmacopoeia*."[25] As David Swenson has illustrated, this characterization of physicians prescribing proprietaries with seemingly little concern about the veracity of the manufacturers' claims was a central driver in the reorganization of American medicine.[26]

Physicians' equivocality in discussions about proprietary medicines indicates a persistent challenge in the delineation between harmful and beneficial medicines. Medical leadership encouraged their confreres to lean upon reliable evaluations of the therapeutic benefits of new remedies, but without the extensive knowledge of pharmacology and chemistry, the time to peruse the medical literature on new remedies, and the ability to delineate paid advertising content from trustworthy assessments of medicines, many doctors were unwittingly traversing a therapeutic minefield. Moreover, the uneasy relationship with pharmacists might mean that a physician was not necessarily prepared to rely upon a pharmacists' perspective, not to mention many pharmacists might be self-interested when pushing their own remedies rather than those "trade marked and fancy named preparations." It was a challenge the pharmacists also recognized. When deliberating whether pharmacists should even carry proprietaries, editor George Evans reminded readers of the *Canadian Druggist* that the best approach was to offer their own ethical alternatives, but to make every effort to show physicians "that we are not usurping or interfering any way with the work of the physicians and that on no account whatever shall we attempt to diagnose." Nevertheless, he insisted, "no reasonable physician will deny that there are numbers of

23 Gabriel discusses the complexity in *Medical Monopoly*, especially Chapter 3, "In the Shadow of War," and Chapter 4, "Therapeutic Reform and the Reinterpretation of Monopoly."

24 Joseph Emery, "Prescribing Proprietaries," *British Columbia Pharmaceutical Review* (March 1907): 184.

25 Emery, "Prescribing Proprietaries," 184.

26 Swenson, *Disorder*, especially Chapter 3, "Therapeutic Chaos and Commercial Conquest."

medicines which druggist may legitimately sell direct to the public."[27] Those ethical proprietaries, compounded, as BCPA president John Cochrane had contended, from the best ingredients and with reliable outcomes, should supplement, not replace, medical treatment.

In arguing that retail druggists' preparations are superior to prefabricated medicines, however, pharmacists faced an embarrassing problem. Between 1899 and 1906, routine "bulletins" issued by the Dominion Analyst repeatedly suggested that medicines compounded by retail druggists tended to be of lower quality than those from wholesale pharmaceutical companies.[28] Most notably, an 1899 report compared preparations of tincture of opium, a commonly prescribed medicine, obtained from pharmacies across the country. Dominion analysts found that few compounded by retail pharmacists met the standard set down in the *British Pharmacopoeia*, while preparations manufactured by wholesale drug firms such as Montreal's Lyman Brothers, were usually compounded accurately. Reviewing the report of 1899, Andrew MacPhail, editor of the *Montreal Medical Journal*, argued that it was entirely reasonable that a physician might prescribe a specific manufacturer's version of a known remedy such as tincture of opium.[29] A 1903 analysis of 294 samples of drugs from pharmacists across the country, a project that looked specifically for arsenic adulteration, thirteen were adulterated and twenty-nine "doubtful." (For comparison, analysis of 182 samples of milk found thirty adulterated and thirty-six "doubtful" so these results were not in themselves unusual.)[30] It was difficult for pharmacists to avoid the fact that the bulletins issued under the authority of the Dominion Adulteration Act indicated that mass produced remedies, rather than those "put up" by retail druggists, were reliable, consistent, and pure, in contrast to the arguments of pharmacy leaders like John Cochrane and George Evans.

Pharmacists thus faced a two-headed dilemma. First was the demonstrated inconsistency in their own compounding practices, something that could not easily be argued away. It might be sufficient to sell a prefabricated

27 George A. Evans, "Should Druggists Handle Patent Medicines?," *Canadian Druggist* (May 1907): 261.

28 The provisions of the Adulteration Act were an expansion of federal powers originally delineated in the Inland Revenue Act and assigned through orders in council between 1873 and 1875. Stand-alone legislation covering analysis was passed in 1884. See Dan Malleck, "Pure drugs and professional druggists: Food and Drug Laws in Canada, 1870s–1908," *Pharmacy in History* 48, no. 3 (2006): 103–15.

29 Andrew MacPhail, "Proprietary Preparations," *Montreal Medical Journal* 32 (May 1903): 359–62. See Malleck, *When Good Drugs Go Bad*, 172–73.

30 "Report Returns and Statistics of the Inland Revenues of the Dominion of Canada... Part III Adulteration of food" (1902).

tincture of opium or citrate of iron, but pharmacists were also required to compound prescriptions conjured up by physicians. This led to the second challenge, which came from many prescriptions written by doctors themselves. As noted earlier, many doctors did not write good prescriptions, a fact that led them to rely increasingly upon proprietary remedies of varying quality and effectiveness. Seeing their professional reputation being challenged by such factors outside of their control, the pharmacy leadership sought to refocus the issue. They decided to use the foundations upon which they built their professional status (knowledge of pharmacy and chemistry, proper care and assessment of drug potencies, and responsible keepers of dangerous drugs) to offer alternatives to doctors who were living in the conflicted state of using proprietaries while decrying their necessity. To the physicians, then, the pharmacists offered standardization.

The *Canadian Formulary* as a Pharmacist-Sponsored Solution

The *Canadian Formulary* was an initiative of the Ontario College of Pharmacy (OCP), but from the outset was intended to be a collaboration of pharmacists across the country. At the OCP's council meeting in August 1902, John Hargreaves proposed the College adopt "some plan of original investigation and research and endorsing and recommending certain standard formulas."[31] A year later the council formally created the Pharmaceutical Research Committee, placing Hargreaves as its chair and giving it an ambitious mandate. [32] The original plan was to work with the Ontario College of Physicians and Surgeons with an eye to "publishing 'an official book of formulae.'" This development excited pharmacists like William Dyas of the *Canadian Druggist* who reminded his readers that the creation of a "Canadian Pharmacopoeia" had been a topic of interest to its readers from the earliest years of the *Druggist*'s publication. Dyas argued that the mandate of the committee should be expanded to allow it to communicate with pharmacy associations across the country, "which might eventually meet together as a committee for the preparation of the Canadian Pharmacopoeia."[33] Whether the council of the OCP heeded the editorial is uncertain, but at the

31 OCP council meeting minutes, August 1902, 13. Original copies of the OCP minutes from 1902 to 1915 have been digitized by the Internet Archive, which deserves your support.

32 OCP council meeting minutes, August 1903, 17.

33 William Dyas, "A Canadian Pharmacopoeia," *Canadian Druggist*, March 1903: 121.

next report of the committee Hargreaves noted that its mandate had been expanded to confer "with other interested bodies." Hargreaves' committee envisioned distributing this *Canadian Formulary* to all pharmacists, and "several interested bodies" including physicians' groups.[34]

The idea of the *Formulary*, although less ambitious than a full national pharmacopoeia, saw widespread support from pharmacists across the country. Pharmacopoeias were normally volumes of comprehensive descriptions of drugs used in medical (and pharmacy) practice. They were important to pharmacists not only because they provided authoritative information about accepted drugs and combinations, but also because they were sometimes embedded in the legal restrictions to which pharmacists were held.[35] Notably, however, the two major pharmacopoeias to which Canadian pharmacists referred (and deferred), the *British Pharmacopoeia* and *United States Pharmacopeia*, had been the initiatives of physicians who, although consulting with pharmacists, led the projects. So creating a Canadian Pharmacopoeia would be a remarkable achievement for Canadian pharmacists, but one that inverted traditions of medical authority. Advocating a Canadian *Formulary* had thus both practical and symbolical value. It would list real, well-tested, and standardized remedies, but by not connecting them to conditions they treated it would not usurp the prescribing authority of physicians. As a result, if the pharmacists could convince physicians to participate in constructing the *Formulary*, they could show their genuine collaborative intent while simultaneously demonstrating their expertise in pharmaco-medical knowledge.

Pharmaceutical societies across the country supported the initiative. When the BC Pharmaceutical Association's council received Hargreaves' letter asking for feedback, it immediately struck a committee to "look into the matter."[36] Although no record exists of this committee's report, Emery of the BCPR reported his hearty approval "of the movement" towards a formulary. In the eastern provinces (Nova Scotia, New Brunswick, and Prince Edward Island), it appears that Hargreaves' letters were misplaced or ignored, since the OCP published its formulary "without any assistance or resistance from the maritime provinces."[37] The Pharmaceutical Association

34 "Report of Special Committee on Pharmaceutical Research," OCP council minutes, August 1903, 15.

35 For example, the Ontario Pharmacy Act (*Statutes of Ontario* (1871) Cap. 34 Sec. 24) set the British Pharmacopoeia as the standard but gave the OCP council the power to choose a different standard.

36 Minutes of the BC Pharmaceutical Association council, December 8, 1904. Minute books in UBC archives, 173.

37 Minutes of the Council of the Nova Scotia Pharmacy Association, April 20, 1908, 292. This was part of a report of the representative on the Canadian Pharmaceutical Association Committee on the Formulary, so it is likely that his

of the North-West Territories (NWT), which at the time included the newly formed provinces of Alberta and Saskatchewan, was most enthusiastically supportive in its records. A committee struck by its council reported that it "heartily endorse the proposal" recognizing the practical and professional advantage of such a volume.

> The multiplicity of preparations, similar in composition offered for sale by many wholesale manufacturing chemists and sampled to physicians and occasionally prescribed entails upon the retail druggist the necessity of keeping an amount of stock of those compounds which, in many cases, their limited use does not warrant and as there is no standard formula of officinal preparations many of which are prescribed largely, the issue of an Authoritative Compendium would standardize many of such compounds, ensure to the physician throughout the Dominion the same dosage and thus the same therapeutic action, be of increased gain to the druggist and tend to preserve the professional aspect of Pharmacy.

It recommended that all druggists of the NWT "bring the proposed compendium to the attention of the Physicians, and send the committee formulae to assist in the work."[38] The only provincial association that did in fact join the OCP in actively constructing the *Formulary* was the Pharmaceutical Association of the Province of Quebec (PAPQ).

Of course, the *Formulary* was not merely an exercise in either demonstrating the unity of the pharmaceutical profession or displaying the chemical knowledge of its members: a key goal was to encourage physicians to follow specific recommended formulae, developed and assessed as optimal for the needs of practitioners and patients across the country. It would address the problems with the sort of bizarre polypharmaceutical prescriptions which had "floored" the *Dominion Medical Monthly*, but more importantly, offer alternatives to proprietary remedies. When informing the OCP that it was inviting pharmacy associations across the country to submit "at least six new formulas" before the end of 1906, the Research Committee specifically

---

statement was a complaint about the apparent disinterest of Maritime societies. There is no evidence in the records of the NB Pharmaceutical Society that an invitation or discussion relating to the formulary was taken up by that society.

38 "Report re Ontario College of Pharmacy," Pharmaceutical Association of the North-West Territories (PANWT) Council minutes 1892–1911, July 10, 1907, in W. C. MacAulay fonds, University of Saskatchewan Archives, MG43-V-1. Until 1905, the North-West Territories had included the area covered by modern day Alberta and Saskatchewan. When these two provinces were carved out of the NWT, the pharmaceutical association remained in action as a PANWT until individual provincial pharmacy legislation was passed in 1910.

mentioned the need for "preparations that will acceptably take the place of proprietary pharmaceuticals with coined names, for which there is an increasing local demand."[39] This purpose was no secret. When the *BCPR* noted its hearty support of the effort, it expressed its "trust [that] physicians may be influenced to prescribe these preparations instead of nostrums the composition of which is decidedly uncertain and often unknown."[40] Providing suggestions to physicians from a profession often seen as subordinate to the medical fraternity was no small task, and it is for this reason that, from the outset, the OCP research committee sought feedback from the Ontario College of Physicians. In the preface of the 1908 publication of the *Formulary*, the Research Committee recommended, as had the Pharmaceutical Association of the North West Territories a few years earlier, that copies be made available to physicians and pharmacists encourage them to use it as an authoritative reference.[41] As the *Canadian Druggist* declared in 1908: "let this be recognized as the standard throughout Canada, and physicians will quickly adapt themselves to using the CF preparations."[42]

It was indeed a hopeful utterance because physicians were not eager to adopt the recommendations of pharmacists, however authoritative, as it affected their professional autonomy, and most especially when it came to the treatment of their patients. Although some medical associations were happy to collaborate with pharmaceutical societies to facilitate, for example, chemistry classes for medical students or to support their legislative efforts, telling a physician what to prescribe undermined a key pillar of the medical profession: the skill, knowledge, and ability to treat illness based upon individual conditions and professional capacity. This is likely why the physicians showed little interest in collaborating on assembling the volume. When reporting on its initial entreaties to the Ontario College of Physicians, Hargreaves and his committee reported that their request "has not met with the expected approval of that body, chief, we believe, for the reason that they misunderstood our objects and desires, and appear somewhat prejudiced."[43] Whether the work of the OCP and the PAPQ in assembling the *Canadian*

39 "Report of Research Committee," OCP council minutes, June 1906, 18.

40 Compendium of Canadian Formulae," *British Columbia Pharmaceutical Review* (November 1905): 70.

41 *Canadian Formulary of Unofficial Preparations* (Ontario College of Pharmacy, 1908), 1. Depending on how you view it this may be the first or second edition. The OCP published a "Compendium of Canadian Formulae" in 1905 but it appears this was intended to generate support by pharmacy and medical societies with a view to compiling a final version. I think 1908 is that final version, even though the research committee calls it the second edition in the introduction.

42 "Canadian Formulary Preparations," *Canadian Druggist* (October 1908): 589.

43 "Report of the Research Committee," OCP council minutes, August 1905, 20.

Formulary ever benefitted from collegial feedback from physicians is difficult to determine. Neither the introduction to the original document, circulated for feedback in 1905, nor the introductions to the subsequent three editions (published 1908–15), mention physicians as members of the committee that compiled the work.

Physicians' apparent lack of interest is not surprising since it mirrors physicians disdain towards the *United States Formulary* assembled by the American Pharmaceutical Association, criticisms of which were also reproduced in Canadian medical journals. As the OCP was seeking feedback for the first edition of the *Canadian Formulary*, the *Maritime Medical News* reproduced an article from *Clinical Medicine* that derided any attempt at redirecting medical attention to national formularies (or even pharmacopoeias). The unsigned article, which appeared in the "Therapeutic Notes" column in the journal (and appeared alongside articles that were clearly advertising copy) argued that the problem with encouraging physicians to reject proprietaries is that "nothing has been done to provide satisfactory substitutes." Probably intentionally missing the point of a *Formulary*, the article's author observed that proponents of such compendia "forget to add that a very large share of these 'official' preparations are old proprietaries under other names. In other words, the great 'reform' consists in the denunciation of such remedies as antiphlogistine, arsenauro, bromidia [etc.] .... While the use of practically the same things under other names is suggested or advised." The article concludes by promoting the value of proprietaries to medical practice, claiming they "have enabled the average physician to secure results more satisfactory to himself and his patients than he was able to secure without them." Providing an alternative to the problem of complex prescriptions which formularies were designed to solve, the author observed that "[v]ery, very few medical men are able to extemporize prescriptions which at the same time are effective, palatable and not uselessly poly-pharmacal" so proprietaries filled a known gap.[44] Another article reproduced from an American medical journal described an analysis of *The United States Formulary* by W. H. Harrison of the Northwestern University School of Pharmacy. Harrison's results showed little patience for standardized recipes that were designed to replace proprietaries:

> some of the preparations were absolutely rank, disgusting, and I could but feel contempt, mixed with indignation, against certain high moguls of pharmacy, who mislead the poor retail druggist and the unsophisticated physician into the belief that their careless, imperfect, theoretical, extemporaneous formulae will yield products 'just as good' as the standard products.

44 "Therapeutic Notes: Another Phase of the Proprietary Question," *Maritime Medical News* (September 1906): xii–xiii. Articles in advertising pages looked like regular articles and were numbered with Roman rather than Arabic numbers.

Harrison concluded by arguing against what he called "National Formulary Propaganda": "Instead of elevating, it tends, as we have shown, to degrade both pharmacy and medicine. It is purely a money-making proposition."[45] That this virulent opposition was a combination of patent medicine propaganda and general resistance by physicians to encroachments by pharmacists is made more stark when we consider that, in 1904 the American Medical Association had struck a "Council on Pharmacy and Chemistry ... to report on the many non-official drugs and combinations on the market for physicians' use" with the intention of publishing a book of approved remedies.[46] The British Medical Society undertook a similar project, publishing in 1909 the first of two volumes that provided the recipes of popular secret remedies.[47] In offering alternative prescriptions for physicians, the pharmacists would see that the problem was neither the medium nor the message: it was the messenger.

The Advent of Dominion Patent and Proprietary Medicine Legislation

The development of the *Canadian Formulary* was coterminous with the shift from the provincial to Dominion action to regulate proprietary medicines, and here again, unity among the pharmacists was essential. After several provinces began unsuccessful attempts to pass proprietary or patent medicine legislation, numerous commentators noted that the effort was more appropriately an issue for the federal government. It made sense both practically and legally. It was practical because such legislation would likely place specific packaging requirements on the products, insisting upon certain language on the labels and possibly even specific requirements for bottles of remedies containing scheduled poisons. Expecting manufacturers to produce different labels for each province and the territories was costly and potentially fatal to small manufacturers. The shift to the federal forum was also legally appropriate because, although few if any of the commentators mentioned constitutional jurisdiction, the Dominion government had the constitutional authority to regulate manufacturing, under provisions of

45 W. H. Harrison, "Miscellaneous –The Proteid Iron Preparations of the National Formulary, or the N. F. Propaganda, with some Queries and Conclusions," *Canadian Practitioner and Review* (September 1908): 602–10.

46 "New and Non-official remedies," *Canada Lancet* (May 1905): 834–35.

47 See *Secret Remedies, What They Cost and What They Contain, Based on Analyses Made for the British Medical Association* (BMA, 1909) and *More Secret Remedies, What They Cost and What They Contain. Based on Analyses Made for the British Medical Association* (BMA, 1912).

the British North America Act that assigned to Dominion authorities the right to pass laws on "Trade and Commerce."[48] Thus the unusual situation arose of professions who were licensed provincially needing to weigh in on a federal law that had the potential to significantly constrain their work. Not surprisingly, pharmacists' and physicians' perspectives on how the legislation should work were notably different.

Pharmacists sought a balance between commercial freedom and protecting the public. This tricky balancing act is illustrated in a letter from the Nova Scotia Pharmaceutical Society to William Fielding, a member of parliament who was asked to help shepherd a law against "fraudulent and injurious nostrums" through the legislature and into law. "The members of [the NSPS] ... are vitally interested in this matter, while on the one hand they desire not to be agents of injurious or fraudulent nostrums, on the other they are anxious that such legislation as may be enacted, may not unnecessarily hamper manufacturers, or the trade generally." The letter outlined two main features of such a law. First, it needed to ensure that "preparations purporting to be medicinal compounds, be required to be such, and not merely alcoholic stimulants." Second, that "preparations containing habit forming drugs ... be required to have a statement of such ingredients."[49] This approach would allow consumers to know whether they were purchasing restricted poisons, while still allowing manufacturers to retain control over the formula of their product. The NSPS approach may have been overly simplistic, but it did reflect the challenge pharmacists faced when balancing their financial interests against their professional reputations.

The balance physicians sought was somewhat different. They insisted that they needed to know what was in any proprietary remedy they might prescribe with the understanding that listing so-called poisons on the label should caution customers about its dangers. Many physicians, well before the revelations of *Colliers* and *The Ladies Home Journal*, understood that some proprietary remedies contained excessive doses of restricted substances, and this admission complicated the understanding of the value of proprietaries. Writing to the *Dominion Medical Monthly* to express its support for a federal committee to investigate the patent medicine issue, the Vancouver Medical Association called the problem "so complex that a proper solution can be arrived at only by competent disinterested persons":

> the drugs that are commonly used in patent medicines are opium or its derivatives, as found in consumption or colic cures and soothing syrups;

48 An Act for the Union of Canada, Nova Scotia, and New Brunswick, and the Government Thereof; and for Purposes Connected Therewith, 30 & 31 Vict. (UK), c. 3 (commonly known as the British North America Act) Section 91 (2).

49 NSPS AGM, June 26, 1906, manuscript book, 37.

> cocaine in catarrh mixtures, acetanelid in headache powders, chloral hydrate in drink cures; belladonna, ergot and cotton root in preparations recommended as abortafacients; [*sic*] and alcohol which is used in medicines represented to cure all diseases .... Yet these are the drugs which are sold in a secret way and without license.[50]

The *Maritime Medical News* looked with favor upon the "better class journals" that were leading the agitation against proprietaries, since "we have the satisfaction of knowing that quackery in its more vicious phases is being brought under the search light."[51] Arguing for the need for physicians to assess for themselves the usefulness of a remedy, many medical commentators contended that the best approach was simply to require all propri etary remedy manufacturers to put the complete formula on the label of their product, thereby allowing physicians to know whether this was something they wanted to recommend to their patients. This, of course, was the practice that had been accepted as an indication of an "ethical" remedy for decades. This approach also would allow customers to know if they were taking something that had a problematic substance like opium, cocaine, or alcohol in excessive volumes. Physicians' interest was both financial and professional. They wanted to be sure that, when they prescribed a proprietary, they knew what their patient was getting, but also wanted to protect their reputations by limiting any blame that might come from the outcome of prescribing problematic substances.

In the initial push for Dominion proprietary medicine legislation, the physicians' lobbying seemed to be more effective, but pharmacists fought a successful rear-guard action. Most bills presented in provincial legislatures included the requirement of the full recipe on the label, acquiescing to the physicians' arguments that only such light would dispel the shadows of secrecy. Pharmacists and their manufacturing chemist colleagues pushed back. They argued that not only was this an unnecessarily and illiberal attack on their proprietary rights, but it also would not achieve what was needed. Taking the perspective of the purchaser rather than the prescriber, they argued that few customers, or patients, had the kind of pharmaceutical knowledge that would benefit from having the entire recipe on the label. A better way, they argued, was to require manufacturers to list products that were on a limited schedule of drugs, not unlike the list of substances restricted by provincial pharmacy laws. Indeed, some thought such a list should encompass the entire poison schedule of most pharmacy acts. Others argued that the proprietary drug schedule should include only the

50 Correspondence, *Dominion Medical Monthly and Ontario Medical Journal* (April 1906): 210.

51 "War Against Quackery," *Maritime Medical* News, February 1906: 47.

most egregious products. At the provincial level the issue was unresolved because no provincial legislature passed a proprietary medicine law in the period under examination.[52] The complexity of the issue, as noted earlier, thrust the issue into the hands of the Dominion government.

Discussion about the Dominion government's role in regulating proprietary medicines had begun at least a decade earlier, but it was a 1904 motion in Senate that began a process leading to legislation.[53] This motion, by physician Senator Michael Sullivan, was made on behalf of the Ontario Medical Council, and asked the government to investigate the patent medicine industry. The motion had wide support in the Senate, and led to a report by A. E DuBerger, an analytical chemist and member of the Pharmaceutical Association of the Province of Quebec (PAPQ). DuBerger's mandate had been to determine how to modify the existing Adulteration Act to deal with proprietary remedies. DuBerger's report was suitably balanced but favored the priorities of his pharmaceutical brethren and their manufacturing colleagues. He argued that formulae needed to be protected, since requiring manufacturers to make them public would undermine "the fruit of long work and … several years of experience and observation" on the part of the vendor. Moreover, making formulae public would be "unfair" and "favour indelicacy and abuses on the part of unscrupulous persons."[54] His recommendation was to form a committee of two physicians, two pharmacists, and "the chief of the pharmaceutical or drug section of the Department of Inland Revenue," which would evaluate the formulae of preparations that were submitted to this committee. It was a solution that protected the intellectual property of the manufacturers, allowed the existing mechanisms to continue to function, and limited the impact on the industry, while, hopefully, diminishing the amount of duplicity and shenanigans of the most egregious secret medicine manufacturers. Creating an oversight board would deputize a government agency to separate the harmful from the beneficial, while doing as little damage as possible to the industry.

It is difficult to determine whether and how DuBerger's perspective influenced ensuing legislation since the report was not discussed in parliament and subsequent events may have muted its impact. Soon after the report was presented to the House, a parliamentary special committee was struck

52 In 1885, Quebec passed an amendment to the pharmacy act that gave pharmacists some control over proprietary medicines. It did not last long. See Malleck, *When Good Drugs Go Bad*, 195–97.

53 Malleck, *When Good Drugs Go Bad*, 204–10.

54 Malleck, *When Good Drugs Go Bad*, 207. For the full text, see A. E. DuBerger, "Return to an Order of the House of Commons, Dated April 23, 1906, for a Copy of the Report of A.E. DuBerger, on the Drug and Proprietary Medicine Trade of Canada," *Sessional Papers of the Dominion of Canada* 125 (1906): 22–23.

to investigate the best way of dealing with the patent and proprietary medicine issue. The records of this committee have been lost, but it appears that DuBerger's report was but one of a number of competing perspectives that came to play in subsequent discussions. Lobbying was certainly ramped up. The Quebec pharmacists wrote to Prime Minister Wilfrid Laurier endorsing (not surprisingly) DuBerger's report as representing the best way to deal with the issue.[55] When an amendment to the Adulteration Act was presented in the House, the Proprietary Articles Trades Association wrote in protest to Laurier, saying their "important industry ... would be injuriously affected thereby."[56] Physicians' groups also wrote, indicating that the formula on the label approach remained their preferred method of dealing with the issue. [57] Parliamentarians, it appears, were being lobbied from all sides.

The attempt to modify the Adulteration Act did not proceed far in the legislature, and Minister of Inland Revenue William Templeman opted instead to draft a new Proprietary or Patent Medicine Act and present it at the next parliamentary session. The first iteration of the law was widely decried. It established an assessment process such as DuBerger suggested and required manufacturers submit samples of all remedies to be submitted for evaluation. It also exempted from its provisions any remedy that was found in the British or US *Pharmacopoeias*, the *Codex Medicamentarius* of France, or "any foreign pharmacopoeia."[58] What drew the ire of the pharmacists and the pharmaceutical industry was the provisions requiring each sample that was submitted for assessment be accompanied by a fee of two dollars, and every package sold thereafter to be subject to a stamp tax. This meant that every retail druggist who put up his own remedy would have to pay two dollars to have it assessed and then charge a stamp tax. It was, as the *BCPR* described it, "an immense piece of departmental machinery" and, not surprisingly, faced concerted pushback.[59]

Although it did not require the formula on the label, the proposed bill, with its stamp tax, drove the pharmacists apoplectic. Emery of the *BCPR* attempted to rally his readers to write their members of parliament and unite across the country in opposition to the law. In October 1906, with a rallying title of "Up, Druggists!" Emery exhorted his fellow pharmacists to pay attention "there must be an end of this idea that 'it does not

55 Tremblay and Muir to Laurier, March 28, 1906, Laurier files, 108895.

56 Watson to Laurier, April 6, 1906, Laurier files, 109256.

57 "Extrait du Proces Verbal de l'association medico-chirurgiale do Distcit to Joliette Reunition du 11 Juin 1906," Laurier files, 111775.

58 Copy of bill in Laurier files 116397–116405. Templeman to Laurier, December 6, 1906, 116397.

59 "Now is the time for action," *British Columbia Pharmaceutical Review* (December 1906): 115–16.

concern us' – for the health of the public is at stake, and an insidious foe more deadly than alcoholism even is sapping the character, energy and life out of the nation." The problem, he saw, was lack of a central motivating agency, "some governing spirit, some definite reliable instructions."[60] As Templeman's law sputtered through parliament, Emery argued that "[w]e cannot ... afford to be independent isolated units; we must get together, decide upon a line of action, appoint committees and act. We wish some energetic men in each city would take this matter up and push it to a complete organization."[61] Others echoed this call. In April 1907, editor Dyas of the *Canadian Druggist* published "A Call For Action" arguing that "[n]o disjointed, unorganized body (if it can be called a body) of men can accomplish satisfactory results, especially in time of strenuous competition and it is only through perfect organization and an unanimity of purpose that any material success may be obtained." Like Emery, Dyas saw the current federal legislation as a serious problem and argued that it was exacerbated by the lack of national unity among pharmacists who "in their present unorganized condition and without a general executive to control and watch over any contemplated incursions on registered rights, ... are unable to successfully combat these encroachments."[62]

These calls appear to have been heard, and when representatives of pharmacy associations met in Ottawa to lobby against the proprietary medicine act in early 1907, George Burbidge, president of the Nova Scotia Pharmaceutical Society, proposed pharmacists unite to create a Dominion Pharmaceutical Association to address issues of national importance to the druggists of the country.[63] The idea was not only to deal with legislative matters, but also to navigate the tricky issue of interprovincial licensing and educational standards, which were hindering pharmacists trained in one province from setting up shop elsewhere. These issues had been contentious since the creation of pharmacy licensing laws, but it was the significant threat presented to druggists by the proprietary medicine legislation that spurred pharmacists out of the lethargy that Emery lamented, and into the offices of the Ontario College of Pharmacy in September 1907. There, in an impressively brief meeting, representatives from pharmaceutical societies across the country formed the Canadian Pharmaceutical Association,

60 "Up, Druggists!," *British Columbia Pharmaceutical Review* (October 1906).

61 Joseph Emery, "The need of Organization," *British Columbia Pharmaceutical Review* (March 1907): 181.

62 William Dyas, "A Call for Action," *Canadian Druggist* (April 1907): 193–94.

63 George Burbidge, "Patent Medicine Legislation and Canadian Pharmaceutical Association," *Canadian Pharmaceutical Journal* 40 (May 1907): 475–76. Burbidge was credited with initiating the process. See "Canadian Pharmaceutical Association," *Canadian Pharmaceutical Journal* 41 (August 1907): 16.

drafted a constitution and bylaws, elected officers, and formed committees to deal with the most contentious issues facing pharmacists at the time. It also endorsed the *Canadian Formulary* "as the standard for preparations not found in official formularies."[64] By this time the first proprietary medicine bill had failed to move through the legislature, so the Canadian Pharmaceutical Association was also poised to influence the shape of the next iteration. When the Patent or Proprietary Medicine Act became law in 1908 it contained several elements that were a direct influence of the Canadian Pharmaceutical Association's work. First, the fee for assessment of every formula was changed to a one dollar charge per manufacturer (rather than per remedy), something most pharmacists could afford. Second, the stamp tax disappeared. Third, no product would be subject to the fee if the full recipe were on the label. Finally, the bill retained the provision that exempted any product manufactured according to the list of official pharmacopoeias, but added to that list "any formulary adopted by any properly constituted pharmaceutical association representing the Dominion of Canada, approved by the Minister." In other words, the *Canadian Formulary*, recognized as authoritative by the Canadian Pharmaceutical Association, was elevated to represent authoritative Canadian pharmaceutical knowledge even if physicians continued not to voice support for its contents.[65]

Conclusion: Risks and Benefits, to the Public and the Profession

The agitation and legislation to deal with the concerns over the proprietary and patent medicine issue demonstrate the intricate contextual nature of ideas of risks and benefits in medicines. Such concepts were debated and shifted based upon political, economic, professional, and philosophical perspectives. To physicians, any remedy was risky if the physician did not know its ingredients or did not prescribe it. The physician's experience and authority delineated benefit from risk. For pharmacists, their expertise in pharmacology, combined with their experience and knowledge of adequate prescription formulation, mitigated some of the risks associated with the mystery behind some remedies when prepared by ethical manufacturers. Yet pharmacists' perspective was influenced (and, doctors may have argued, corrupted) by their liminal situation between profession and trade. With their

64 "Dominion Pharmaceutical Association Organizational Meeting," *British Columbia Pharmaceutical Review* (October 1907), 71–79.

65 "An Act Respecting Proprietary or Patent Medicines," *Statutes of Canada* (1908), Cap. 56, Sec. 2(b).

need to sell products to make a living, pharmacists' views of regulation and restriction were attentive to the effect such actions would have on the market. This was not necessarily a negative feature. Protecting the integrity of the market from the worst excesses of government overreach would safeguard the reputation of the pharmacy profession while simultaneously limiting the opportunties of disreputable companies, driven by profit, to engage in unsavoury activities while purporting to act for the benefit and health of their customers. Balancing the risks of specific government regulations against the benefits of such oversight remained a complex process, nearly as complicated as determining the risks and benefits of the drugs themselves.

Chapter Two

Ehrlich's Dangerous Magic: Salvarsan and the Fantasy of Pharmaceutical Innovation

Joseph M. Gabriel

In 1914, eight people died after a physician at the Los Angeles County Hospital named Albert T. Charlton treated them with the arsenical drug Neo-Salvarsan for, as one newspaper put it, an "unspeakable disease." Charlton resigned from the hospital soon after and was legally charged with their deaths. Yet whether he was actually responsible was an open question. According to some observers, Charlton might have been at fault due to administering the drug incorrectly; others pointed out that the hospital had purchased a batch of the drug on the open market for the lowest price available and that the deaths might have resulted from a poorly made product. The Grand Jury in Charlton's case eventually determined that the drug had decomposed and become poisonous, although they were unable to determine why – it might have been Charlton's handling of the drug, or a crack in the vial, or some problem with the manufacturing process. Whatever the reason, the Grand Jury recommended that charges against Charlton be dropped due to the difficulty of assigning responsibility. They also called on federal authorities to exercise "more stringent supervision" over the market to forestall a public backlash against the drug so that "society may not lose this great boon." Physicians across the country came to a similar conclusion: some blamed the manufacturer, some blamed Charlton, some blamed both. Whoever was responsible, observers pointed out that unreliable Salvarsan was part of the broader problems of poorly trained clinicians, poor manufacturing, counterfeit goods, and drug peddlers.[1] No one blamed the drug

1 "Grand Jury to Seek Flaws," *Los Angeles Times* (March 11, 1914); "'Death' Medicine Proved Innocent," *Los Angeles Times* (September 25, 1914), II1;

itself. The supposed "death medicine," as one newspaper put it, had been "proved innocent."[2]

Salvarsan is well known to historians of medicine.[3] First synthesized in 1907 in the laboratory of German scientist Paul Ehrlich, Ehrlich dubbed the chemical a "magic bullet" because of its supposed ability to act on the specific microorganism that caused syphilis without harming the rest of the human body.[4] Salvarsan was commercially introduced by the German manufacturer Fabwerke Hoechst AG soon after. Ehrlich also developed a more

---

"Eight Treated; Seven Dead and one Dying," *Los Angeles Times* (March 9, 1914), II1; "Fault Found in Technique," *Los Angeles Times* (April 3, 1914), II1; Edward H. Marsh, "The Dangers Accruing from Drugs Purchased from Peddlers," *The Medical Times* (April, 1914): 102–4; "Deaths Following Injection of Neo-Salvarsan in Los Angles," *Journal of the American Medical Association* (March 21, 1914): 935–36; "Seven Deaths following the Interspinal Injection of Neo-Salvarsan in the Los Angeles County Hospital," *Indianapolis Medical Journal* (1914): 157–58.

2 "'Death' Medicine Proved Innocent," II1.

3 Among other topics, historians have examined Salvarsan's role in public health campaigns, Ehrlich's importance in the broader history of chemotherapy and tropical medicine, the drug's role as a precursor to the latter development of antibiotics, and efforts to market the drug through what scholars have called "scientific marketing" and "scientific commercialism." Allan M. Brandt, *No Magic Bullet: A Social History of Venereal Disease in the United States since 1880* (Oxford University Press, 2020); John Parascandola, *Sex, Sin, and Science: A History of Syphilis in America* (Praeger, 2008); Steven Riethmiller, "From atoxyl to salvarsan: searching for the magic bullet," *Chemotherapy* 51, no. 5 (2005): 234–42; Deborah Neill, *Networks in Tropical Medicine: Internationalism, Colonialism, and the Rise of a Medical Specialty, 1890–1930* (Stanford University Press, 2020); William Rosen, *Miracle Cure: The Creation of Antibiotics and the Birth of Modern Medicine* (Penguin, 2017); J. E. Lesch, ed., *The First Miracle Drugs: How the Sulfa Drugs Transformed Medicine* (Oxford University Press, 2006); Axel C. Hüntelmann, "A different mode of marketing? The importance of scientific articles in the marketing process of Salvarsan," *History and Technology* 29, no. 2 (2013): 116–34; Axel C. Hüntelmann, "Making Salvarsan: experimental therapy and the development and marketing of Salvarsan at the crossroads of science, clinical medicine, industry, and public health," in *Ways of Regulating Drugs in the 19th and 20th Centuries*, ed. Jean-Paul Gaudillière and Volker Hess (Palgrave Macmillan UK, 2013), 43–65; Jonathan Liebenau, *Medical Science and Medical Industry: The Formation of the American Pharmaceutical Industry* (Palgrave Macmillan UK, 1987), 109–24.

4 Ehrlich appears to have first used the phrase "magic bullet" in 1906 to refer to antiserum rather than a chemical substance. See "Address delivered at the dedication of the Georg-Speyer-Haus," in *The Collected Papers of Paul Ehrlich*, ed. F. Himmelweit, 4 vols. (Pergamon Press, 1960), vol. 3, 53–63. See also N.

soluble and easier to prepare version of the drug, which Hoechst marketed under the name "Neo-Salvarsan" around 1912.[5] Over the course of the next three decades, Salvarsan and Neo-Salvarsan became common treatments for syphilis in the United States. At the same time, the so-called "magic bullet" framework became an important part of both the popular and scientific understanding of the relationship between pharmaceutical interventions and disease. "The dream of a chemical agent which will destroy pathogenic microörganisms … and which at the same time is harmless to the body organism has been a guiding force of a host of medical scientists for many decades," noted the physician Frederick C. Smith in his 1944 book on sulfanilamide therapy. "Ehrlich had it and was indefatigable in his search for such a medicament, finally bringing forth salvarsan, which with its modification, neosalvarsan, is still a standard treatment for syphilis."[6]

This chapter is about how we imagine innovation and cure.[7] It is also about how we imagine innovation and harm. I use the widespread adoption of Salvarsan, Neo-Salvarsan, and later sulfanilamide in the United States to tell a story about how we invest our fantasies of cure in the development of new pharmaceuticals and how we manage the sad fact that these products both heal and harm us. I argue that we do so through a narrative process that separates the scientific and the social into distinct domains. Salvarsan and Neo-Salvarsan were conceptualized not only as tremendous scientific advances through the conjoined dreams of military precision and therapeutic promise; they were also imagined as dangerous substances that should be investigated and managed through medical science and expertise

S. Mayo, "Intravenous Therapy" in *The Abbott Laboratories: Helpful Hints for the Veterinarian* (1926): 1.

5 The company secured patents and trademarks on both drugs and their names; during World War I, however, the US government seized Hoechst's property rights on the chemicals as part of its broader seizure of German assets; the drugs were then given the non-commercial names "arsphenamine" and "neo-arsphenamine" by federal authorities. Due to space constraints, I have left this issue aside in this chapter, but see Dale Cooper, "The Licensing of German Drug Patents Confiscated during World War I: Federal and Private Efforts to Maintain Control, Promote Production, and Protect Public Health," *Pharmacy in History* 54, no. 1 (2012): 3–32; Kathryn Steen, "Confiscated commerce: American importers of German synthetic organic chemicals, 1914–1929," *History and Technology, an International Journal* 12, no. 3 (1995): 261–84.

6 Frederick C. Smith and George Morris Piersol, *Sulfonamide Therapy in Medical Practice* (F. A. Davis Company, 1944), v.

7 This sentence intentionally echoes the opening line of Bharat Jayram Venkat, *At the Limits of Cure* (Duke University Press, 2021).

so that their benefits might be expanded and their risks reduced. Yet such efforts would not be enough: the risks of this "dangerous magic," as one observer called sulfanilamide, were also conceptualized as a function of ignorance, greed, sexual immorality, and other problems reformers associated with irrational forms of belief and behavior supposedly characteristic of racial minorities, prostitutes, disreputable pharmacists, and other parties. These problems required more than scientific investigation and professional expertise: from the perspective of numerous reformers, they also needed to be managed through legislative and other means so that the therapeutic potential of pharmaceutical discovery might be fulfilled. The risks and benefits of Salvarsan, Neo-Salvarsan, and later sulfanilamide were thus divided into distinct domains subject to different, but overlapping, types of investigation and management.

What might be called the boundary work of Salvarsan – the demarcation of scientific from social practice and meaning – was an imaginative act narrated along temporal lines.[8] I argue that this articulation of the longing for cure grew out of changes in the conceptual foundations of scientific medicine that developed over the course of the late nineteenth and early twentieth centuries. It was also linked to the commercial development of new products through collaborative relationships with pharmaceutical manufacturers during this time. As an almost endless flood of new products were introduced to the market during the interwar period, an iterative system of drug development was then established in which the new tended to replace the old; at the same time, pharmaceutical risk and benefit were divided into scientific and social domains with the latter seemingly operating as a barrier to the former. The progress of experiment thus encountered the limits of cure and yet, while frustrated, continued to promise a future better than the past through the commercial introduction of new types of magic.[9] Ehrlich's discovery, in

8 Thomas F. Gieryn, "Boundary-work and the demarcation of science from non-science: Strains and interests in professional ideologies of scientists," *American Sociological Review* 48, no. 6 (1983): 781–95. On narrative and imagination in medical science, see the collection of essays on epidemics and Charles Rosenberg's work published in *Bulletin of the History of Medicine* 94, no. 4 (2020), including Keith Wailoo, "Spectacles of difference: the racial scripting of epidemic disparities" (602–25) and Samuel K. Cohn Jr., "The dramaturgy of epidemics" (578–89). See also Sari Altschuler, *The Medical Imagination: Literature and Health in the Early United States* (University of Pennsylvania Press, 2018); Charles E. Rosenberg, *Explaining Epidemics* (Cambridge University Press, 1992).

9 I am invoking Harry M. Marks, *The Progress of Experiment: Science and Therapeutic Reform in the United States, 1900–1990* (Cambridge University Press, 1997).

turn, was rearticulated as a part of history, an important moment in the story of humanity's battle against disease that has now gone by, even as the narrative structure that it helped advance continued – and continues – to shape our fantasies of cure.

Specificity and Wonder

Charlton's fateful administration of Neo-Salvarsan in 1914 reflected a profound transformation in medical thought about how drugs work. In the early nineteenth century, outside of a small number of what were called "specifics," drugs were not assumed to operate on disease in the same way across distinct clinical cases. Case reports provided examples of a remedy's general utility but did not imply effectiveness for any particular patient's ailments due to the distinctiveness of the individual under humoral and other medical theories and the general lack of ontologically discrete disease categories. Medical science was therefore based on the testimony of individual physicians about their experiences testing substances on their patients, and the job of the physician was to integrate this body of knowledge with the specific characteristics and problems of the patient he sought to treat.[10] Manufacturers of so-called quack remedies contradicted this approach by keeping the ingredients of their products secret and otherwise monopolizing their goods for their own, supposedly, selfish ends, thereby limiting the physician's ability to tailor treatment to the individual patient's needs.[11] They also advertised to the public and claimed generalized utility for their goods, a practice which reformers in the orthodox medical community saw as deeply irrational and conflicting with the unique nature of each case. Orthodox physicians thus critiqued the monopolization of new remedies as a form of quackery and juxtaposed it to both the "professional character" needed to make trustworthy scientific claims and with the utility of medicines themselves.[12]

10 John Harley Warner, *The Therapeutic Perspective: Medical Practice, Knowledge, and Identity in America, 1820–1885* (Harvard University Press, 1986), 11–82; Charles Rosenberg, "The Therapeutic Revolution: Medicine, Meaning, and Social Change in Nineteenth-Century America," *Perspectives in Biology and Medicine* 20, no. 4 (1977): 485–506.

11 Joseph M. Gabriel, *Medical Monopoly: Intellectual Property and the Origins of the Modern Pharmaceutical Industry* (University of Chicago Press, 2014), esp. Chapter 1.

12 Gamma, "On the Inexpediency and Invalidity of Granting Patents for Medicines, Considered in a Medico-Legal View," *Boston Medical and Surgical Journal* 13 (1835): 218–21, 218.

As historians have long noted, in the decades following the American Civil War orthodox physicians began to rely on laboratory science to warrant their knowledge claims and to consider disease as a vast collection of discrete ontological entities that are the same across each instantiation regardless of the case at hand. This growing specificity of disease was, in turn, matched with the growing specificity of drug action, and while specific drugs might have a variety of effects, each of these effects was itself increasingly understood as specific in nature. Investigating the relation between drug and disease in the laboratory depended upon an array of experimental conditions which themselves might or might not be comparable. The increasing specificity of disease and drug was thus matched with the increasing specificity of laboratory practice and, at least ideally, the recognition that laboratory investigations should be roughly equivalent to one another regardless of the scientist who conducted them. By 1900 the assumption that "physiological standardization" should be practiced in laboratory science had attained at least some currency, a phrase that applied not only to substances but also to laboratory practices themselves. Roughly standardized laboratory practice, in turn, appeared to be a precondition upon which knowledge of drug action might be generated.[13]

Similar principles applied to clinical research. In the early nineteenth century orthodox physicians knew that drugs worked because they had certain physical effects, such as causing people to vomit or sweat, that appeared to be correlated with their patients feeling better and that could, after sufficient repetition, be predicted to at least some degree. These results were also reported in the medical press or shared among colleagues, with the assumption that such case reports should inform a physician's treatment of his patients but also that they were not dispositive. By the end of the nineteenth century, however, the effects of drugs on the human body were rapidly being rendered into categories that extended beyond the individual case

13 On the development of laboratory science and what John Harley Warner has called "physiological therapeutics," see William Rutherford, *An Experimental Research on the Physiological Actions of Drugs* (Macmillan and Co., 1880), 89–162; Cay-Rüdiger Prüll, "Paul Ehrlich's Standardization of Serum: *Wertbestimmung* and Its Meaning for Twentieth-Century Biomedicine," in *Evaluating and Standardizing Therapeutic Agents, 1890–1950*, ed. Christoph Gradmann and Johnathan Simon (Palgrave Macmillan, 2010), 13–29; John Harley Warner, *The Therapeutic Perspective: Medical Practice, Knowledge, and Identity in America, 1820–1885* (Princeton University Press, 2014); John Harley Warner, "The Fall and Rise of Professional Mystery: Epistemology, Authority and the Emergence of Laboratory Medicine in Nineteenth-Century America," in *The Laboratory Revolution in Medicine*, ed. Andrew Cunningham and Perry Williams (Cambridge University Press, 1992), 110–41.

and instead linked the action of specific drugs to relatively predictable outcomes regardless of the patient in question. At the heart of this halting process was a complex transformation in which experimental knowledge about drug effects was separated from the testimony of individual physicians and instead cast as the result of dis-interested collective investigation; this process of abstraction was, in turn, dependent on efforts to standardize dose, group experimental subjects into categories based on shared trait, and otherwise control experimental factors in order to render clinical experiment legible across case.[14] By World War I it was widely recognized that both collective investigation and controlled trials legible across case were necessary to meaningfully warrant claims to effectiveness.

Manufacturers in the so-called ethical wing of the industry played an important part in this process. During much of the nineteenth century, reputable manufacturers had largely refrained from making therapeutic claims about their goods and commercially developing what today we might call "innovative" products due to the assumption within the medical community that doing so would infringe on their scientific prerogatives and was driven by self-interest. Beginning in roughly the 1880s, however, companies such as Parke, & Company and Frederick Stearns & Company began to argue that commercially introducing new medicines and describing the therapeutic effects of these goods contributed to the development of medical science; they also began to invest in in-house laboratories and to develop clinical testing programs based on collaborative relationships with clinicians. This type of scientific infrastructure served both commercial and scientific goals and was based on shared sets of assumptions about the importance of collective investigation, disinterest as an epistemic virtue, and the standardization of evidence. Manufacturers thus played an important part in the transformation of medical science during this period as they worked with the medical community to reorient drug development along the newly emergent epistemological lines; they also worked to render pharmaceutical patenting as ethically legitimate through the now-familiar logic of investment and both commercial and therapeutic return. This took place along lines of social and institutional relationships in which manufacturers, physicians in clinical practice, and – beginning in the late nineteenth century – academic scientists overlapped and established themselves as distinct social and scientific class

14 "New Inhalation Treatment for Phthisis," *Northwestern Lancet* (1899), 96–97. On clinical science and medical epistemology, see Eli Osterweil Anders, "'A Plea for the Lancet': Bloodletting, Therapeutic Epistemology, and Professional Identity in Late Nineteenth-Century American Medicine," *Social History of Medicine* 29, no. 4 (2016): 781–801; Steve Sturdy, "Looking for Trouble: Medical Science and Clinical Practice in the Historiography of Modern Medicine," *Social History of Medicine* 24, no. 3 (2011): 758–75.

with overlapping and often reinforcing norms, or what manufacturer H. K. Mulford called in 1906 “the charmed circle.”[15]

There was an incredibly important racial component to all this. Orthodox medicine had long been practiced almost exclusively by white, male physicians and, with a handful of exceptions, systematically excluded both white women and racial minorities of both sexes. A preoccupation with the supposed physical and social differences between races was a central part of the development of medical science over the course of the nineteenth century – although this changed somewhat following the Civil War with the establishment of Black medical schools and the development of Black professional networks – and the social and institutional structures of orthodox medicine remained both highly segregated and racially exclusionary during the late nineteenth and early twentieth centuries.[16] The same can be said for pharmaceutical manufacturing: although more research on the issue needs to be done, occasional efforts by formerly enslaved people to establish manufacturing companies along the new epistemic lines appear to have failed due to a lack of financial investment and exclusion from developing scientific and commercial networks dominated by whites.[17] As the turn toward laboratory

15 H. K. Mulford to Francis E. Stewart, Stewart Papers, University of Wisconsin. On the development of pharmaceutical science and collaborative relationships between the medical community and industry before World War I in the United States, see Gabriel, *Medical Monopoly*; Joseph F. Spillane, *Cocaine: From Medical Marvel to Modern Menace in the United States, 1884–1920* (Johns Hopkins University Press, 2000); Jonathan Liebenau, *Medical Science and Medical Industry: The Formation of the American Pharmaceutical Industry* (Springer, 1987).

16 Christopher Willoughby, *Masters of Health: Racial Science and Slavery in US Medical Schools* (UNC Press Books, 2022); Rana A. Hogarth, *Medicalizing Blackness: Making Racial Difference in the Atlantic World, 1780–1840* (UNC Press Books, 2017); W. Michael Byrd and Linda A. Clayton, *An American Health Dilemma: A Medical History of African Americans and the Problem of Race: Beginnings to 1900* (Routledge, 2012); Todd Lee Savitt, *Medicine and Slavery: The Diseases and Health Care of Blacks in Antebellum Virginia* (University of Illinois Press, 2002).

17 This claim should be considered tentative. For one example of an effort to start a Black-owned manufacturing company, see “Negroes Organize Wholesale Drug Co,” *Atlanta Constitution* (April 13, 1910); “Short Items of Interest,” *Atlanta Constitution* (August 19, 1909), 5. More scholarly work needs to be done on Black pharmacy and drug manufacturing before World War I, but see John Elbert Clark, *Early Education of African American Pharmacists 1870–1975* (Bookstand Publishing, 2021); Gregory Bond, “Recovering and expanding Mozella Esther Lewis’s pioneering history of African-American pharmacy students, 1870–1925,” *Pharmacy in History* 58,

science and collective clinical research took place it thus did so largely along the lines of white institutions and claims; the explanatory framework for understanding supposed differences in the distribution of increasingly specific diseases was, in turn, constituted in two distinct ways within white medical science. On the one hand, disease appeared to operate in different groups of people in complex ways that eluded easy explanation but often seemed linked to physical differences, including supposed differences between racial groups. At the same time, however, the presumed equivalence between cases at the heart of the new drug and disease ontologies suggested similarity across racial difference and, perhaps, what some social theorists have since posited as an overdetermined universal body based on the norms of the white subject.[18]

Connected to this process was a growing bifurcation between drug action and what we now call social context. The rendering of both disease and treatment along lines of ontological specificity produced not just a vast and ever-growing array of distinct ailments and medicines; it also worked to abstract the intersection of drug and body from the broader array of relationships that constitute the world. In doing so, the scientific and the social were increasingly rendered into distinct domains, although – as Bruno Latour makes clear – never fully so.[19] This too was intertwined with race and other marks of difference: during the early nineteenth century, orthodox physicians had often considered enslaved and Indigenous peoples to possess secret therapeutic knowledge that might be revealed and exploited through the process of scientific discovery and the circulation of medical knowledge. The transformation of medical science along the new epistemic and collaborative lines thus took place in the context of resource extraction and the scientific geographies of race as orthodox physicians and their manufacturing colleagues worked to convert the cosmologies of Indigenous and formerly enslaved peoples into commercially profitable and scientifically legible forms

---

nos. 1–2 (2016): 3–23. On debates about racial capitalism as an analytic category, see Justin Leroy, "Racial capitalism and black philosophies of history," in *Histories of racial capitalism*, ed. Destin Jenkins and Justin Leroy (Columbia University Press, 2021), 169–84; Michael Ralph and Maya Singhal, "Racial capitalism," *Theory and Society* 48, no. 6 (2019): 851–81.

18 On medical epistemology as a "collective agreement," see Owen Whooley, *Knowledge in the Time of Cholera: The Struggle over American Medicine in the Nineteenth Century* (University of Chicago Press, 2012). See also Emily August, "Medicine's Cultural Power: The Textbook Case of *Gray's Anatomy*," in *Embodied Difference: Divergent Bodies in Public Discourse*, ed. Jamie A. Thomas and Christina Jackson (Lexington Books, 2019), 167; Anirban Das, "Medical Knowledge of the Body. Colonial Encounters," *Rethinking Marxism* 13, no. 2 (2001): 109–31.

19 Bruno Latour, *We Have Never Been Modern* (Harvard University Press, 2012).

of knowledge.[20] At the same time, beliefs and practices that did not conform to the changing scientific framework were increasingly interpreted as misguided and fundamentally irrational, whether due to ignorance, superstition, greed, or some other characteristic that supposedly did not align with the developing therapeutic framework. As a result, over the course of the late nineteenth and early twentieth centuries, orthodox medical science both excluded Black and brown perspectives at a structural level and characterized other perspectives on health and healing – perspectives often understood in racialized terms – as both irrational in nature and, perhaps, concealing some kernel of truth that might be exploited through scientific investigation and development. Medical science was thus reformulated not just through changing scientific epistemology and its collaboration with commercial forces but also through the language and changing institutional structures of racialized epistemology; so too was the growing distinction between the social and the scientific.

One result of all this was that discovery was increasingly narrated in dramatic terms. Orthodox physicians had long understood the progress of medical science as slow, methodical, and based on individual investigation and testimony – but also, in an important way, as collective in nature since it depended on a community of reputable physicians dedicated, at least in theory, to investigating disease and sharing their results with one another to advance the common good. From this perspective, dramatic tales of sudden discoveries and wonderous cures were the domain of quackery.[21] As drugs were increasingly understood as having specific actions on disease, and as disease was transformed into discrete and specific clinical entities, however, it became increasingly meaningful to understand specific new drugs as having not just specific effects, but *dramatic* specific effects. The transformation of disease into discrete clinical entities – whether linked to bacteriology or to what Charles Rosenberg has called "the therapeutic revolution" more broadly – was thus intertwined with the possibility of dramatic medical progress and wonderous descriptions of drug effects.[22] Indeed, by the

20 For a discussion of one aspect of this dynamic, see Joseph M. Gabriel, "Indian Secrets, Indian Cures, and the Early History of the United States Pharmacopoeia," in *Drugs on the Page: Pharmacopoeias and Healing Knowledge in the Early Modern Atlantic World*, ed. Matthew Crawford and Joseph M. Gabriel (University of Pittsburgh Press, 2019), 240–62.

21 Stephanie P. Browner, *Profound Science and Elegant Literature: Imagining Doctors in Nineteenth-Century America* (University of Pennsylvania Press, 2005), 15–38.

22 Bert Hansen, "America's First Medical Breakthrough: How Popular Excitement about a French Rabies Cure in 1885 Raised New Expectations for Medical Progress," *American Historical Review* 103, no. 2 (1988): 373–418;

early twentieth century a wide variety of scientific advances had led to the development of numerous products that seemed remarkable in their therapeutic powers, including vaccines and serums, antipyretics such as phenacetin and aspirin, and glandular products such as adrenalin. Many of these products were first developed in Europe – particularly in Germany – but as these goods were tested and marketed in the United States they were folded into the developing institutional and social systems that made up American medical science. They also became part of, and contributed to, developing narratives of wonder and discovery in which commercially developed pharmaceuticals were intertwined with the dream of precision and cure. "The most perfect therapeutic agents which can be produced or even imagined are the antiserums," noted one scientist in 1911. "This follows from the fact that they are strictly specific agents which act only on the parasites."[23] Adrenalin chloride, noted manufacturer Parke, Davis & Company around the same time, "acts more like a miracle than a medicine."[24] Still, the connection between scientific epistemology and the white racial imagination was never far from the surface; a 1904 advertisement for adrenalin makes the point – it pictures a beautiful white goddess, bringing the boon of the miracle cure to those who suffer.[25]

Descriptions of the "amazing" power of new medicines were also accompanied by the dream of military precision and targeted destruction in the "war" against disease.[26] Ehrlich's discovery of Salvarsan was the most important example of this; as Lorenzo Servitje points out, the military metaphor has long been connected to the act of healing and was deeply embedded in Ehrlich's thinking about the effects of dye staining and bacterial identification.[27] At the same time, by the late nineteenth century – even as clinical investigation began to be rendered distinct from individual physician testimony and dispersed through the scientific effort to achieve legibility across case – discovery and invention in the medical domain were also, perhaps

---

Charles E. Rosenberg, "The therapeutic revolution: Medicine, meaning, and social change in nineteenth-century America," *Perspectives in Biology and Medicine* 20, no. 4 (1977): 485–506.

23 Charles Hunter Dunn, *Animal Experimentation in Relation to Epidemic Cerebrospinal Meningitis* (American Medical Association, 1911), 5.

24 Parke, Davis & Company advertisement, *Pharmaceutical Archives* 5, no. 6 (1902): back matter; "New Wonder Drug Worth $7,000 a Pound," *Saint Paul Globe* (April 20, 1902), 19.

25 Adrenalin advertisement, *Pharmaceutical Era* (August 11, 1904), 8.

26 "Making War on Diphtheria: Health Department Engaged in a Fight Against the Disease," *The Sun* (Baltimore, November 1900), 7.

27 Lorenzo Servitje, *Medicine is War: The Martial Metaphor in Victorian Literature and Culture* (SUNY Press, 2021).

paradoxically, increasingly described according to narratives that centered individual creativity and labor.[28] Ehrlich's use of the phrase "magic bullet" encapsulated both these trends, linking wonder at its healing power to the dream of precision and military victory.[29] It also worked to abstract the process of discovery into a creative act centered on Ehrlich's supposed brilliance, thereby subsuming the contributions of others with whom he worked.[30] As one physician in New York put it in 1911: "we have added to our therapeutics, through the immortal genius of Ehrlich, the most powerful weapon in the fight against syphilis that civilization has ever known."[31]

Yet this beautiful and violent dream faced numerous troubles. Perhaps most importantly, Ehrlich's initial claim that a single, large dose of Salvarsan would safely kill all spirochaete in a person's body quickly proved inaccurate. Physicians soon realized that Salvarsan could actually be quite dangerous, that multiple doses were usually necessary, and that the preparation and intravenous administration of the product were burdensome and brought their own risks of harm.[32] By the outbreak of World War I, critics in the medical community were speaking of the "miracle madness" that had

28 Louis Pasteur, for example, was an important example of this process with his "inspiring genius" and "sublime studies" that, apparently, "laid the scientific foundation for all the modern therapeutic achievements in surgery as well as medicine." "Pasteur," *Medical Review* (July–December 1895): 281. On how Pasteur worked to create this myth of himself, see Gerald L. Geison, *The Private Science of Louis Pasteur* (Princeton University Press, 1996). See also, for example, Mark A. Lemley, "The myth of the sole inventor," *Michigan Law Review* 110, no. 5 (2011): 709; David A. Mindell, "Opening Black's Box," *Technology and Culture* 41, no. 3 (2000): 405–34; George Slusser, "The perils of experiment: Jules Verne and the American lone genius," *Extrapolation* 40, no. 2 (1999): 101–15.

29 Paul Ehrlich, "The Harben Lectures on Experimental Researches on Specific Therapeutics," *The Lancet* (1907): 351. The quote is from 1906 lecture, translated, from *Collected Papers of Paul Ehrlich*, vol. 3, 59. He also used equivalent phrases in German in earlier work to describe, as one translated version later put it, "magic bullets which seek their target of their own accord."

30 This included not just the Japanese scientist Sahachiro Hata, with who Ehrlich worked closely, but also the other people who worked in Ehrlich's laboratory and whom he collaborated with in other ways. See, for example, Jonathan Liebenau, "Paul Ehrlich as a commercial scientist and research administrator," *Medical History* 34, no. 1 (1990): 65–78. On Hata, see Ichiro Kawamura, "Sahachiro Hata (1873–1938) and his contributions to the birth of antimicrobial chemotherapy," *Journal of Infection and Chemotherapy* 29, no. 5 (2023): 546–48.

31 Quoted in "Salvarsan in Syphilis," *American Journal of Urology* (1911): 224.

32 For example, see "Therapeutics of Salvarsan," *Journal of the American Medical Association* (1911): 1353.

initially surrounded the drug and describing its passing.[33] There were also a seemingly endless number of questions and scientific debates about how to properly use both Salvarsan and Neo-Salvarsan to maximize the benefits and minimize the harms of these powerful substances. Experimental work thus took place in a narrative structure that linked past knowledge to poten tial futures and articulated risk and promise as laying at the interaction of therapeutic agent and the human body. Physicians also began to suggest that the complexity of these debates, and the potentially tragic results that might occur if these drugs were improperly used, meant that Salvarsan injections should only be administered by competent physicians that are, as one textbook put it, "accustomed to such surgical procedures."[34]

There were other troubles as well. The introduction of both Salvarsan and Neo-Salvarsan seemed to evoke numerous dangers that lay beyond the narrow scope of laboratory research and clinical experiment. According to some critics, for example, the widespread use of these drugs would lead to increased promiscuity among poor Blacks, members of the military, and other groups by turning syphilis into a disease that no longer needed to be feared. Other critics pointed to the proliferation of what they considered poorly manufactured substitutes, counterfeit and adulterated versions, and disreputable "peddlers" and retailers of the drugs.[35] Still others warned of quack physicians who incompetently administered these dangerous goods; as one critic noted in 1911, disreputable "medical institutes" sprang up in the wake of the advertising campaign by Hoescht for the drug, and "as a consequence many sufferers have been victimized."[36] Such problems grew out of the transformation of both disease and treatment along lines of specificity, but they also pointed toward an emergent domain of concern that seemed both distinct from, yet intertwined with, laboratory and clinical investigation. Laboratory investigations might reveal the presence of adulterated products on the market, for example, but they were not enough to prevent them. Other approaches were needed.

33 For example, Edward L. Keyes, "Notes on Salvarsan," *Cornell University Medical Bulletin* (1912): 1.

34 James Tyson and M. Howard Fussell, *The Practice of Medicine: A Textbook for Practitioners and Students with Special Reference to Diagnosis and Treatment* (P. Blakiston's Son & Co., 1913), 189.

35 Edward H. Marsh, "The Dangers Accruing from Drugs Purchased from Peddlers," *Medical Times* (April 1914), 102–4.

36 "Fraudulent Exploitation of Salvarsan," *American Druggist and Pharmaceutical Record* (April 10, 1911).

Dangerous Drugs and the Bifurcation of Risk

In 1917 a social reformer named Frank Osborne gave a talk at the Annual Meeting of New York Conferences on Hospital Social Service about "community control of syphilis," in which he bemoaned the failure of society to keep pace with the promises of scientific advancement. "Modern science," he noted, "has provided methods of isolation and identification of the invading organisms," and "specific treatment properly administered holds out the greatest promise of cure that has ever existed." Despite such progress, however, "it is a question whether there is not as much syphilis among us today as there was before these discoveries were made and these methods developed." He thus argued for the establishment of a series of dispensaries to treat venereal disease, the need for "rigid" social work to ensure that patients would return for follow-up treatment, and that authorities keep the public "constantly informed" about the disease. He also argued that

> Before any attempt should be made to attack the problem constructively on the medical side, a well-directed destructive campaign should be carried out. By this is meant the destruction of all sources of misinformation and falsehood circulated by so-called "advertising specialists. ... It goes without saying that a strenuous movement for law enforcement should also be carried out in the community for the vigorous repression of prostitution and the careful regulation of saloons, hotels, dance halls, etc."

Osborn thus embraced the magic bullet framework, but he did so in a way that suggested that society needed to be changed in order for it to fulfil its promise.[37]

Osborn was not alone in this. As historians have long noted, by the outbreak of World War I therapeutic reformers in the United States had begun to establish a complex and overlapping set of laws, professional organizations, and activist groups dedicated to regulating the manufacture, buying, and selling of drugs.[38] As Osborn's comments indicate, these reformers

37 Frank Osborn, clipping in American Social Hygiene Association papers, 4

38 There is now an extensive body of scholarship that examines different aspects of this movement, including Richard Del Rio, "Expanding Our Scope: Pharmaceuticals and Criminal Justice," *History of Pharmacy and Pharmaceuticals* 61, nos. 3–4 (2019): Terry S. Coleman, "Early developments in the regulation of biologics," *Food and Drug Law Journal* 71, no. 4 (2016): 544–607; James Harvey Young, *Pure Food: Securing the Federal Food and Drugs Act of 1906* (Princeton University Press, 2014); Joseph M. Gabriel, "Restricting the Sale of 'Deadly Poisons': Pharmacists, Drug Regulation, and Narratives of Suffering in the Gilded Age," *The Journal of the Gilded Age and Progressive Era* 9, no. 3 (2010): 313–36; David E. Lilienfeld, "The first pharmacoepidemiologic

tended to divide the potential benefits and harms of drugs into two distinct types that I will, for the sake of convenience, refer to as the "medical" and "social" domains. On the so-called medical side, the risks and benefits of drugs were increasingly understood in ways that grew out of the turn toward both physiological and clinical science and the transformation of disease into ontologically discrete entities that could be studied, tracked, and intervened in. This was a type of risk that – physicians and other parties increasingly assumed – could be managed within the clinical relationship and through the process of scientific investigation; the reduction of risk and the heightening of benefit were thus a matter of professional expertise, laboratory and clinical investigation, epistemic and ontological standardization, and acts of calculation in which future promises and threats were rendered legible across imagined instantiation – often, and perhaps typically, along lines of presumed racial difference and white racial epistemology.[39] These efforts often included what might be called social questions, yet such questions – although considered potentially important – were secondary to the research task at hand; they thus appear as fragments and gestures, asides and speculations, brief explanations that stop abruptly. "As in other series of clinic syphilitics," noted the authors of a 1929 study of how to "fight against" congenital syphilis, "the difficulty of convincing the parents of the importance of the treatment routine, in spite of the child's reluctance, is quite apparent." The authors then briefly – very briefly – discuss the need for parent education and "follow-up work," noting that "the solution of such problems is chiefly in the domain of the public health nurse and other workers in social hygiene." Yet, despite the assertion that "the importance of their solution cannot be overemphasized," the authors spend the rest of the paper discussing the symptoms and lesions of the disease, the amount, type, and effects of the treatments they administered, and other such issues.[40] Problems in the social domain are left to others.

As the ghostly traces of the social within the medical suggest, not all danger could be addressed through scientific investigation and medical expertise; Osborn's call for a "destructive campaign" against those who

investigations: national drug safety policy in the United States, 1901–1902," *Perspectives in Biology and Medicine* 51, no. 2 (2008): 188–98; David T. Courtwright, *Dark Paradise* (Harvard University Press, 2009;) Michael M. Cohen, "Jim Crow's drug war: race, coca cola, and the southern origins of drug prohibition," *Southern Cultures* 12, no. 3 (2006): 55–79.

39 For example, see "Arsphenamine Poisoning occurring among negro women," *Journal of Disease Information*, summarizing an article by Grosbeck Walsh and Courtney Strckley, *American Journal of Syphilology* (June 1935): 323

40 Lloyd B. Dickey and Leonard T. Sutton, "Combatting Congenital Syphilis," *California and Western Medicine* (October 1929): 245.

spread "misinformation" points to these types of concerns and solutions. Historians are most familiar with efforts to criminalize the illicit use of intoxicating goods such as opium and cocaine, yet physicians and other therapeutic reformers also assumed that numerous other dangers circulated on the therapeutic market that could not be addressed solely through laboratory or clinical investigation. Adulteration and product secrecy, for example, raised the specter of therapeutic disequivalency, as did a confusing and ever-expanding universe of pharmaceutical nomenclature. At the same time, many people simply did not use drugs as they should; some used them too much or in inappropriate ways, while others failed to use them when and how they should, whether due to ignorance or superstition, distrust of physicians, or some other reason that operated as a barrier to rational and efficient care. Addressing these types of problems might depend on the types of knowledge that laboratory and clinical investigation provided – laboratory testing of products on the market, for example – but they were not enough: these problems required interventions that went beyond the medical domain, including educational efforts for the public; the suppression of counterfeit, adulterated, and quack medicines; mechanisms to enforce the standardization of nomenclature and limit the consumption of dangerous products to medical use; and law enforcement efforts that targeted illicit and disreputable forms of distribution and use.

The fantasy of cure that accompanied the widespread adoption of Salvarsan was thus narrated through the binary between medical and social domains, on the one hand, and the overlaps between them on the other. Yet there was also a significant amount of tension between the two in the imaginations of therapeutic reformers. Despite the widespread use of Salvarsan and other treatments, public health authorities and other worried observers noted with alarm the widespread prevalence of the disease in the two decades following World War I.[41] "In spite of a remarkably increased efficience and number of antisyphilitic remedies during the last quarter of a century, and in spite of the developments in method of early diagnosis," noted two worried observers in 1934, "no corresponding diminution of syphilis and its destructive effects can be noted."[42] Physicians and other reformers assumed that the continued dangers of syphilis were intertwined with a wide range of problems in the social domain, including deviant sexual behavior, lack of patient education

41 David Willmoth, "Surgical Aspects of Syphilis with Esepecial Reference to the gastro-Intestinal Tract," *International Journal of Surgery* (December 1920): 370; For example, "Prevalence, Incidence and Trend of Syphilis" *Journal of Venereal Disease Information* (1936): 125–33.

42 George W. Raiziss and M. Severac, "Experimental Chemotherapy and the Destuction of Spirocheta Pallida in the Brain," *Journal of Chemotherapy* (April 1934): 3.

and poor attitudes toward treatment, the predatorial behavior of disreputable retailers, and the widespread use of so-called quack remedies.

The fantasy of cure, and its limits, were deeply shaped by racialized epistemology. White physicians and other reformers often investigated and explained the apparently high rate of syphilis among poor Blacks as a result of natural inferiority and physical difference, for example, but they also assumed that supposedly higher degrees of ignorance and gullibility, superstition, sexual promiscuity, and resistance to white medical authority played a central role in both the prevalence of the disease, the dangerous use of both Salvarsan and quack treatments, and other problems.[43] One white physician in Cleveland, for example, made the following statements in 1927 when interviewed by investigators for the American Social Hygiene Association:

> Ninety-eight per cent of the Negroes infected with syphilis or gonococcal infections are self-treated. They go to a drug store because they consider the local pharmacist their friend. They want to save money … I find the Negro patients, even after they come to me for treatment early, become delinquent and as soon as a discharge stops they feel that they are cured. The reasons, I believe, for the self-treatment or no treatment among the colored people is due to the fact that they do not consider a venereal disease infection serious enough. Syphilis, for instance, they do not call by name. They call it "pock," "skin trouble," and "blood sickness," and many pharmacists in this locality, in order to make money, push and advertise the sale of certain blood specifics and blood tonics of which many are asked for and sold.[44]

Such behavior, white reformers believed, pointed to the dangers of rampant commercialism and the failures of the developing regulatory system; they also pointed to the supposed ignorance, gullibility, and sexual immorality of Black communities. Not surprisingly, Black physicians and social reformers

43 For example, see Ernest L. Zimmermann, "A Comparative Study of Syphilis in Whites and in Negroes," *Arhcives of Dermatology and Syphilology* (July 1921): 79; "Robert H. Foster, "Paresis in the Negro," *American Journal of Psychiatry* (April 1926): 631–40. See also Christopher Crenner, "The Tuskegee Syphilis Study and the scientific concept of racial nervous resistance," *Journal of the History of Medicine and Allied Sciences* 67, no. 2 (2012): 244–80; Bradford Charles Pelletier, "An Ill-bred Culture of Experimentation: Malaria Therapy and Race in the United States Public Health Service Laboratory at the South Carolina State Hospital, 1932–1952," *Journal of the History of Medicine and Allied Sciences* 80, no. 1 (2025): 67–91.

44 "Report on the Extent of the Sale of Nostrums and Prescribing for and Treatment of the Venereal Diseases by Druggists & Irregular Practitioners in the City of Cleveland," University of Minnesota Twin Cities, Social History archive, American Social Health Association Records [ASHA], box 101, folder 11.

disagreed. They too operated within the developing epistemic framework that separated the scientific from the social, and they too invested their dreams in the fantasy of pharmaceutical cure. Yet not surprisingly they came to different conclusions about the saliency of race, rejecting the relationship between racial difference and purported racial inferiority, on the one hand, and the supposed role of some social characteristics, such as sexual behavior, in their explanations of the difference in disease prevalence between the races. They instead pointed to a lack of educational opportunities, poverty and deleterious living conditions, medical racism, and other problems in the social domain that led members of their race to be especially vulnerable to illness, the lure of quack treatments, and other dangers.[45] Yet despite their differences, both black and white therapeutic reformers dreamed of a world in which pharmaceuticals could do their work. They dreamed of a world in which the power of medical science to fight disease was set free.

Dangerous Magic: Regulatory Reform and Narratives of Pharmaceutical Innovation

In 1936 Franklin D. Roosevelt's son came down with an acute case of septic sore throat, a life threatening ailment since, as one news account put it, there was "danger that the *streptococcus haemolyticus* might get into his blood stream ... in such a situation, a rich and robust Harvard crewman is no safer from death than anybody else." Fortunately, young Franklin was treated by a "fashionable and crackerjack" Boston physician with a "specific cure for all streptococcic infections." It was a new drug called "Prontosil," and "under its influence young Roosevelt rallied at once." This was a widely reported and dramatic story, and while this particular newspaper article retained a somewhat muted response to the new drug – simply calling it "notable" – such restraint was soon replaced by statements attesting to its remarkable effects as news of the drug spread and physicians used it to cure

45 Preston M. Edwards, "President's Address," *Journal of the National Medical Association* (January–March 1923): 39–40; Dennis A. Bethea, "Some Significant Negro Movements to Lower Their Mortality," *Journal of the National Medical Association* (April–June 1930): 85–88; Samuel M. Auerbach, "Quackery," *Journal of Negro Life* (December 1929): 373–76; "Dr. D.L.T. Wright Demands Fight Continue on Health Centers," *Cleveland Call and Post* (July 8, 1937), 1. See also Ayah Nuriddin, "Liberation Eugenics: African Americans and the Science of Black Freedom Struggles, 1890–1970" (PhD dissertation, Johns Hopkins University, 2021), esp. 29–86; Thomas J. Ward, *Black Physicians in the Jim Crow South* (University of Arkansas Press, 2003).

gonorrhea, scarlet fever, and other ailments. Prontosil, argued one physician, is "the most amazing drug in the history of medicine in my time."[46]

Prontosil was just one among a seemingly endless number of new pharmaceuticals on the therapeutic market during the interwar period. Ethical firms had long based their business strategies on manufacturing familiar remedies that were widely acceptable to the orthodox medical community – indeed, doing so had traditionally served to distinguish them from what they considered their unscrupulous competitors in the so-called "patent medicine" wing of the industry – and such goods remained an important part of their core business strategy during this period. At the same time, however, manufacturers in the so-called ethical wing of the industry increasingly based their financial success on what is now a familiar system of investment in scientific research, collaboration with academic research scientists and physicians in clinical practice, and extensive promotion of these new products within the medical and pharmacy communities. They also fully embraced the use of patents as a core part of their business strategy in a way that would have been unthinkable sixty or seventy years earlier, including by investing significant resources in the legal and scientific management of patent rights.[47]

Investment was thus linked to commercial success through the creation of new therapeutic goods that carried the promise of cure. Yet this process of investment also limited the horizon of possibilities for manufacturers and the academic scientists and clinical researchers they worked with. Sunk costs tended to constrain future choices through path dependency: the expense of investing in new machinery, for example, had to be balanced against the potential future earnings of products – and sometimes imagined products –

46 "Prontosil," *Time* (December 28, 1936), 21; "E.P. Physicians Cure Scarlet Fever with Prontosil, Amazing new Red Dye," *El Paso Herald Post* (June 15, 1937); Constance Foster, "New Miracles in Healing," *Parents' Magazine* (November 1940), 14–15. For another example, see "New Medical Victory Cited: Development in Use of Sulfanilamide Held Age's Greatest Miracle," *Los Angles Times* (February 1940).

47 For example, see N. A., "Memo. Lilly Research and Control Staff" (January 5, 1937), Pfizer/Upjohn Papers, AC-2007-157, A-3149, box 8 of 11, folder "Departments – Medical Department, 1935–1938." On the American pharmaceutical industry during the interwar period see David Herzberg, *White Market Drugs: Big Pharma and the Hidden History of Addiction in America* (University of Chicago Press, 2020); Nicolas Rasmussen, "The drug industry and clinical research in interwar America: three types of physician collaborator," *Bulletin of the History of Medicine* 79, no. 1 (2005): 50–80; John Patrick Swann, *Academic Scientists and the Pharmaceutical Industry: Cooperative Research in Twentieth-Century America* (Johns Hopkins University Press, 1988); C. Weiner, "Patenting and academic research: Historical case studies," *Science, Technology, & Human Values* 12, no. 1 (1987): 50–62.

that were increasingly assumed to generate substantive profits for a limited amount of time; this recognition reflected both the limited time that firms enjoyed market exclusivity due to patent rights and the more general dynamic that successful products tended to decrease in profitability over time as other firms introduced competing goods. One result was that patentable compounds that represented significant investment in both scientific and legal development costs tended to drive a process whereby the substance was tested for a variety of problems until a commercially viable therapeutic use could be discovered.[48] More generally, firms increasingly strategized about how to maintain high profit margins on new products for as long as possible so that investment costs could be recouped and profits reinvested in equipment, labor costs, or other needs. A similar process took place among academic scientists and – to a lesser extent – clinical researchers, where scientific path dependency and financial investment in research capability were increasingly linked to both professional and reputational success and to narratives of progress in which scientific work held the potential for dramatic therapeutic and commercial breakthroughs.[49]

One result of all this was the development of an iterative system of drug development in which new medicines were increasingly narrated in wonderous terms; as time passed, and other products entered the market, these medicines tended to be either replaced or transformed from exceptional to ordinary goods in the stories that people told about them. An expanding domain of truth claims about the risks and benefits of drugs within what I have been calling the "medical" domain were thus linked to both scientific and commercial processes, on the one hand, and – on the other – to cycles of enthusiasm and hope that spread beyond the daily work of scientists, clinicians, and drug manufacturers.[50] At the same time, new drugs often

48 Rein Voss, *Drugs Looking for Diseases: Innovative Drug Research and the Development of the Beta Blockers and the Calcium Agents* (Springer, 1991). See also Justin Barr, "A short history of dapsone, or an alternative model of drug development," *Journal of the History of Medicine and Allied Sciences* 66, no. 4 (2011): 425–67; Toine Pieters, *Interferon: The Science and Selling of a Miracle Drug* (Routledge, 2005).

49 This set of arguments is based on my current research project, tentatively titled "Pharmaceutical System," and archival work in a variety of collections. See, for example, the discussion between Gordon Alles and Francis Boyer related to securing rights to Alles's patent on amphetamine for commercial development by Smith, French & Kline in Gordon Alles Papers, California Institute of Technology Archives, box 1, folder 8. See also Nicolas Rasmussen, *On Speed: The Many Lives of Amphetamine* (NYU Press, 2008).

50 Snelders and Kaplan make a similar argument in relation to the "careers" of cannabis indica and chloral hydrate in the nineteenth century. See Stephen

became wrapped up in longstanding concerns about risk in the social domain. Therapeutic reformers during the interwar period considered the drug market to be fraught with danger; they thus worked to reform drug the market along what they considered rational and benevolent lines – including efforts to standardize the manufacture of medicines and the names under which they are sold, suppress the sale of counterfeit and adulterated goods, limit the sale and use of narcotics and other dangerous products to medically-sanctioned forms of consumption, and educate and – when necessary – punish and control racial and ethnic minorities, the poor, working class youth, disreputable women, and other parties for the benefit of the common good. The separation of risk into medical and social forms was at the heart of these efforts.

The story of Prontosil illustrates many of these dynamics. The antimicrobial power of the drug was discovered by a German bacteriologist named Gerhard Domagk while working in the laboratories of Bayer AG, at that time part of the pharmaceutical and chemical conglomerate IG Farben. Domagk and his colleagues also discovered that the active ingredient in Prontosil was a substance that Bayer scientists had previously manufactured – and patented – called sulfanilamide. It rapidly gained a reputation as a powerful treatment for a variety of common infections, including pneumonia, scarlet fever, and gonorrhea.[51] Bayer was unable to successfully monopolize Domagk's discovery, however, and in the United States soon faced a highly competitive market as numerous types and preparations of sulfa drugs were introduced by competitors – some made with secret ingredients. There was a significant amount of ambiguity about the relationship between "sulfanilamide," "Prontosil," and other goods sold under other names; indeed, "sulfanilamide" itself was an unstable therapeutic object since it was not always clear if different versions made by different manufacturers were, in fact, the same thing. Yet the idea that there was *a* drug called sulfanilamide that had curative effects on a variety of specific diseases was a powerful one and deeply intertwined with the narrative of discovery and triumphant science. Still, this enthusiasm was tempered by the dangerous nature of the drug and, not surprisingly, by the effort to contain its risks within both the medical and social domains. In New Jersey, for example, the Board of Pharmacy passed a resolution condemning the sale of the drug for self-medication and warned pharmacists that the unsupervised sale of sulfanilamide preparations

Snelders, Charles Kaplan, and Toine Pieters, "On cannabis, chloral hydrate, and career cycles of psychotropic drugs in medicine," *Bulletin of the History of Medicine* 80, no. 1 (2006): 95–114.

51 For example, Frederick E. Reuter, "The Use of Sulfanilamide in the treatment of Gonorrhea," *Venereal Disease Information* (August 1937). 302; "The Use of Sulfaniladmie in Scarlet Fever," *New England Journal of Medicine* 219, no. 24 (1938): 947–53.

was against the public interest.[52] "In a great many instances these drugs are more dangerous than the malady they are supposed to cure," noted one account. Sulfanilamide, it seemed, was "dangerous magic."[53]

These dangers were articulated in racially laden terms. In September 1937 reports began to appear of deaths linked to a preparation of the drug marketed under the name "Elixir Sulfanilamide," and by October at least seventy-three deaths had been linked to the drug. Reformers quickly seized on the tragedy to pass the 1938 Food, Drug, and Cosmetic Act. As Daniel Carpenter has argued, one of the keys to the passage of the law was that during its lobbying efforts the FDA successfully created a public narrative for the disaster that focused on white victims. In particular, FDA efforts centered on the story of a woman named Maise Nidiffer from Oklahoma who had lost her six-year-old daughter to the drug. Nidiffer's picture of her smiling daughter became a staple of newspaper articles about the tragedy and, in promoting this narrative, FDA shifted the emerging focus on the disease away from Black men and the self-treatment of venereal diseases and toward the failures of the regulatory system to protect innocent white victims. As Carpenter notes,

> Maise Nidiffer's letter and the photograph of her daughter impelled and expressed the conversion of episode to tragedy. Together, the text and image took what had been a series of scattered deaths among "patients" – faceless subjects who in the American racial imagination were syphilitic black men – and purged it of blackness, of sexual maturity, and of social isolation. The victim of American policy failure was now a daughter connected to a mother and a loving family, a smiling white child who could not be said to have courted the agony that sulfanilamide wreaked upon her body.[54]

This shift in narrative from social risk associated with Black users toward the failure to properly mitigate medical risk to innocent white users was at the heart of the effort to press for comprehensive legislation. Doing so depended on rhetorically and conceptually separating the diethylene glycol that had been used in the preparation of "Elixir Sulfanilamide" from sulfanilamide itself, rendering the former a "deadly chemical" foolishly added to the

52 H. A. Tarbell, "Sulfanilamide must be used with Care; a case report," *Journal of the Medical Society of New Jersey* (1937): 506–7. See also *Journal of the American Medical Association* 109 (October 2, 1937):1128.

53 J. D. Ratcliff, "Dangerous Magic," clipping in ASHA, box 135, 15.

54 Daniel Carpenter, *Reputation and Power: Organizational Image and Pharmaceutical Regulation at the FDA* (Princeton University Press, 2010), 98–99.

product and the latter a "valuable drug" that still deserved its wonderous reputation.[55] The law passed soon after.

The 1938 law has been extensively studied by historians and other scholars, and rightly so: as Carpenter notes, it established the foundation for the growth of the FDA into what is now the world's largest and most powerful regulatory body. The most important provision of the law was the creation of a new legal category – the "new drug" – and the establishment of a system of premarket review for drugs that fell into this category by the FDA.[56] The law required manufacturers of "new drugs" to supply the FDA with the results of "investigations which have been made to show whether or not such drug is safe for use," as well as other requirements, that created both the "new drug" and the "experimental drug" as legal objects that were distinctive from other objects.[57] It also required that evidence about these objects be accumulated, organized, and presented to the FDA for evaluation before commercial sale and that new drugs be given distinctive names. Manufacturers were also required to include a variety of information on their product labels, such as dosing information and the names of various dangerous ingredients, although the law provided that "a drug dispensed on a written prescription signed by a physician, dentist, or veterinarian" was exempt from these requirements. Soon after, the FDA issued regulations clarifying that that any product labeled with the phrase "Caution: to be used only on the prescription of a physician" was exempt from the labeling sections of the law – but also that pharmacists were not allowed to sell such products unless a physician had prescribed them.[58]

Taken together, the law can be understood as an effort to manage both medical and social forms of risk by bringing together the assumption that pharmaceuticals should be subject to premarket review, that manufacturing and use should be standardized via a stable system of pharmaceutical nomenclature, that adulterated and counterfeit drugs should be prohibited from the market, and that access to dangerous drugs should be mediated through medical authority via prescription law. The latter aspect of the law, however, was soon beset with difficulties: the clause authorized manufacturers to designate their products as requiring a prescription for purchase, but there was no requirement that they do so and different manufacturers might

55 "Elixir Fatalities Arouse Demand for Drug Control," *Atlanta Constitution* (November 26, 1937), 1.

56 Carpenter, *Reputation and Power*, 73.

57 Carpenter, *Reputation and Power*, 113–14; Harry M. Marks, *The Progress of Experiment: Science and Therapeutic Reform in the United States, 1900–1990* (Cambridge University Press, 1997), 89–97.

58 See Harry M. Marks, "Revisiting 'The Origins of Compulsory Drug Prescriptions'," *American Journal of Public Health* 85, no. 1 (1995): 109–15.

or might not apply the requirement to the same, or to very similar drugs, differently. Other manufacturers appear to have simply ignored this part of the law, since applying the prescription-only legend tended to reduce sales, and many pharmacists probably sold products marked with the legend without being presented with a prescription. This seemed particularly dangerous to many authorities: properly used, sulfanilamide "is one of the wonders of modern medicine," as Surgeon General Thomas Parran put it in a 1939 *Los Angeles Times* article. Used outside of the direction of a physician, however, "the treatment may lead to results far worse than the disease," including "extreme muscle weakness, vomiting, insanity, and even death."[59] Voluntary compliance with the 1938 law on the part of druggists seemed inadequate to meet the danger; other measures were needed. In the District of Columbia, for example, authorities warned druggists that selling the drug without a prescription could result in a $10,000 fine, or three years in jail, or both.[60]

Conclusion

In 1940, the film *Dr. Ehrlich's Magic Bullet* was released. Starring Edward Robinson and directed by William Dieterle – who had recently won an Academy Award for Best Picture for *The Life of Emile Zola* – the biographical film told the story of Dr. Ehrlich as a sympathetic genius who improved the world through the power of science. The film cast the discovery of Salvarsan in heroic terms and positioned the discovery as part of the broader story of the progress of medical science. However, the film also placed the dangers of the drug at the center of its narrative. According to the film, shortly after the discovery of Salvarsan thirty-eight patients die after receiving treatment. After another physician publicly denounces the drug, Ehrlich then sues him for libel. In the resulting trial Emil von Bering dramatically testifies that the drug killed not thirty-eight but thirty-nine, including syphilis itself. "True, thirty-eight individuals are dead," von Bering declares, "but those dead should be thought of as sacrifices. As martyrs if you will, to the public good."[61] Ehrlich tragically dies soon after the trial due to the strains of the episode on his health, but not before lecturing his colleagues about the need to fight not just diseases of the body but diseases of the soul, including

59 Thomas Parran, "Sulfanilamide – Miracle or Menace?," *Los Angeles Times* (October 29, 1939), H4.

60 "Ruhland Cautions Druggists on Sulfanilamide 'Peddlin'," *Washington Post* (September 1, 1940), 4. For another example, see "7 Druggists Face Arrest," *San Francisco Examiner* (February 2, 1940), 30.

61 *Dr. Ehrlich's Magic Bullet*, dir. William Dieterle (1940), Warner Bros., 1:36.

greed, hate, and ignorance. Harm to patients is thus narrated as unfortunate and regrettable, but also a part of the ongoing process of scientific discovery and triumph; medical forms of risk are brought to the forefront of the story but submerged under a narrative of triumph and sacrifice, while other forms of risk are either ignored or cast as enemies of scientific reason and virtue.

It was a moving statement of the power of medical science to heal – and, simultaneously, to harm. Yet it also subtly recast Ehrlich's discovery as something that seemed a part of the present into something that seemed a part of the past even as Salvarsan and Neo-Salvarsan continued to be widely prescribed. Dramatic narratives associated with the sulfa drugs made salvarsan much less wonderous in comparison; indeed, narratives of medical progress from the late 1930s and early 1940s continued to describe Ehrlich as a brilliant scientist and pioneer in chemotherapy – but also as someone who's theories had limited utility in our "war against germs."[62] A 1940 article published in the *Bulletin of the History of Medicine* is a good example; it tells the story of "Paul Ehrlich, the genius" and puts salvarsan in the context of later developments in chemotherapy, including the development of Prontosil. "The work so auspiciously begun by Ehrlich and his associates has continued," the author notes. "The most epoch-making discovery was that of Domagk in 1935 of the effect of a drug called prontosil in the treatment of streptococcic infections. But let us go back to pick up the thread of the story chronologically."[63] Here, Domagk occupies the place that Ehrlich had occupied in earlier narratives: the genius inventor, the culmination of history, the brilliant and epoch-making scientist after whom nothing is ever the same. Ehrlich is cast as a part of the past, an earlier episode in the grand and unfolding story of medical science.

We know, of course, that sulfanilamide was not an ending. Indeed, in many ways the sulfa drugs were a beginning – the first miracle drugs, as John E. Lesch has put it.[64] The introduction of the next wonder drug Penicillin continued the story, transforming the treatment of bacterial infections. As it did, stories about this new wonder drug solidified Ehrlich's status as a brilliant scientist – yet also describing him as one who had failed in his task. "Penicillin is the most promising weapon against syphilis ever found," noted a 1943 account published in *Collier's*. "It looks like the magic bullet which Doctor

62 John Pfeiffer, "Sulfanilamide," *Harper's Monthly Magazine* (December 1, 1938), 392. For another example, see Iago Galdston, "Newest Progress in Our Chemical Warfare on Germs," *Nashville Tennessean* (February 25, 1940), 49.

63 Maurice S. Jacobs, "Paul Ehrlich and his Relation to Modern Chemotherapy," *Bulletin of the History of Medicine* 8 (1940): 956–64.

64 John E. Lesch, ed., *The First Miracle Drugs: How the Sulfa Drugs Transformed Medicine* (Oxford University Press, 2006).

Ehrlich sought and failed to find."[65] Over the next two decades Penicillin, and later Streptomycin and other antibiotics, became the archetypal magic bullets, populating both our fantasies and our scientific, therapeutic, and scholarly practices even as Ehrlich and his brilliant discovery faded from view except as a matter of scholarly interest. Of course, as historians such as Alan Brandt have suggested, the fantasy of the magic bullet has never been able to fully address the reality of how disease – and people – actually operate, in part due to the complex relationship between disease and what we now call the social determinants of health.[66] The specter of antibiotic resistance hovers over our fantasies as well, blending them with nightmares of epidemic disease run amok and our lingering fears of the past. These and other difficulties cast the dream of the magic bullet in doubt, but they do so along temporal lines in which the future promises to be better than the past through scientific, technological, and commercial innovation. They also do so through the racialized bifurcation of risk into medical and social domains, including the troubling binary between licit and illicit markets and the horrors that this binary has unleashed. There is always another magical bullet to redeem our world, it seems, even as the ones we have continually fail us.

65 J. D. Ratcliff, "Victory over Syphilis," *Collier's* (November 6, 1943), 73–74.

66 Brandt, *No Magic Bullet*, 161.

Chapter Three

A Non-Linear History of Side Effects: Risk Management, Pharmaceutical Innovation, and the WHO's Adverse Drug Reaction Monitoring, 1945–1980[1]

Nils Kessel

Introduction: Three Terms and a Translation Problem

This chapter has its origins in a translation problem that I encountered more than ten years ago. In English, French, and German sources on side effects of drugs from the 1960s onwards, I came across a coexistence of the term "side effect/effect secondaire/ Nebenwirkung," on the one hand, and the term pairs "Adverse drug event/reaction" or "événement/effet indésirables" and "unerwünschte(s) Arzneimittelereignis/wirkung" on the other. The question therefore arose as to what motivated this exchange of terms and how comprehensive it was. Even today, the same situation can still be found in all three languages: in colloquial language, but moreover also in

1 All my thanks to David and Joe, two wonderful colleagues I have the pleasure to work with. My sincere gratitude goes to them and to all contributors. I would also like to thank the two anonymous reviewers for their comments on earlier versions of this chapter.

official and scientific texts, the term "side effect" can be found.[2] The term "adverse drug reaction" (ADR) remains largely reserved for specialized contexts, especially in adverse drug reaction monitoring. "Adverse drug event" (ADE) is also found in pharmacological literature and the associated fields of drug regulation and monitoring, as there the distinction between the observed event and the proven effect is relevant. The medical literature usually explains this shift from side effect to ADE/ADR as a necessary step forward towards better drug safety. Following the thalidomide disaster in 1961, in which sleeping pills containing thalidomide were discovered to cause malformations in fetuses, it would have been necessary to build international and national ADR monitoring from scratch.[3]

Starting from my initial observation that terminological change occurred during the 1960s, with the introduction of the new terminology of ADE/ADR, my hypothesis to be developed in the beginning of this chapter is that "side effect" and ADE/ADR are no longer the same epistemological "thing." For my argument, I first show how side effect management was already on its way as practitioners' clinical approach for individual patients. I then describe how WHO clinical experts from academic medicine used thalidomide as an opportunity to promote comparative prescription and consumption studies that followed both public health and healthcare budget objectives. Thus, the emergence of modern ADR monitoring translates a change in scale between clinical side effects and a potential public health problem that is called ADR. This change in scale also reconfigured the objectives of side effect management. It was not individual medical risk that was central, but the prevention of disasters that would severely affect large populations. As a consequence, focus was given to clinical research in hospitals and on severe consequences of "essential" medications for hospital care. I conclude with a short look at the reconfiguration of an epidemiological

2 Adrianus Cornelis van Grootheest, "Improving Pharmacovigilance and the Role of the Pharmacist" (PhD dissertation, University of Groningen, 2003), 36. In Dutch, "Schadelijke nevenwerkingen van geneesmiddelen" means harmful side effect of medicines. In "Improving Pharmacovigilance," Van Grootheest translates the terms as "harmful effects of prescription drugs" (53).

3 An example of a linear history of pharmacovigilance is Thierry Buclin, Rose-Anna Foley, and Françoise Livio, "Pharmacovigilance, hémovigilance, vaccinovigilance, tératovigilance... : quelles retombées imprévues pour les patients, les intervenants de santé et les systèmes de soins?," *Anthropologie & Santé* 19 (2019), http://journals.openedition.org/anthropologiesante/4937. A google Ngram viewer diagram for the term "adverse drug reaction" (English, case insensitive, 1800–2022) shows such a curb, the term being mentioned around 1955, rising sharply from 1960 onwards with the periods 1964–1973, 1980–1991, and 2001–2008 as times of increasing numbers of publications.

surveillance model into a clinical trial-focused model for identifying and managing side effects in hospital settings. ADR research would ultimately become disinterested in population screening for medically dubious uses or products because they were excluded de facto.

Thus, the story this chapter tells uses the introduction of ADE/ADR terminology as a starting point for a different, non-linear history of side effects, their investigation, and their management. It is less about success and more about failure, less about the foresight of pioneers and more about desperate attempts to control uncontrollable quantities of drugs and their effects on society.

Leopold Meyler and Practitioners' Management of Side Effects

In 1951, Dutch physician Leopold Meyler (1903–1973) published a book on side effects, which was translated into English the following year under the title *Meyler's Side Effects of Drugs*.[4] Within a few years, *Meyler's Side Effects of Drugs* had become a standard work about side effects.[5] The first edition of 1952 offered an overview of the side effects described in the medical literature, organized according to therapeutic drug classes and substances. In contrast to medical handbooks or student manuals, his therapeutic caveats were limited to brief references that were neither explained in more detail nor organized according to general principles. *Meyler's Side Effects* was a compendium for physicians, a list system to be updated regularly. These were based on a systematic evaluation of the medical literature. To this end, Meyler evaluated English, Dutch, and German-language literature and drew on abstracts of articles in other languages.

Meyler relied on a specific, broad understanding of side effects, as the entry on "barbituric acid derivatives" shows. In it, he distinguished between three types of symptoms, which he subsumed under the term side effect, but differentiated precisely with regard to their physiological origin. First, he dealt with reactions to overdoses or particular physiological sensitivities of patients, which he did not yet differentiate from each other at the time:

> Overdose, or when the dose is normal, the patient is particularly sensitive to the drug, as happens in anoxia (asthma, marked anaemia) ... and in patients with liver disease .... Both cases may show the picture of acute barbituric acid poisoning: confusion; drowsiness; coma; secondary infections.[6]

4 Van Grootheest, "Improving Pharmacovigilance," 36.

5 *Meyler's Side Effects* is still published and has reached its sixteenth edition (2016).

6 Leopold Meyler, *Side Effects of Drugs*, trans. Ph. Vuijsje and W. Mulhall Corbet (Elsevier Press, 1952), 4.

This was followed secondly by allergy symptoms and thirdly by manifestations of chronic poisoning. Under the third heading, there were comments on addiction as a side effect and on the difficulties of barbiturate withdrawal.[7]

Meyler's *Side Effects of Drugs* was intended to help the practicing physician to interpret the patient's complaints or a deterioration in the patient's condition.[8] Meyler himself explained the aim of his book as follows:

> In this book we have endeavored to collocate all the known facts regarding the side effects of the various drugs, and we hope that it will prove a useful work of reference. We also hope that it will be of use in investigating whether "new" symptoms in the course of certain diseases are due to the disease itself or to the drugs used in its treatment.[9]

A decade later, in a paper published in 1965, Meyler distinguished now seven forms of side effects that were relevant to the practitioner. First were side effects dependent on toxicity. Those were characterized by threshold values and represented classical cases of intoxications with poisons. Second were side effects caused by what Meyler called "relative overdosage." Relative overdosage referred to toxic effects in humans due to their specific organic conditions. For example, the same molecule that did not harm healthy persons could have toxic effects in those whose liver or kidney function was limited. He also presented the archetypical side effect dependent on a secondary pharmacological action of a drug.[10] Meyler insisted on separating what he called "sensitivity," i.e., the individual (over)sensitivity interpreted as a physiological reaction, from the primarily psychic condition he labeled as being dependent on "hypersensitivity."[11] In modern terminology, we would understand individual (over)sensitivity in terms of allergy as an immune reaction against one or several compounds of a drug, as a ***pharmacokinetic*** reaction to the drug in the body. Physiological oversensitivity was a problem relatively frequently encountered with penicillin,

7 Meyler was later to present a list of seven different forms of side effects. See Leopold Meyler, "Side Effects of Drugs," in *Usus und Abusus von Pharmaka. 4. Internationaler Kongress der Internationalen Föderation für Hygiene und Präventivmedizin* (Verlag der Wiener Medizinischen Akademie, 1965), 2.

8 Front cover of Leopold Meyler and Andrew Herxheimer, *Side Effects of Drugs*, 6th ed. (Excerpta Medica, 1968).

9 Meyler, *Side Effects of Drugs* (1952), vii.

10 Loperamide's constipative effect would be such an example. See Jeremy A. Greene and Avery Gulino's contribution in this volume.

11 Leopold Meyler and M. N. Dukes, *Side Effects of Drugs: Adverse Reactions As Reported in the Medical Literature of the World 1963–1965*, 5th ed. (Excerpta Medica, 1966), 2.

and it had raised awareness for allergies caused by drugs.[12] Sensitivity, in contrast, would refer to a heightened sensitivity to the drug's action in the body (*pharmacodynamics*), for example a stronger effect than expected when given a lower dose than the one usually used for obtaining the therapeutic effect. "Hypersensitivity" in Meyler's sense was understood as caused by psychological condition rather than the drug's measurable effect. Two other types received less interest but still were presented: "drug interactions"; and the side effect depending on suggestion.

By relying on the evaluation of the medical literature, Meyler's book also limited itself to the effects that doctors considered worthy of publication. In specific terms, this meant that the focus was on phenomena requiring treatment and not on all possible observations in connection with the drug. Side effects in Meyler's sense were therefore phenomena that were observable in the use of medication in medical practice and for which medical authors already assumed a possible or even proven causal relationship between the preparation and the (side) effect. At the same time, a side effect in Meyler's 1952 book also included effects that occurred with particular types of use, such as intentional or accidental overdose. Poisoning and addiction were thus included in the concept of side effects.[13]

In Meyler's understanding of drugs, drug interactions, overdosage, and secondary pharmacological actions of a specific drug could *all* be considered as categorically equivalent. Side effects thus covered all undesired effects that can arise when a drug is *in use*, independent of whether the drug is used appropriately or inappropriately. With his practitioner's view, Meyler provided a clinically comprehensive picture of effects a physician would be likely to encounter in his or her daily practice. Yet, Meyler did not provide a precise survey of side effects' frequency or distribution in specific populations. In his 1952 book, he rather insisted on the relative rarity of side effects based on

12 Anne Kveim Lie and Bård Hobæk, "Less is more. Norwegian Drug Regulation, Antibiotic Policy, and the 'Need' Clause," *The Milbank Quarterly* 97, no. 3 (2019): 768. According to several authors, Meyler himself would have suffered allergic reactions to medicines. See Van Grootheest, "Improving Pharmacovigilance," 46; and Jeffrey Aronson, "The history of Meyler's *Side Effects of Drugs* and the *Side Effects of Drugs Annuals*, 1951–2015," in Leopold Meyler and Jeffrey Aronson, *Meyler's Side Effects of Drugs. The International Encyclopedia of Adverse Drug Reactions and Interactions*, 16th ed. (Elsevier, 2016), viii–xxii.

13 For the long history of addiction in Louis Lewin's and others' conceptualization of side effects, see Stephen Snelders, Charles Kaplan, and Toine Pieters, "On Cannabis, Chloral Hydrate, and Career Cycles of Psychotropic Drugs in Medicine," *Bulletin of the History of Medicine* 80, no. 1 (2006): 95–114.

the frequency with which they were mentioned in the medical literature.[14] His focus was on giving practitioners a guide to where to expect and how to identify side effects as a problem of individual practice. His evidence was mostly based on clinical case reports, not on larger epidemiological studies. By the late 1950s, Meyler's approach represented the standard for studying and managing side effects. His book was not the only one of its time devoted to side effects, however. In fact, a whole series of books on side effects appeared in the early 1950s as Adrianus Cornelis van Grootheest has shown.[15] This more general attention to side effects can be explained by decades of serial observations on various groups of drugs, old and new, and their dangerous effects. Owing to the possibility of addiction-related overdose and the development of new preparations, such as the hormones developed since the 1930s or new antibacterial sulfonamides and antibiotics, all psychoactive substances came into focus.[16] However, most authors' scope was on documenting the side effects of substances.[17] In contrast, Meyler moved beyond descriptions centered on drugs or diseases by offering a typology, and instead attempted to classify and ultimately explain side effects as (mostly) physiological phenomena.

14 Meyler, *Side Effects of Drugs* (1952), vii.

15 Van Grootheest, "Improving Pharmacovigilance," 36 cites C. Albahary, *Maladies médicamenteuses d'ordre thérapeutique et accidental* (Masson & Cie, 1953); G. Duchesnay, *Le risque thérapeutique, prévention et traitement des accidents* (G. Doin & Cie, 1954); H. L. Alexander, *Reactions with Drug Therapy* (Saunders Company, 1955); R. Heintz, ed., *Erkrankungen durch Arzneimittel, Diagnostik, Klinik, Pathogenese, Therapie* (Georg Thieme Verlag, 1966).

16 Scott H. Podolsky, *The Antibiotic Era. Reform, Resistance, and the Pursuit of a Rational Therapeutics* (Johns Hopkins University Press 2015). Antibiotics were at the forefront of debates about drug risks since their widespread use raised debate about iatrogenic antibiotic resistance, overprescription, and overconsumption, as well as risks for side effects and drug interactions. See also Claas Kirchhelle, *Pyrrhic Progress. The History of Antibiotics in Anglo-American Food Production* (Rutgers University Press, 2020), who shows the importance of antimicrobial resistance emerging in post-World War II agriculture. For the most important antibiotic drug disaster, relating to Chloramphenicol, see Thomas Maeder, *Adverse Reactions* (William Morrow & Cie, 1994).

17 An important early study was Robert Harlan Moser, *Diseases of Medical Progress: A Survey of Diseases and Syndromes Unintentionally Induced as the Result of Properly Indicated, Widely-Accepted Therapeutic Procedures* (Charles C. Thomas, 1959).

The Age of Multiplication

In his 2008 article about the "multiplication processes," Swiss historian Jakob Tanner pointed out that the industrial modernity of the late nineteenth and twentieth centuries can be understood as an age of unprecedented multiplication of both knowledge and objects. In line with the findings of the history of consumption and technology, Tanner pointed out that an unprecedented number of objects, including a multitude of technologies, characterized the everyday lives of people in the rich countries of the world. New practices of production and consumption, such as the development of disposable items, not only changed the markets in which they were sold and bought.[18] In accounts reminiscent of the decades between approximately 1920 and 1970 as a pharmaceutical Golden Age, these years appeared to be

18 Tanner, Jakob, "Multiplikationsprozesse in der Moderne – Plädoyer für ein Analysekonzept," *Historische Anthropologie* 16, no. 1 (2008), 2–8. The underlying history of technology of these global markets is written by historians of consumer society, innovation, and technology for many consumer goods, and to a lesser degree for pharmaceuticals, too. Literature on specific technologies such as cars is enormous. For more general approaches, see Wolfgang König, "Massenproduktion und Konsumgesellschaft. Ein historischer und systematischer Abriss," in *Die Konsumgesellschaft in Deutschland, 1890–1990. Ein Handbuch*, ed. Heinz-Gerhard Haupt and Claudius Torp (Campus, 2009), 46–61; and the "Making Europe" book series. For pharmaceuticals, see David Herzberg, *White Market Drugs: Big Pharma and the Hidden History of Addiction in America* (The University of Chicago Press, 2020); Andrea Tone, *Age of Anxiety: A History of America's Turbulent Affair with Tranquilizers* (Hachette, 2009); David Herzberg, *Happy Pills in America. From Miltown to Prozac* (Johns Hopkins University Press, 2008); Nancy Tomes, "Merchants of Health. Medicine and consumer culture in the United States, 1900–1940," *The Journal of American History* 88, no. 2 (2001), 519–47; Nancy Tomes "The Great American Medicine Show Revisited," *Bulletin of the History of Medicine* 79, no. 4 (2005), 627–63. Sophie Chauveau, "Malades ou consommateurs? La consommation de médicaments en France (second XXe siècle)," in *Au nom du consommateur. Consommation et politique en Europe et aux Etats-Unis au XXe siècle*, ed. Marie Chessel, Alain Chatriot, and Matthew Hilton (Éditions La Découverte, 2005), 182–98; Rasmussen Anne, "La résistible ascension du comprimé. Pharmaciens, médecins et publics face aux nouvelles formes pharmaceutiques," in *Les nouvelles pratiques de santé. Acteurs, objets, logiques sociales (XVIIIe–XXe siècles)*, ed. Fabrice Bourdelais and Olivier Faure (Belin, 2005), 103–20; Annika Hoffmann, *Arzneimittelkonsum und Geschlecht: eine historische Analyse zum 19. und 20. Jahrhundert* (Franz Steiner Verlag, 2014); Nils Kessel, "Nebenwirkungen der Konsumgesellschaft? Geschichte des Arzneimittelgebrauchs in Westdeutschland, 1950–1980" (PhD dissertation, Albert-Ludwigs-Universität Freiburg im Breisgau and Université de Strasbourg, 2015).

the time of a "therapeutic revolution."[19] Equivocally enthusiastic about many new drugs, Sir Derrick Dunlop, head of the British Committee on the Safety of Drugs, spoke of a "therapeutic explosion," and so did the *British Medical Journal*'s reviewer of the fifth volume of Meyler's *Side Effects of Drugs*, with an interesting, though ambivalent compliment: "Though the book may give a jaundiced view of treatment, as it only discusses the evils of the therapeutic explosion and not its benefits, it will continue to be of the greatest value in helping to determine whether new symptoms arising in the course of a disease are due to the malady itself or to the remedy employed."[20]

Historian Dominique Tobbell has underlined the Cold War framing of such narratives focusing on past innovation for justifying the softer

19 For drug innovation in this period, see Sophie Chauveau, *L'invention pharmaceutique. La pharmacie française entre l'Etat et la société au XXe siècle* (Editions Synthelabo, 1999); Jean-Paul Gaudillière, "Better prepared than synthesized: Adolf Butenandt, Schering AG and the transformation of sex steroids into drugs (1930–1946)," *Studies in History and Philosophy of Biological and Biomedical Sciences* 36, no. 4 (2005): 612–44; Heiko Stoff, *Wirkstoffe. Eine Geschichte der Institutionalisierung, Standardisierung, Aktivierung und Prekärisierung der Hormone, Vitamine und Enzyme, 1920–1970* (Franz Steiner Verlag 2012); Beat Bächi, *Vitamin C für alle! Pharmazeutische Produktion, Vermarktung und Gesundheitspolitik 1933–1953* (Chronos Verlag, 2009); Viola Balz, *Zwischen Wirkung und Erfahrung – eine Geschichte der Psychopharmaka. Neuroleptika in der Bundesrepublik Deutschland, 1950–1980* (Transcript, 2010); Jeremy A. Greene, *Prescribing by Numbers: Drugs and the Definition of Disease* (Johns Hopkins University Press, 2007); Christina Ratmoko, *Damit die Chemie stimmt. Die Anfänge der industriellen Herstellung von weiblichen und männlichen Sexualhormonen 1914–1938* (Chronos Verlag, 2010); Stuart S. Blume, *Insight and Industry. On the Dynamics of Technology Change in Medicine* (Harvard University Press, 1992); Ilana Löwy, ed., *Medicine and Change: Historical and Sociological Studies of Medical Innovation; Proceedings of the Symposium INSERM Held in Paris, 21–23 April, 1992* (John Libbey Eurotext, 1992); Viviane Quirke, *Collaboration in the Pharmaceutical Industry. Changing Relationships in Britain and France, 1935–1965* (Routledge, 2008). From an economic history perspective, see Judy Slinn, "Research and Development in the UK Pharmaceutical Industry from the nineteenth century to the 1960s," in *Drugs and Narcotics in History*, ed. Mikulas Teich and Roy Porter (Cambridge University Press, 1995), 168–86. For a discussion on the "therapeutic revolution," see Jeremy A. Greene, Flurin Condrau, and Elisabeth Siegel Watkins, eds., *Therapeutic Revolutions: Pharmaceuticals and Social Change in the Twentieth Century* (Chicago University Press, 2016).

20 Citation taken from front cover of Meyler, *Side Effects of Drugs* (1968).

regulation of the "Western" pharmaceutical industry, particularly in the US.[21] In those narratives, the uncertainty of side effects was understood as the price to pay for medical progress – an argument historians of technology are very familiar with. In this narrative, pharmaceutical innovation was directly linked to free-market capitalism and its manufacturers who would provide "benefits" in form of new molecular entities and, ultimately, new drugs for curing diseases.[22]

Yet, multiplication was not just about different drugs. As Tanner argues more generally, it was also about more of the same drugs, since production capacity and speed increased dramatically through automatization. Pill machines that could produce far more tablets contributed to a considerable increase in output between 1920 and 1970, moving the industry from manual labor to semi-automated production, and ultimately automated production towards the end of the century. Since the 1930s in the US, and the late 1940s in Europe, the pharmaceutical industry's marketing infrastructure and efforts increased rapidly.[23] After World War II, public healthcare in Europe became available in most countries with the NHS in Britain, and the Assurance-maladie de la Sécurité sociale in France. In both German states, the existing healthcare systems were considerably expanded and included most citizens. In the US, the creation of Medicare and Medicaid contributed to the expansion of pharmaceutical markets, too.[24] Thus, the technological, economic, and social policies' base of multiplication fundamentally changed drug markets between approximately 1920 and 1970. More individual substances than ever before were available and, in contrast to other sectors, the pharmaceutical industry regularly used old compounds for making new combination products. New, less well-known substances had arrived on the market in large number thanks to screening practices with the help of which

21 Dominique A. Tobbell, *Pills, Power, and Policy. The Struggle for Drug Reform in Cold War America and Its Consequences* (University of California Press, 2011).

22 Recent historiography has quite nuanced the narrative of such a "revolution" by asking what it actually encompassed and who benefitted from it. Jeremy A. Greene and Elizabeth Siegel Watkins, eds., *Prescribed: Writing, Filling, Using and Abusing the Prescription in Modern America* (Johns Hopkins University Press, 2012); Greene, Condrau, and Watkins, eds., *Therapeutic Revolutions.*

23 Jean-Paul Gaudillière and Ulrike Thoms, eds., *The Development of Scientific Marketing in the Twentieth Century* (Pickering & Chatto, 2015).

24 On France, see Bruno Valat, *Histoire de la sécurité sociale. Histoire De La Securite Sociale (1945–1967). L'État, l'institution et la santé* (Editions Economica, 2001); on Germany, see Bundesministerium für Arbeit und Soziales und Bundesarchiv, eds., *Geschichte der Sozialpolitik in Deutschland seit 1945*, 11 vols. (Bundesarchiv, 2002–2008).

manufacturers would diversify their offer even in saturated markets. In West Germany, statistics from the 1960s suggest that, while physicians only used an average of some 150 pharmaceutical products, dosage variations and different application forms as well as package sizes contributed to a pharmaceutical market of some 2,000 singular drugs and some 70,000 different available products.

Drugs are complex technologies, and as such knowledge about their benefits and risks is necessarily situated in their historically specific environment of bodies, interacting natural and synthetic molecules, and the various legal and illegal uses made of them. Not surprisingly, pharmacologists, who rather defended a vision of single-substance drugs and are well known for their skepticism towards combination medicines, became increasingly worried about the number of available drugs on a market. Multiplication made knowledge production about drug use an even more complex endeavor. In 1955, the World Health Organization's (WHO) study group for pharmaceutical preparations stated that the world had fundamentally changed with regard to how knowledge about drugs was managed. While pharmacopoeias, large lists of pharmaceutical substances, had continuously provided health practitioners, particularly pharmacists, but also authorities with useful knowledge about drugs, these technical book series did no longer keep up with the "few hundred new medicinal substances … introduced in the *materia medica* every year."[25]

Indeed, most countries' drug markets in the early twentieth century had been regulated by commercial laws regulating the distribution of drugs, and by pharmacopeia that listed substances available for use in medicines.[26] This list system regulation was then copied for controlling other pharmaceutical substances such as the new regulatory category of "narcotics." Yet, lists as "paper technologies" are flexible because they can be amended but they need to be updated constantly to be up to date.[27] Establishing these lists, printing, and distributing the volumes or at least the updated pages needed

25 *Use of Specifications for Pharmaceutical Preparations. Report of a Study Group* (World Health Organization, 1957), 10.

26 For the US, see: Joseph M. Gabriel, *Medical Monopoly: Intellectual Property and the Origins of the Modern Pharmaceutical Industry* (University of Chicago Press, 2014); and Daniel Carpenter, *Reputation and Power. Organizational Image and Pharmaceutical Regulation at the FDA* (Princeton University Press, 2010). For the German context, see: Wolfgang Wimmer, *Wir haben fast immer was Neues. Gesundheitswesen und Innovation der Pharmaindustrie in Deutschland 1880–1935* (Duncker & Humblot, 1994).

27 Anke Te Heesen, "The Notebook. A Paper-Technology," in *Making Things Public. Atmospheres of Democracy*, ed. Bruno Latour and Peter Weibel (MIT Press, 2005), 582–89.

considerable financial and organizational effort. From the 1930s onwards, German regulators complained about the challenges involved in keeping the pharmacopeia up to date with all the new synthetic substances developed.

Instead of welcoming the many new drugs on the market based on these substances, the above-mentioned WHO study group was concerned about the genuinely new risks these new drugs created in use:

> This large number of new substances presents a certain hazard to public health, especially as a relatively short time may now elapse between the production of a new substance and its use in therapeutics. Twenty years ago this interval could be as much as five to ten years, and today it may be as short as six months. Side-reactions and toxicity cannot possibly be well determined during such a short time. New preparations may be very widely used shortly after introduction, and it is important to have means for their immediate supervision.[28]

In the 1950s, therefore, it was not so much the fact that side effects existed and should be monitored by doctors that changed, but rather the level at which the side effects of medicines were now understood. Previously, they had been seen as an inherent risk of every drug therapy that had to be weighed against the benefits. Drug risks from the producer's side were often associated with fraudulent quack preparations and dubious, small producers. It was against them that the research-intensive pharmaceutical companies had built their reputation as "serious" and "scientific."[29] Yet "quacks" generally acted on a limited regional or even local level. Of course, there had already been drug scandals before, which illustrated the potential dangerousness of drugs on a populational level. But disasters such as the 1930 BCG vaccination catastrophe in the North German city of Lübeck, the sulfanilamide crisis in the USA in 1937, or the Stalinon intoxication of some 100 children in France in 1954 were attributed to faults in drug manufacturing.[30]

28 *Use of Specifications for Pharmaceutical Preparations*, 11. On the quantification problems of drug consumption and rising levels see Kessel, "Nebenwirkungen," chapters 5, 6, and 7; as well as Nils Kessel and Christian Bonah, "Revolutionary Markets? Approaching therapeutic innovation and change through the lens of West German IMS Health data, 1959–1980," in *Therapeutic Revolutions*, ed. Greene, Condrau, and Siegel Watkins, 97–125.

29 On scientific marketing, see Jean-Paul Gaudillière and Ulrike Thoms, "Introduction," in *The Development of Scientific Marketing in the Twentieth Century*, ed. Gaudillière and Thoms, 1–14; and Kessel, "Nebenwirkungen."

30 On Stalinon, see Christian Bonah and Jean-Paul Gaudillière, "Faute, accident ou risque iatrogène? La régulation des événements indésirables du médicament à l'aune des affaires Stalinon et Distilbène," *Revue française des affaires sociales* 2007/3: 127–37; on Sulfanilamide and thalidomide in the US, see the

What changed in the 1950s, though, was the idea that consumption on such a large scale itself would become a public health risk. Correctly prepared drugs would themselves become dangerous either because of individual bodily reactions, for example drug allergies, or because of possible interactions in medical treatment with several medications. While none of the known risks were new, the scale had changed, and experts knew it.

Side effects as a populational risk in an epidemiological understanding needed other tools than the management of clinical medicine individual physicians relied on. For this reason, at the end of the 1950s, medical or state authorities in Europe and the USA set up offices to record side effects.[31] In the Federal Republic of Germany, the Drug Commission of the German Medical Association, which had been in existence since 1952, began collecting side effects around 1960. In the Netherlands, a government agency was even set up in 1958 under the influence of physicians, the MEB.[32] In the US, the American Medical Association Council on Drugs set up its own Registry on Blood Dyscrasias between 1952 and 1955.[33] In the 1960s the US FDA got its own Office of Drug Safety.[34]

Although many experts had recognized that side effects were no longer solely an individual problem of clinical therapy, but also one of public health in view of mass consumption after World War II, the market mechanisms underlying the multiplication of substances and products remained unquestioned. The increase in the number of drugs on the markets was uncritically

---

relevant sections in Carpenter, *Reputation and Power*, 85–87, 230–44. On the BCG vaccine used in Lübeck see Christian Bonah, "'As Safe as Milk or Sugar Water'. Perceptions of the Risks and Benefits of the BCG Vaccine in the 1920s and 1930s in France and Germany," in *The Risks of Medical Innovation*, ed. Thomas Schlich and Ulrich Tröhler (Routledge, 2004), 71–92.

31 Carpenter, *Reputation and Power* provides a useful overview of regulation authorities in developed countries (724–25), but does not include post-market surveillance in the table.

32 R. H. B. Meyboom, "Detecting Adverse Drug Reactions: Pharmacovigilance in The Netherlands" (PhD dissertation, Katholieke Universiteit Nijmegen, 1998).

33 Harry M. Marks, "Making Risks Visible: The Science, Politics, and Regulation of Adverse Drug Reactions," in *Ways of Regulating Drugs in the 19th and 20th Centuries*, ed. Jean-Paul Gaudillière and Volker Hess (Palgrave Macmillan UK, 2013), 107. The notable exception is the US, where surveillance had already been initiated in the 1950s by the American Medical Association. See Beulah Lee and Wayne M. Turner, "Food and Drug Administration's Adverse Drug Reaction Monitoring Program," *American Journal of Hospital Pharmacy* 35, no. 8 (1978): 35.

34 For the US institutional setting of post-market regulation, see Carpenter, *Reputation and Power*, 587–94.

seen as a phenomenon out of reach by most physicians, by the WHO study group, and by most scientific authors. Metaphorically, it was described in terms of natural disasters, as a flood overwhelming humanity rather than the result of economic and regulatory decisions.[35] Although the WHO study group members recognized that market forces, namely increasing competition in increasingly saturated markets, were at least partly responsible for the high number of pharmaceuticals, they did not question them and did not (yet) call for their regulation:

> The Group noted that keen competition forced the manufacturers to produce new pharmaceutical specialties at frequent intervals. For the protection of the users, it is necessary that arrangements should be made to obtain as early as possible sufficient knowledge of the toxicity, pharmacological and clinical action, and side effects of these preparations.[36]

In this view, side effects became an unavoidable evil of new market conditions. They could only be monitored but not be entirely prevented without strongly organizing the market, for example via a strict comparative benefit-risk evaluation as practiced in Norway. In this sense, drug monitoring would only observe evolving free markets. Ideally, it would then identify risks soon enough to alert physicians.[37] The reason for this fatalistic view of side effects becomes clear if you look through the medical literature on side effects at the time.[38]

Despite being himself a whistleblower on phenacetin risks, Swiss anatomist Ulrich Zollinger illustrates a vision that can be found in many European and

35 This critique is not new, however. Contemporaries had already complained about "drug floods" in the 1870s. See Gabriel, *Medical Monopoly*; and Kessel, "Nebenwirkungen," chapter 4.

36 *Use of Specifications for Pharmaceutical Preparations*, 10–11.

37 Regulation in this sense was thought as purely professional, in Jean-Paul Gaudillière's and Volker Hess' sense as one "way of regulating." Jean-Paul Gaudillière and Volker Hess, "General Introduction," in *Ways of Regulating Drugs in the 19th and 20th Centuries*, ed. Gaudillière and Hess, 1–16.

38 Similar examples can be found in Nils Kessel, "Beyond Innovation: The Marketing of 'Old Drugs'," in *The Development of Scientific Marketing in the Twentieth Century*, ed. Gaudillière and Thoms, 15–27, including a short discussion of Derrick Dunlop's point of view. The relationship with the industry divided the medical communities in both Europe and North America. As Harry Marks has noted, "[t]hese narratives reflect a long-enduring conflict within the medical profession itself, between reformers who regard commercial influences as inherently corrupting 'nearly all abuses arise because someone profits thereby' – and practitioners committed to the conjoined principles of therapeutic innovation and professional autonomy" (*Making Risks Visible*, 102).

North American countries, particularly in Switzerland and West Germany. He considered it absurd to hold painkillers responsible for any addiction phenomena, and, rhetorically, compared it to tobacco: Doing so would be as absurd as blaming the tobacco industry for a smoker's lung cancer.[39] Instead, medical criticism blamed consumer behavior, particularly the "abuse" of psychotropic drugs such as hypnotics, tranquillizers, and painkillers.[40] In West Germany, "consumption" of medicines became synonymous for medically unjustified self-medication. Psychiatrists worried about new patient groups in psychiatric hospitals whose profile and suffering challenged traditional concepts of addiction and dependence. Since the late 1950s, German physicians saw women in particular falling victim to "modern consumer society," in which abuse of psychotropic drugs such as hypnotics and painkillers was both a symptom of societal pathology and a factor driving the "overuse" of medicines. [41] As David Herzberg points out through his book *White Market Drugs*, different groups of users of psychotropic drugs were either branded as deviant agents of drug abuse or seen as innocent victims of disease.

Despite moral panics about legal drug consumption, there was not much quantitative evidence for such an idea, and even less for its presumably epidemic dimensions.[42] These moral panics were largely based on what I called elsewhere "amalgams," inseparable connections of clinical cases from psychiatry, pathologists' evidence for organic harm caused by certain drugs, and economists' appropriation of clinical evidence for supporting cost-cutting in public health care.[43]

39 Hans Ulrich Zollinger, "Chronische interstitielle Nephritis bei Abusus von phenacetinhaltigen Analgetika (Saridon usw.)," *Schweizerische Medizinische Wochenschrift* 31/1955: 746, discussed in Kessel, "Nebenwirkungen."

40 Herzberg, *Happy Pills in America*; Tone, *Age of Anxiety*; Kessel, "Nebenwirkungen."

41 Phenacetin, but also acetanilide, another active ingredient used in anti-inflammatory drugs and painkillers, were just as central as morphine derivatives, but also the frequently used sleeping pills made of bromides and barbiturates. On Phenacetin, see Kessel, "Nebenwirkungen"; and Nils Kessel, "Le problème de l'ignorance," in *Sciences humaines, médecine et santé. Manuel du Collège des enseignants de SHS en médecine et santé*, ed. Christian Bonah et al., 2nd ed. (Les Belles Lettres, 2021), 468–78.

42 Kessel, "Nebenwirkungen." For a short discussion in English, see Kessel and Bonah, "Revolutionary Markets?"

43 While the undertones of decline and cultural critique caused by psychopharmaceuticals proved to be wrong, overall consumption of medicines increased since 1945 for various reasons. Discussions about the global rise of pharmaceuticals are complicated though since they are mostly calculated based on expenses, which do not allow serious estimations of actual drug intake. For a discussion about the consumption quantification problem, see Kessel, "Nebenwirkungen."

The multiplication of drugs also made monitoring and regulation of new risky products more difficult. The WHO study group concluded that "the amount of literature and the diversity of the sciences involved make it difficult or impossible for those responsible for the control of pharmaceutical preparations to keep abreast of the flood of information or data being issued."[44]

In times of the internet and smartphones, this argument has to be put back into its technological context. Publication information was usually sent around either by mail, while important information could be transferred by telegram or phone; but bibliographic information was usually collected via mail. The time from publication of a journal article about a drug's effect and its arrival in a center in charge of data collection on drugs could take days if not weeks. WHO experts would rely on librarians for data collection, but they still needed to survey the data which, even with assistance from other personnel, could take weeks or even months. Yet the rhythm with which new products arrived on the market made it necessary to increase the number of experts in charge.

The solutions that were found to tackle this issue varied and are worth looking at, since they show differences in managing side effects. Throughout the 1950s and 1960s, Meyler's *Side Effects of Drugs* was regularly re-edited, reaching its sixth edition in 1968. *Side Effects of Drugs* illustrates well the accumulation of knowledge about individual substances and drug groups but also the increase in drugs on the market. It grew steadily in size and format. Meyler's first edition in English had been a comparatively small book in the so-called digest format (14 x 21.6 cm) of 268 pages with a font size of 12 points. The sixth edition measured 19x24cm and had 579 pages. The font size was reduced to 10 points and the available space was utilized to the maximum with the help of a two-column system in order to leave only little empty space.

However, Meyler's series was not a completely new edition of the same volume but rather an ongoing review of the previous last two years of medical literature, as indicated the added subtitle "A Survey of Unwanted Effects of Drugs reported in 1965–1967" to the sixth edition. Thus, Meyler's *Side Effects* provided an updated, continuous book series in which each volume never got outdated and which allowed its compilers to manage the increasing number of products by focusing on the most recent information of the last two years. Later, the series was once again modified and the *Side Effect of Drugs Annual* (SEDA) split from *Side Effects of Drugs*.[45] These formal changes are not mere adaptations to editorial requirements but refer to the

44 *Use of Specifications for Pharmaceutical Preparations*, 11; see also footnote 35.

45 Aronson, "The history of Meyler's *Side Effects of Drugs*."

fundamental problem of multiplication doctors and regulators were increasingly concerned with.

Above all, they made the manual collection and processing of information on side effects more difficult.[46] Existing paper technologies, namely vade-mecums and literature collections, were already outdated by the time they appeared, as medical publishing practice and the processing of literature by experts was done manually: the author in question compiled the literature that had appeared over several years, analyzed it and wrote a concise description of each substance.[47] The result was useful for medical prescribers who were looking for experience with the drugs mentioned in the reference period. However, there was no claim to completeness. Each volume therefore had to be read in the context of the other volumes. In 1968, however, the entire collection of six volumes already comprised several thousand pages, which is why the 1968 edition was the first to attempt to link information from the older volumes with the new ones. The single author Meyler had meanwhile surrounded himself with a team of thirty mainly Dutch and British university authors. He published the 1968 volume for the first time with the British pharmacologist Andrew Herxheimer. In the foreword, the two editors explained the changed form and the expanded authorship as a consequence of the "mass of new information".[48] The team of authors now consisted almost exclusively of doctors from hospitals and university clinics.[49] Such a work corresponded to the classical encyclopedia and thus belonged to the risk regulation via printed list systems that characterized the first half of the twentieth century.

Put simply, *Side effects of Drugs* corresponded on the clinical side to the use of drugs in the pharmacopoeia on the manufacturing side. Knowledge about drugs (pharmacopoeias) and observed effects attributed to drugs (side effects of drugs) were found in these lists. In both cases, however, nothing was said about what actually happened on the markets and in use. Pharmacopoeias did not provide any information on the quantities actually produced or used, and the Side effects of Drugs series remained vague and sometimes even

46 I have studied elsewhere the power imbalance between pharmaceutical companies and regulators but also public health insurance in West Germany regarding access to market data and more generally knowledge about pharmaceutical markets. See Nils Kessel, "Étudier les marchés du médicament: les entreprises pharmaceutiques et la transformation du marketing en Allemagne de l'Ouest (1960–1980)," in *Les marchés de la santé*, ed. Bruno Valat (Presses Universitaires du Midi, 2021), 173–98.

47 Te Heesen, "The Notebook."

48 Meyler and Herxheimer, *Side Effects*, v.

49 See Meyler and Herxheimer, *Side Effects*, vii–viii for its list of contributors.

silent when it came to the frequency of side effects. However, these two aspects played a role in the case of the thalidomide catastrophe.

The Thalidomide Shock, Mass Consumption, and Its Regulation

Now it could be assumed that the biggest drug disaster of the twentieth century fundamentally changed medical experts' and practitioners' views on drug risk. On November 26, 1961, manufacturer Grünenthal AG withdrew its sleeping pill containing thalidomide from the West German market.[50] Months later thousands of newborn children whose mothers had used the medication against nausea during pregnancy or for better sleep were identified as potential victims of the drug's teratogenic effects. Many industrialized countries – with some notable exceptions such as France or the US – have been affected by it. Outside of West Germany, the thalidomide disaster produced victims in Sweden, Switzerland, and the UK and its global history is only about to be researched.[51] During this period, more than 5,000 children in West Germany were born with malformations and an unknown number of adults suffered irreversible neurological defects. The thalidomide events were in many respects an exceptional catastrophe. It not only led to the premature death of embryos, but produced the rare syndrome called phocomelia in the newborn, which, ironically, made it visible compared to other drug risks.[52]

The regulatory consequences of the thalidomide scandal have been extensively discussed by political scientists, law scholars, sociologists, and

50 Beate Kirk, *Der Contergan-Fall. Eine unvermeidbare Arzneimittelkatastrophe? Zur Geschichte des Arzneistoffes Thalidomid* (Wissenschaftliche Verlagsgesellschaft, 1999); Alexander von Schwerin, "1961 – Die Contergan-Bombe. Der Arzneimittelskandal und die neue risikoepistemische Ordnung der Massenkonsumgesellschaft," in *Arzneistoffe im 20. Jahrhundert. Historische Skizzen von Lebertran bis Contergan*, ed. Nicholas Eschenbruch, Viola Balz, Ulrike Klöppel, and Marion A. Hulverscheidt (Transcript, 2009), 255–82; Thomas Großbölting and Niklas Lenhard-Schramm, eds., *Contergan: Hintergründe und Folgen eines Arzneimittel-Skandals* (Vandenhoeck & Ruprecht, 2017); Trent Stephens and Rock Brynner, *Dark Remedy: The Impact of Thalidomide and its Revival as a Vital Medicine* (Perseus Publishing, 2001); Carpenter, *Reputation and Power*; Kessel, "Nebenwirkungen."

51 Ludger Wimmelbücker and Anita Kar, "A history of thalidomide in India," *Medical History* 67, no. 3 (2023): 228–46.

52 See Solène Lellinger's contribution on Mediator in this volume.

historians.[53] In most works, thalidomide figures as the starting point for new regulation.[54] Yet, Daniel Carpenter has already shown that the US pre-market regulation model stems from the late 1930s experience with sulfa drugs rather than from thalidomide, which was not even marketed in the USA.[55] In most European countries, on pre-market regulation regarding side effects, new forms of toxicity testing were successively introduced on both a pre-clinical and a clinical level.[56] Controlled clinical trials and quickly randomized clinical trials (RCT) were introduced for testing in humans. Existing legislation was reviewed in the larger context of the creation of a Common European Market for which market admission standards were harmonized.[57] This process took considerable time, particularly in West Germany, where the new (second) drug law passed parliament only in 1976.[58] Premarket regulation did block substances considered too toxic but in West Germany, the USA, Switzerland and many other countries it did little if nothing to

53 Marks, *Making Risks Visible*; Stefan Timmermans and Valerie Leiter, "The Redemption of Thalidomide. Standardizing the Risk of Birth Defects," *Social Studies of Science* 30, no. 1 (2000), 41–71; for Germany, see Kirk, *Contergan-Fall*; Arthur Daemmrich, *Pharmacopolitics. Drug Regulation in the United States and Germany* (University of North Carolina Press, 2004); Carpenter, *Reputation and Power*.

54 Current scholarship still depicts the thalidomide disaster as the starting point of modern drug regulation and modern drug testing. However, scholars such as political scientist Daniel Carpenter have argued that, although the disaster certainly has contributed to tightening drug regulation, drug regulation processes are much older. Yet, there is no doubt that it has accelerated the spread of the American model of drug testing in countries such as West Germany. The thalidomide disaster also encouraged initiatives for better "drug safety" on both national and international levels.

55 Carpenter, *Reputation and Power*.

56 Carpenter, *Reputation and Power*; for Germany, see Ute Stapel, *Die Arzneimittelgesetze 1961 und 1976* (Deutscher Apotheker Verlag, 1988); Axel Murswieck, *Die staatliche Kontrolle der Arzneimittelsicherheit in der Bundesrepublik und den USA* (Westdeutscher Verlag, 1983). Several governments, such as West Germany and Britain, came under pressure to tighten their drug laws and effectively/consequently implemented the American model of drug regulation and its phasic testing procedures.

57 Scandinavian countries such as Norway already had quite comprehensive market control mechanisms since the 1920s. After World War II the American liberal market model was taken over by the key European manufacturing countries. A central motor became the project of a common European market following the Treaty of Rome in 1957.

58 Kirk, *Contergan-Fall*; Murswieck, *Kontrolle*.

control the benefits of a drug regarding competing products.[59] Capitalist markets and their consumers, more frequently physician prescribers rather than patients, should influence the commercial success of medicines. The limits of such a model have been widely studied, especially regarding the influence of marketing.[60]

It is true, however, that post-market surveillance of pharmaceutical markets accelerated in the wake of the thalidomide disaster. Manufacturers such as Geigy in Switzerland created "[s]ide effect [monitoring] offices" and state agencies either started ensuring surveillance themselves such as in the Netherlands or delegated official surveillance missions to the medical profession or institutions. In the US, the FDA's internal efforts to promote post-market surveillance through epidemiological collection of data about risks took off from the early 1960s.[61] The World Health Organization (WHO) tried to standardize side effect monitoring and identification and became a key player for international side effect monitoring. The WHO's approaches were about the standardization of methods, tools, and terminologies. From the WHO's point of view, international comparison was crucial for knowledge production about health and, of course, for the WHO's legitimacy as a unique reference institution. Yet, drugs were difficult to standardize beyond their molecular form. Brand names and international naming standards were one problem.[62] But dosage, package size, prescription habits, prices, and many other elements also varied from one country to another.[63] Pharmaceutical markets proved to be too complex to allow comparison between them without any common standard of measurement. Yet

59 In the US, from 1967 the Drug Efficacy Study (DESI) did offer such comparison. See Carpenter *Reputation and Power*, 346–54. In France and Germany, comparison between therapeutic benefits of drugs was only introduced more recently.

60 Sergio Sismondo, "Key Opinion Leaders and the Corruption of Medical Knowledge: What the Sunshine Act Will and Won't Cast Light On," *Journal of Law, Medicine and Ethics* 41, no. 3 (2013): 635–43; John Abraham and G. Lewis, *Regulating Medicines in Europe: Competition, Expertise and Public Health* (Routledge, 2000); Gaudillière and Thoms, eds., *Scientific Marketing*.

61 Carpenter, *Reputation and Power*, 590–94.

62 See Jeremy A. Greene, *Generic: The Unbranding of Modern Medicine* (Johns Hopkins University Press, 2014).

63 Per Knut M. Lunde, Ingerid Baksaas-Aasen, M. Halse, Ivar Halvorsen, B. Stromnes, and K. Øydvin, "The Methodology of Drug Utilization Studies," in *Studies in Drug Utilization: Methods and Applications*, ed. Ulf Bergman, A. H. W. Wahba, Barbro Westerholm, and Almar Grímsson (World Health Organization, 1979), 20.

comparison was the essential methodology to establish averages and potential norms for international concertation.

Since 1964, the WHO had two programs going on: the WHO adverse drug reaction monitoring; and the Scandinavian-dominated WHO Drug Utilization Research Group (DURG).[64] Both groups coexisted but followed different paths of managing drug-related risks while targeting different types of benefits. DURG was more ambitious in its goals since it undertook to study consumer behavior from both physicians and patients on an international level.[65] This group took seriously the argument that widespread use of pharmaceuticals had been an essential condition for thalidomide's catastrophic dimension, affecting tens of thousands of people.[66] For DURG members, consumption and prescription as drug risk factors had even gained importance since the 1950s because of an increasing number of new compounds put on the market. Long-term drug use for more frequent chronic diseases let the experts expect that additional risks due to drug interactions would increase in the future. Experts, such as the British researcher Owen Wade and his Scandinavian colleagues, knew that book series such as Leopold Meyler's were useful tools for educating practitioners about side effects, but these books would not provide a tool for surveillance and prevention. The Drug Utilization Research Group's programmatic article summarizes the committee's objectives:

> Cost and prescription figures have indicated that 'consumption' of drugs in Europe, and probably in many other areas, has been increasing over the last two decades. It has also become increasingly evident that drugs are frequently not used to their full potential, nor according to generally accepted criteria. This has led to an enhanced interest among research workers,

64 A first portrait of this group has been provided by Anne Kveim Lie (2016, unpublished working paper) who generously shared her manuscript with me.

65 Kveim Lie and Hobæk, "Less is more." This also confirms broader historical observations from historians of technology who insist on the expert's perspective and its tendency to attribute technological risk and failure to users. See, for example, Ruth Oldenziel and Mike Hård, *Consumers, Tinkers, Rebels: The People Who Shaped Europe* (Palgrave Macmillan, 2013).

66 There was strong evidence to support this idea: thalidomide had been identified when physicians in Australia and Germany observed a higher frequency of phocomelia – the specific malformations thalidomide can provoke. For months physicians believed they resulted of nuclear radiation due to secret atomic bomb testing. Only the fact that all victims' mothers had taken thalidomide enabled them to link the drug to the pathology. What if thalidomide had not shown those visible malformations, but instead provoked long-term disease or organ failure, such as in the case of certain analgesics? Would it have been identified in time then?

> health administrators, and members of the health professions in surveying the drug utilization pattern and following its development with time. Major quantitative and qualitative differences in the prescribing pattern have been detected between countries and regions within individual countries. This calls for a more systematic, precise, and comprehensive description and follow-up of drug utilization after the drugs have been marketed, to evaluate the clinical consequences of the sometimes widely different drug therapy traditions.[67]

Comparing prescriptions, expenses, but also drugs and their clinical phenomena, as intended by the Adverse Drug Monitoring Reaction Group at the WHO, was supposed to standardize concepts, methods, and measurement units. While DURG could produce its own data, at least in Scandinavia, by simply standardizing existing comprehensive datasets such as public health insurance annual reimbursements, the adverse drug monitoring program had to rely on reporting physicians, manufacturers, or state agencies.

A key problem in side effects was of epistemological nature. How to know that a phenomenon was linked to a drug, especially if it was reported by third parties such as practitioners? So, one of the first steps of the DURG and the adverse drug monitoring experts was terminological standardization. The very term "side effect" became an object of discussion, because of its polysemy. While Meyler had considered the term a perfect umbrella for undesired phenomena associated with the clinical use of drugs, WHO experts were reluctant to keep it. It was simply impossible to have a category that was so ambiguous with regard to causality. "Side effect" suggested a causal link between a drug and a symptom or syndrome occurring in patients. However, academic, and more broadly political and media discussions about drugs dangerousness was if observation could be attributed to a drug based on the available evidence. Yet in cases such as phenacetin, thalidomide, or the contraceptive pill's possible thrombotic side effects, controversy broke out about the validity and stability of the knowledge available.

In 1968, the WHO abandoned the term "side effects" and removed it from its official vocabulary. WHO commissions on Drug Monitoring had developed a new, more differentiated understanding of drug risks. In the revised version of the 1968 reports, "side effect" was replaced by the new conceptual set "adverse drug event" (ADE) and "adverse drug reaction" (ADR). Both were technical categories that could be distinguished as to their level of proof. An ADE was an *ex post*-defined observation that could be related to the use of a specific drug but was neither classified in terms of causality nor related to specific user behavior. In contrast, an ADR was defined as "[a]ny noxious change in a patient's condition which a physician

67 Lunde et al., "The Methodology of Drug Utilization Studies," 18.

believes to be due to a drug, which occurs **at dosages normally used in man**, and which 1) requires treatment, or 2) indicates **decrease or cessation of therapy** with the drug, or 3) suggests that future therapy with the drug carries an **unusual risk** in **his** patient. [emphasis is mine]."[68]

The WHO's therapeutic reformers shared with their American colleagues Harry M. Marks has studied a deep mistrust in medical practitioners and, of course, patients. They did not believe that observation made outside the hospital, by general practitioners insufficiently trained in pharmacology could provide a sufficient base for recognizing side effects. Instead, they thought that these practitioners needed to be understood as providers for raw data that had to be analyzed by qualified experts.

The final judgement of a causal link was taken out of practitioners' hands: an observation actually being recognized as an effect of the drug then remained in experts' hand, and more importantly, it was based not just on qualitative clinical judgement but on a sufficient number of similar observations. WHO intended to build up a new global reporting system for ADR which should collect data from all countries, then analyze them in order to have sufficient data for probabilistic calculations.[69] An ADR was necessarily a probabilistic calculation. As such it should contribute to more objectivity in drug risk assessment. The new concept set ADE/ADR should better reflect the institutional separation of practices of use and identification of drug characteristics than the term side effect. ADR excluded any excessive or illicit use of a drug. Side effects could result from inappropriate use, whether an ADR could not. In consequence, all observations made by practitioners that were based on patients who overused or misused a drug had to be excluded by the clinical experts who evaluated forms of ADE and clinical report collections for identification of potential ADRs. For instance, a side effect could be the result of an addiction to hypnotics with an increased dosage. It would not be considered an ADR because addiction to specific drugs included and was defined by their therapeutically inappropriate use.

Yet, the ADR monitoring program never succeeded in producing the ambitious data its founders had dreamt of.[70] The WHO international

68 WHO definition in J. Koch-Weser, E. M. Sellers, R. Zacest, "The Ambiguity of Adverse Drug Reactions," *European Journal of Clinical Pharmacology* 11, no. 2 (1977): 75–78. Emphasis in the original.

69 Van Grootheest, "Improving Pharmacovigilance," 38f. For the larger picture, see also David Demortain, "Les heurts de la transnationalisation. L'OMS, l'International Conference on Harmonisation et la régulation internationale du médicament," in *La mondialisation des risques. Une histoire politique et transnationale des risques sanitaires et environnementaux*, ed. Soraya Boudia and Emmanuel Henry (Presses Universitaires de Rennes, 2015), 109–21.

70 Marks, *Making Risks Visible*, 98.

monitoring center, initially located in Virginia before moving to Uppsala in Sweden, was not successful.[71] It collected 16,000 reports in 1977, which is not much neither.[72] National reporting systems were considered inefficient by WHO experts.[73] In West Germany, for example, only some hundred cases of suspected ADs were reported to the national surveillance board. These were far too few compared to the country's more than hundred million prescriptions per year. Reasons for insufficient reporting were various, ranging from bureaucratic paperwork and fears of legal consequences to ignorance about the system.

Controlling through Clinical Trials

In consequence, clinical pharmacologists set up clinical trials in hospitals instead of collecting data from non-specialized practitioners throughout the country. When retreating into the better controlled conditions of a hospital environment, medical experts hoped to create the most accurate experimental conditions. It was hoped that these would allow pharmacologists to exclude all potential effects in the patient's body that, for example, were due to diet, life and work rhythm, or secret addictions.

Even in the controlled space of the hospital, ADR identification remained a very difficult task. This owed too to the methodological complications that arise when commonly used drugs receive focused attention: "a slightly elevated risk for a common medical condition requires studying many more patients than demonstrating an increased risk for an unusual side effect."[74]

In the late 1970s a clinical pharmacology research group published an analysis of 500 so-called "untoward clinical events" which had been identified as adverse drug reactions by practitioners in the US.[75] The results

71 Demortain, "Les heurts de la transnationalisation."

72 *WHO Chronicle*, 31, no. 10 (1977): 419. The 1977 number provided for collected ADRs are: 130,000 for 3,000 substances in 10,000 products; 16,000 reports on average; and 1,000 drug names. On the failure of the WHO's Uppsala Center and the role of ICH, see also Demortain, "Les heurts de la transnationalisation."

73 William N. Wardell, Michael C. Tsianco, Sadanand N. Anavekar, and Henry T. Davis, "Postmarketing Surveillance of New Drugs: I. Review of Objectives and Methodology," *The Journal of Clinical Pharmacology*, 19, nos. 2–3 (1979): 86: "No such [comprehensive post-marketing surveillance] system yet exists in any country [in 1979]." See also Demortain, "Les heurts de la transnationalisation."

74 Marks, *Making Risks Visible*, 98.

75 Koch-Weser, Sellers, and Zacest, "The Ambiguity of Adverse Drug Reactions," 75.

showed that not only general practitioners diverged in their assessment of what could be considered as an ADR, but also the experts interpreted differently many of the ADR reports.[76] The article authors concluded that "[t]he divergence of judgments suggests that suspected ADRs are usually ambiguous clinical events, and that incidence, severity, medical consequences and cost of ADRs can only be estimated."

In consequence, ADR research led by clinical pharmacologists such as Koch-Weser tried to obtain more control on the soundness of observations and evaluations by not only narrowing ADRs to normal behavior but by focusing on medications primarily used in hospital therapies rather than those therapies used in outpatient care. The final restriction applied was the focus on "severe" ADRs: post-marketing surveillance (PMS) studies were isolated studies of problematic drugs.[77]

This set of methodological choices has had important consequences on the ways "side effects" were managed once they had become "adverse drug reactions." Focusing on "severe" ADRs meant to weigh different risks against each other and to lend greater importance to acute reactions that emerge in hospital care. In contrast, side effects emerging after mid- or long-term use in outpatient care were neglected. Thus, the benefit of post-market surveillance was distributed unevenly among consumers and patients. Regulators and their advisors from clinical pharmacology tended to think about patients without paying attention to class, race, and gender as long as it did not matter for biological processes related to the drugs, as for example in the case of the pill. Yet, the history of phenacetin, thalidomide, and more recently Mediator in France, or the opioid epidemic in the US shows that drug users were differently affected because of their socially, racially, and gendered consumption patterns.

Side effect monitoring through reporting systems continue to this day and are part of attempts to improve the quality of data. Throughout the 1980s, however, criticism of post-market surveillance continued to focus on the structural limits, as analyzed by Daniel Carpenter.[78] Until most recently, when big data calculation capacities, deep-learning AI, and patient-based

76 Among the 500, the three experts qualified between 14.4 and 28.2% as valid ADRs; 26.4 and 38.0% as probable ones; 21.4 and 31.0% as possible; and 8.4 to 14.5% as no ADRs. Most controversial was the contribution of drug effects to fatalities. The clinical pharmacologists' assessment varied by 71% from 10 (examiner A) to 28 (examiner B).

77 Wardell et al., "Postmarketing," 86. For the Type A, B, and C adverse drug reaction classifications replaced by the DoTS (Dose, Time, Susceptibility) scheme, see Jamie J. Coleman and Sarah K. Pontefract, "Adverse drug reactions," *Clinical Medicine* 16, no. 5 (2016): 481–85.

78 Carpenter, *Reputation and Power*, chapter 9.

alert documentation are beginning to offer new possibilities, drug epidemiology has not influenced conceptual change but followed the adoption of clinical pharmacology's priorities and authority.[79]

Conclusion

How do we explain that Meyler's established definition of side effects was replaced by a much narrower understanding of what a side effect was? In German sociologist Niklas Luhmann's terms, such a change would eventually appear as just another example of the need of highly complex societies to manage complexity through differentiation and reducing incompatibilities. While Meyler's concept encompassed many different medical and social spheres, and its various social realities, an ADR is narrowed down to the sphere of clinical pharmacology, which is the only scientifically legitimate space for validating an ADR. Only clinical pharmacology's studies can "prove" that an ADR exists and thus turn an ADE into an ADR. Following Luhmann's lead, therefore, we can understand that it is the specific code of the subsystem of clinical science that allows it to recognize the existence of ADRs as "true." Yet, following Dominique Tobbell, this specific process of differentiation is not a mere result of scientific logics but must be placed back into the relatively short period between the 1950s and the mid-1970s during which the political front lines between the West and the East were particularly visible. The ADR concept was a technocratic response to a social problem. Side effects should remain in the hands of practitioners, but medical science done by clinical pharmacologists should produce true knowledge about effects in order to avoid conflict between drug safety and their authorities, and pharmaceutical companies who would defend legally and politically their products.

Yet, there is no straightforward story to tell from side effect to ADR. There has not been a sudden awareness for drug risks after thalidomide. Drug risks were known before, both by general practitioners and clinicians, as well as by regulators, companies, and media bodies. What changed in the late 1950s – and thalidomide was its strongest catalyst in late 1961 – was that the impact of multiplication became obvious. National and international

79 On patient-centered alerts and the problems of anecdotal evidence, see Antoine Lentacker, "Just stories. Side effects and the patient voice online," in *Technology, Health, and the Patient Consumer in the Twentieth Century*, ed. Rachel Elder and Thomas Schlich (Manchester University Press, 2025), 137–64; as well as Antoine Lentacker, "Epistemology of the side effect: anecdote and evidence in the digital age," *BioSocieties* 19 (2024): 84–111.

epidemiological early-warning systems were built around pharmaceuticals as hazardous chemicals and, just as with other hazards, they were managed inside continuing free markets.

If these various systems of managing risks of medicines proved often less successful than expected, this is often due the enormous costs the material infrastructures, machines, and data collectors and analysts produced. Therefore, a look at the material base is essential, and it can explain why traditional paper technologies such as updated compendia like Meyler's *Side Effects of Drugs* might have turned out more effective than the ambitious but underfunded WHO ADR monitoring program.

ADR monitoring, today often integrated in pharmacovigilance systems, and patient-centered side effect management continue to coexist; indeed, they were never intended to substitute one another. Ironically, the side effect management undertaken by physicians perpetuates Meyler's vision of side effects as problems emerging with a drug in use that a physician can attribute to a drug.

The conceptual change from side effect to ADR initiated by the WHO had two important consequences for the management of pharmaceutical risks. First, on a socio-political and therapeutical level it contributed to devaluing individual practitioners' judgment and observation in comparison with the medical "objectivity" of clinical trials. It did so in the same way as Harry Marks has described therapeutic reformers' efforts to establish the clinical trial for the admission of drugs to the market. However, while clinical trials became the exclusive path of market admission, side effect management remained shared between two levels, that of individual therapy on the one hand, and that of national as well as international risk surveillance on the other. By doing so, it produced permanent tensions between different forms of knowledge: clinical observation; and statistical evidence from clinical trials. Ironically, due to lack of resources, the scientific method failed in practice in surveilling drug risks efficiently.

Secondly, on a technical and political level it reconfigured concepts that oriented research about drug risks but also drug risks as a socio-political object. With ADR, uses had to be "normal", and the ADR redefinition of the side effect thus simplified the complex relationship that characterizes a drug in practical use. Instead of including forms of medical or patient error, of voluntary or involuntary overuse (or more rarely underdosage), it standardized both use and its users. People with addictions could still suffer side effects due to their consumer behavior, but excessive consumption leading to intoxication would not be classifiable as an ADR although addiction itself became later introduced as an ADR. As such, the boundary between side effect and intoxication became hermetic. The complex realities of practice, though, continued quite undisturbed by the new risk management system. As such, it did what defenders of pharmaceutical innovation had asked for: it should neither further restrict regulation nor change the perspective of new drugs as genuinely positive.

Part Two

Narrating Risk and Benefit

Chapter Four

What's in a Substance? LSD and the Impending Decline of the West[1]

Beat Bächi

Try to forget everything you know about LSD.[2] In the spring of the year 1943, Albert Hofmann is the first human being to experience the power of the substance LSD-25. As there are no models for describing its effects, he simply does not know what is happening to him. While on the other side of the Swiss border, directly opposite on the other bank of the Rhine from

1 I would like to express my sincere thanks to Magaly Tornay for the many years of extremely interesting and valuable discussions we have had about drugs, especially LSD.

2 To quote just some of the numerous important contributions to the history of LSD apart from Albert Hofmann's own account in his bestseller *LSD – Mein Sorgenkind*, published in 1979, see Erika Dyck and Chris Elcock, eds., *Expanding Mindscapes: A Global History of Psychedelics* (MIT Press, 2023); Erika Dyck, *Psychedelic Psychiatry: LSD from Clinic to Campus* (Johns Hopkins University Press, 2008); Dieter Hagenbach and Lucius Werthmüller, *Albert Hofmann und sein LSD (mit einem Vorwort von Stanislav Grof)* (AT Verlag, 2011); Jeannie Moser, *Psychotropen: Eine LSD-Biographie* (Konstanz University Press, 2013); Jakob Tanner, "'Doors of perception' versus 'Mind control'. Experimente mit Drogen zwischen kaltem Krieg und 1968," in *Kulturgeschichte des Menschenversuchs im 20. Jahrhundert*, ed. Birgit Griesecke et al. (Suhrkamp, 2009), 340–72; Magaly Tornay, *Zugriffe auf das Ich: Psychoaktive Stoffe und Personenkonzepte in der Schweiz, 1945 bis 1980* (Mohr Siebeck, 2016).

Basel, the Nazis are literally "on speed,"[3] Hofmann compares the "symptoms of poisoning" he experiences with the symptoms "observed after excessive use of pervitin" or similar (meth)amphetamines. The fact that Hofmann believes that LSD-25 is somehow similar to these amphetamines was due to contingent circumstances. CIBA, the local competitor to his employer Sandoz, already had a successful circulatory and respiratory stimulant on the market under the brand name Coramine (nicotinic acid diethylamide). And the chemical structure of lysergic acid diethylamide was similar to that of Coramine. Hence, Hofmann was hoping to manufacture a competing product. Another decisive factor was his physician, who had been called in after Hofmann had come home with severe signs of poisoning, and interpreted them against the background of his own experiences. The doctor had "accidentally conducted experiments with Pervitin himself" and experienced similar symptoms, such as motor restlessness, impaired vision, and color visions.[4]

While we are used to stories of LSD as a "subversive" substance, at least since the 1960s, over the course of its biography it has experienced a wide variety of attributions and appeared in various guises and garments. Hence, before coming to the quite contemporary question of whether this substance might be a risk or a benefit (for individuals or social groups), this contribution tries to illuminate the collective biography of LSD and its inventor Albert Hofmann.[5] The seemingly infinite roles LSD has played at different stages of its life and in different cultural settings make it obvious how many insights are missed if one assumes that substances stand outside history. But can substances and materials be imbued with meanings at will, or is there something essentialist in matter that resists social construction?[6]

3 See Hans-Christian Dany, *Speed: Eine Gesellschaft auf Droge* (Nautilus, 2007); Norman Ohler, *Der totale Rausch: Drogen im Dritten Reich* (Kiepenheuer & Witsch, 2015); and Nicolas Rasmussen, *On Speed. The Many Lives of Amphetamine* (New York University Press, 2008).

4 Archiv IMG, N Hofmann 148.1: Berichte von Selbstversuchen mit d-Lyserg-säure-diäthylamid-tartrat, 1943–1946: Dr. med. Walter Schilling, Prakt. Arzt, Bottmingen, Bericht an Hr. Prof. Stoll, Beobachtungen bei Dr. A. Hofmann nach Einnahme von 0,25 mg des Diaethylamids der Lysergsäure am 19.4.43, 22. 4. 1943 (gez. Beerle). (All quotes from sources in German: own translation.)

5 For the broader argument of this text see Beat Bächi, *LSD auf dem Land. Produktion und kollektive Wirkung psychotroper Stoffe* (Konstanz University Press, 2020; 2nd ed., 2024).

6 The classic text on this question is Emilie Gomart, "Methadone: Six Effects in Search of a Substance," *Social Studies of Science* 32, no. 1 (2002): 93–135.

In the Field: LSD and the Birth of the Mind[7]

When Albert Hofmann composed a first draft on the history of the discovery of LSD in 1952, he stated that LSD had been discovered "by chance." However, it was "not a pure coincidence," but "the occurrence of the event leading to the discovery" was "given a distinct chance."[8] For the nearly immaterial effects of LSD to become visible, large material flows were necessary. Only when ergot (the natural raw material for LSD) was produced on an industrial scale in Switzerland during World War II, and thus became cheaper, was Hofmann enabled to experiment again with LSD-25 in 1943. When he had developed it for the first time in 1938, a small quantity was reserved for animal testing. It failed to demonstrate any particular vasoconstricting properties on the uterus of rabbits, and consequently the new substance risked falling into oblivion until it emerged anew in 1943, when the situation regarding the resource ergot had fundamentally changed.

Solving the resource problems by industrializing ergot production eventually paved the way for Hofmann's serendipitous discovery of LSD. But the substance produced effects that were neither easily classifiable nor easy to study. What is special about LSD is not so much what it does (many other toxins do the same), but how it does it. LSD seemed to work in purely psychic regions. This might also explain the extremely tiny dose necessary to trigger unprecedented effects. In view of a dose that lies beyond human perception thresholds, the almost immaterial LSD promised to illuminate the body-mind problem. While the US chemical giant Du Pont had created one of the most concise slogans in advertising history, "better living through chemistry," the psyche was about to be opened up to chemical methods as well.

But how should these new phenomena be interpreted, the effects of novel substances be described, objectified or even measured? From the substances to the effects, collectively shared or at least communicable patterns of interpretation, horizons of experience, and chains of association were needed. It was not only the rye fields producing ergot that played a crucial role here, but also the military field that provided a first backdrop for interpretation.

7 Parts of his section were published in Beat Bächi, "Psychotropic Drugs from and in the Fields. Rural Roots and Collective Effects of LSD," in *Expanding Mindscapes. A Global History of Psychedelics*, ed. Erika Dyck and Chris Elcock (MIT Press, 2023), 215–37. For a more comprehensive version of the idea developed in this section, see Magaly Tornay and Beat Bächi, *Drogen. Zur Einführung* (Junius, 2025), 91–122.

8 Archiv IMG, N Hofmann 148: "LSD LA 111," Mappe 148.4: Beilage zum Brief von Albert Hofmann an Ruedi Bircher, Sandoz Pharmaceuticals, New York, "Wie das Phantasticum LSD 25 entdeckt wurde," Basel, 12. Dezember 1952, 1 and 4f.

Hofmann was drafted into the army several times in the eventful year 1943. During his time of service, he continued to deal with LSD in a very practical way. During his military service in Claro (Tessin), he conducted a total of three self-experiments. He took LSD on September 28 after dinner, then went to an inn with his "comrades," drank coffee with grappa, and played "footballino and billiards." During all this, he felt completely turned in on himself with a "feeling of warm security within himself." On October 2, he took LSD after a coffee and a glass of "Grogg" and the following night had nightmares, where he saw a "madly mutilated woman, with arms cut off and eyes burned out." He was equally horrified by his fellow servants considering him "insane" and, above all, by his realization that he could not convince them otherwise.[9]

Despite these terrible dreams, Hofmann wanted to continue working to solve the mystery of this strange substance, so wrote "from the field" to his superior Arthur Stoll, Sandoz's head of the pharmaceutical department in Basel. Even though he found it comforting that the chemical questions around LSD were "problems for the long term," he was impatient that clinical research was lagging behind. "To make up for this backlog soon, I would like to propose that d-lysergic acid diethylamide be clinically tested without waiting for further results from animal testing," he wrote to Stoll. Hofmann suggested that Stoll's son Werner, who worked in the psychiatric clinic Burghölzli (now the Psychiatric University Hospital in Zurich), might be enthusiastic about such experiments.[10] At a time when psychiatry mainly used somatic cures directed at the body, it was an excellent coincidence that Arthur Stoll's son worked in psychiatry.

It was Arthur Stoll who then raised ethical concerns and wrote to Hofmann that "a certain pharmacological and toxicological basis" had to be created for clinical studies – "if one did not want to risk too much." In his view, this was required by the "responsibility towards the sick" on whom the substance was to be tested. Furthermore, his son Werner was also in military service for a longer period of time. In view of these circumstances, Stoll wrote: "we must in any case have a little patience if we want to get him to test the diethylamide on humans."[11]

Probably because of Stoll's negative reply, on October 31, 1943, Hofmann made another self-experiment during his active service. This time

9 Archiv IMG, N Hofmann 148.1: Berichte von Selbstversuchen mit d-Lysergsäure-diäthylamid-tartrat, 1943–1946: Albert Hofmann an Herrn Prof. Stoll: Bericht über 3 Selbstversuche mit d-Lysergsäure-diäthylamid, 30.XII.1943, 1.

10 FA Novartis, Sandoz, H 105.022 (1940–1947), Brief von A. Hofmann (an Stoll), Im Felde, 27. Oktober 1943.

11 FA Novartis, Sandoz, H 105.022 (1940–1947), Brief von Stoll an Hofmann, Basel, den 29. Oktober 1943.

the effect only set in after three hours and he wondered whether the coffee might have "neutralized" the effect of LSD. But then he felt a "tickle and dizziness in the genital area" and had the "uncanny feeling of no longer being normal." After enjoying sensual visions, he ate rusk and chocolate, as befits a Swiss soldier. Finally, in the evening, as he was back on duty the next morning, he took "3 Optalidon" to sleep well – a barbituric acid derivative by Sandoz containing caffeine that was used as a painkiller and preventive measure against "hangovers" at the time. As a result, Hofmann slept quite well, but the following morning felt a "typical slight Optalidon euphoria."[12]

Finally, on May 2, 1945, the head of the pharmacological laboratory of Sandoz, Ernst Rothlin, sent "20 vials of L.S.D. 25 including 2 pipettes" to Werner Stoll, who was now an assistant at the psychiatric clinic Burghölzli. Parallel to this, preliminary experiments with "healthy" test subjects, mainly Sandoz staff, were conducted in Basel.[13] At that time, it was common practice in Swiss psychiatry that the consent of the patients or their relatives was required for somatic cures such as electro- or insulin shock for the treatment of schizophrenic and depressive patients. The use of pharmacological substances, on the other hand, did not normally require the consent of the patients or their relatives.[14] Pharmaceutical substances were probably considered non-invasive; in addition, somatic shock cures brought with them much greater physical danger. In the so-called insulin coma therapy, which was widespread between the mid-1930s and 1950s as a common treatment for schizophrenia and depression, the administration of insulin artificially induced hypoglycemia and kept the patient in a coma for several minutes or longer. In view of these applications, which are also physiologically not without risk, LSD may have been considered a low-threshold "cure," given the negligible dose that seemed to be effective in immaterial, psychological regions.

Crucially, however, psychiatry proved to be the place where LSD was reframed as a what Werner Stoll called a "phantasticum." Even though its effects on patients were disappointing, in the trials with healthy subjects a new possible use arose: LSD allowed doctors and psychiatrists to experience

12 Archiv IMG, N Hofmann 148.1: Berichte von Selbstversuchen mit d-Lysergsäure-diäthylamid-tartrat, 1943–1946: Albert Hofmann an Herrn Prof. Stoll: Bericht über 3 Selbstversuche mit d-Lysergsäure-diäthylamid, 30.XII.1943, 1f.

13 Regarding LSD's introduction into psychiatry, see Magaly Tornay, "Early Experimental LSD Cultures in the Clinic," in *Expanding Mindscapes*, ed. Dyck and Elcock, 141–64. See also Tornay, *Zugriffe*, 143; and Tornay and Bächi, *Drogen*, 98–109.

14 See Marietta Meier, Mario König, and Magaly Tornay, *Testfall Münsterlingen: Klinische Versuche in der Psychiatrie, 1940–1980* (Chronos, 2019), 279–82; Marietta Meier, Mario König, and Magaly Tornay, *On Trial: Testing new drugs in psychiatry, 1940–1980* (Manchester University Press, 2024).

similar symptoms, notably hallucinations on themselves to the ones their patients had during psychotic episodes.[15] So LSD emerged from psychiatry not only as a "phantasticum," but also as a "psychomimeticum," a drug mimicking the symptoms of psychosis, and thus a potential clue to solving the mysteries of the mind.

"Demons": First Reinterpretations of LSD as a Problem Child

Lysergic acid did not only slip into ever new guises in the field. After the first clinical tests on humans, there were numerous LSD experiments with animals. Experiments were carried out with spiders, mice, dogs, cats, fish, donkeys, snakes, monkeys, rabbits, pigeons, salamanders, rats, hamsters, ants, and an elephant.[16] At the same time, attempts were made to record the "symptomatology" of LSD intoxication in an increasingly standardized way. A corresponding questionnaire is divided into "A. Onset of effects" and "B. General symptomatology." This section is in turn subdivided into "Motor function," "Vegetative symptoms," "Perception," "Higher mental functions," and "Decay of the effect."[17] After the question of the human-animal boundary had receded into the background in favor of phenomenological measurement and statistical evaluation of spider webs, for example, the question now arose as to whether LSD actually only had its effects in the area of "higher and highest psychological and mental functions," as Hofmann repeatedly formulated it, or whether it also produced changes in simple, fundamental behavioral patterns. Finally, LSD made it possible to reformulate the boundaries between humans and animals, so that at the famous Macy conferences the question once arose as to whether neurotic cows could exist.[18]

Also noteworthy is Hofmann's 1952 draft, "Wie das Phantasticum LSD 25 entdeckt wurde," in which he not only adopts Stoll's term "phantasticum" but which demonstrates the small changes to his accounts of the first

15 Bonah, this volume.

16 See Sandoz, "Catalogue of the literature on DELYSID, Juni 1959," in Institut für Medizingeschichte, Universität Bern, Nachlass Albert Hofmann: Schachtel "Diverses," Abstract on LSD.

17 Archiv IMG, N Hofmann 148: "LSD LA 111," Mappe 148.3: Protokolle zu Selbstversuchen mit LSD-Derivaten und Psilocybin 1947–1961: Fragebogen zu LSD-Versuch, ohne Datum, wahrscheinlich um 1951.

18 See Tornay, *Zugriffe*, 47, 52. A Macy conference in 1955 treated the subject of "neuropharmacology."

self-experiments over time. As he noted in a letter to a friend, this report was identical – "with minor additions" – to the one he had given to Prof Stoll at the time. Hofmann now wrote: "At times I wandered back and forth in the room with violent movements, as if I had to tear a terrible demon that had taken possession of me out of me and push it away."[19] The "demon," who would later repeatedly be a central figure in the retrospective description of the first encounter with LSD, only became a constitutive component of Hofmann's stories almost ten years after the first trip. It served as a symbolic figure for the passage through hell as a purification ritual and the subsequent rebirth.[20]

Psilocybe mexicana: Do Substances and their Origins Prefigure their Effects?

Some years after Hofmann's invention of a "demon" in his awakening story, the "flesh of the gods" of the Aztecs found its way into the laboratories of the Swiss pharmaceutical company Sandoz.[21] Hence, Albert Hofmann carried out his first self-experiment with 2.4 grams of *Psilocybe mexicana* at his workplace on July 1, 1957. He tried to express his impressions with the following words:

> After half an hour, the outside world began to transform itself in strange ways. Everything took on a Mexican character. Because I was fully aware that knowing the Mexican origin of these mushrooms I could now imagine Mexican sceneries, I consciously tried to see my environment as I normally knew it. However, all efforts of the will to see things in their familiar shapes and colors remained unsuccessful. With my eyes open or closed, I only saw Indian motifs and colors. When the doctor supervising the experiment bent over me to control the blood pressure, he turned into an Aztec sacrificial

19 Archiv IMG, N Hofmann 148: "LSD LA 111," Mappe 148.4: Beilage zum Brief von Albert Hofmann an Ruedi Bircher, Sandoz Pharmaceuticals, New York, "Wie das Phantasticum LSD 25 entdeckt wurde," Basel, 12. Dezember 1952, 1; 4f.

20 Jeannie Moser, "'The cure is biochemical'. Drogen und die Arbeit am Selbst in den sozialutopischen 1950er- und 1960er-Jahren," in *Handbuch Drogen in sozial- und kulturwissenschaftlicher Perspektive*, ed. Robert Feustel et al. (Springer, 2019), 82.

21 See Bächi, *LSD auf dem Land.* Interesting contributions to the story of Mexican Mushrooms come from Benjamin Feinberg, *The Devil's Book of Culture: History, Mushrooms, and Caves in Southern Mexico* (University of Texas Press, 2003); and Andy Letcher, *Shroom: A Cultural History of the Magic Mushroom* (Faber & Faber, 2006).

> priest, and I would not have been surprised if he had pulled out a knife made of obsidian. Despite the gravity of the situation, I was amused to see how my colleague's Alemannic face had taken on a purely Indian expression.

When this "dream" came to an end after about six hours, Hofmann felt that "re-entering the familiar reality" was like a "happy return from a foreign world experienced as very real to the familiar home [*die altvertraute Heimat*]."[22]

It was Hofmann's correspondence partner Rudolf Gelpke (1928–1972)[23] in particular who was literally driven by these questions about a possible "objective element" in the substance of the drug. Gelpke had studied ethnology, philology, philosophy, history of religion, and Islamic studies in Basel, Berlin, Zurich, and Tehran. Among other things, he was a correspondent of the newspaper *Neue Zürcher Zeitung* (NZZ) in Tehran and dealt in depth with the role of hashish and opium in Iranian intellectual history. In 1960 Gelpke was appointed lecturer for Persian language and literature at the University of California, Los Angeles, but from 1963 he lived mainly in Tehran. His most important contribution to the cultural study of drugs was his book *Vom Rausch im Orient und Okzident* (Of Intoxication in the Orient and Occident), published in 1966. The question of the culturally specific patterns of visions triggered by psychotropic substances preoccupied him in many of his letters to Hofmann. In 1961, Gelpke, who was interested in scientific symbol research, wrote the following lines to Hofmann: "Something of the most mysterious to me seems to be the phenomena of the 'Indian' or 'Oriental' changes in landscape and people, which you and I, for example, have observed on various occasions. Up to now, I have always considered such phenomena to be an expression of my subjective, inner fixation with Persian memory images – but I can hardly doubt now that there is an objective element (in the substance of the drug itself) that is decisive. But if this should prove to be true – wouldn't the effects on our whole world view be of immense consequence?"[24]

Gelpke's wife, Li Gelpke, also took psilocybin. She captured her visions during three self-experiments with psilocybin in ink drawings. She wrote: "When weeks later books about Mexican art came into my hands, I found the

22 Archiv IMG, N Hofmann 151: Mappe 151.8: Vortrag "Mexikanische Zauberpilze" gehalten vor Thurgauische Naturforschende Gesellschaft, Frauenfeld, 25. April 1961, 1 and 7f.

23 For Rudolf Gelpke see Peter-Paul Bänziger et al., *Die Schweiz auf Drogen: Szenen, Politik und Suchthilfe, 1965–2022* (Chronos, 2022), 52.

24 Archiv IMG, N Hofmann 136: Einzel-Korrespondenz Nr. 2, Rudolf Gelpke (1961–1979), inkl. Korrespondenz mit der Witwe von Rudolf Gelpke: Brief von Rudolf Gelpke an Albert Hofmann, Basel, den 13. April 1961.

motives of my visions there again – with a sudden shock."[25] This enchantment of the external reality awaited an explanation. However, Aurelio Cerletti, the director of the Sandoz pharmacological laboratory, had already in 1959 summarized knowledge about the sacred mushrooms in an essay in the *Deutsche Medizinische Wochenschrift*, and the "disenchantment" of the "ancient Aztec drug by modern science" had reached a certain conclusion through the structural elucidation and total synthesis on an industrial scale. At the same time, the focus of interest had shifted from the area of cultural-historical and ethnomycological questions to the field of biochemistry of indole derivatives with central nervous activity. Thus, "the small mushrooms and their inherent magic power had successfully been snatched from the darkness of past centuries and from the spell of magical ideas by the united ethnographic-mycological and chemical-pharmacological research."[26]

This way of speaking about the mushrooms, which was also common in the scientific community and which increasingly pushed back the sacral silence, regarded the visions as hallucinations caused by biochemical reactions of the nervous system. This is a neurophysiological and no longer a metaphysical or sacral discourse. To call the visions that occur during a trance or a trip "hallucinations" means, in Western logic – which bases perceptions on something "objective" outside themselves – to postulate a form of reality that is not shared by the traditional communities that order their lives around the concept of the sacred.

How to Objectify Drug Effects? LSD as a Danger to High Society

While in the 1950s pharmacological innovations such as the introduction of neuroleptics were enthusiastically celebrated, in the 1960s the risks of such substances suddenly revealed themselves to a broad public. The main trigger for this was thalidomide, an over-the-counter drug from the German company Grünenthal marketed under the brand Contergan.[27] In a scandal in 1961/62, its teratogenic effects became widely known, since it caused numerous miscarriages and malformations in newborns.

It also affected Albert Hofmannn, Sandoz, and its handling of psychotropic drugs. In a personal letter to Rudolf Gelpke in 1962, Albert Hofmann

25 Quoted after Hagenbach and Werthmüller, *Hofmann*, 110.

26 Aurelio Cerletti, "Teonanacatl und Psilocybin," *Deutsche Medizinische Wochenschrift* 84, no. 52 (1959): 2318, 2321.

27 See Matthew Oram, *The Trials of Psychedelic Therapy: LSD Psychotherapy in America* (Johns Hopkins University Press, 2018).

described his feelings: "We and especially the Sandoz people in (the) USA" were currently experiencing very unpleasant stories with LSD and psilocybin. The "worst and most dangerous" thing for the company and the substances was the fact that a high-ranking health official in Canada had described "LSD and thalidomide as the two most dangerous drugs," for which an absolute ban should be imposed in the country. According to Hofmann, this showed how uninformed the people responsible often were or how their actions were influenced by an even less well-informed press. If there are two drugs with nothing in common, Hoffman wrote,

> then it is thalidomide, which has caused so many children to be malformed, and LSD. The only thing they have in common is that they have been mentioned frequently in the daily press recently. In order to counter the nonsensical accusations that our company is trying to make money with a dangerous drug (as you know, we have so far distributed almost all LSD and psilocybin free of charge to only qualified investigative bodies) and to force the health authorities to finally create a legal regulation for the distribution of these novel substances, the distribution of LSD and psilocybin was completely stopped.[28]

Many serious researchers could no longer continue their research projects. It was now up to them to exert pressure on the health authorities, Hofmann thought – "this primarily concerns the Food and Drug Administration in the USA" – so that legal regulation could be established as soon as possible. Sandoz had proposed to the FDA that it should take over the distribution of LSD and psilocybin, and Sandoz would provide the necessary substances. "So you see, it's trouble, not progress. It seems to be taking a long time for LSD and psilocybin to reach their rightful place in the world."[29]

The last Sandoz patent for LSD expired in 1963. At the time, LSD was available in pharmacies in Switzerland on prescription under the trademark "Delysid."[30] Nevertheless, the regulatory authorities' increasing demand for "statistical evidence" when introducing new drugs had very specific consequences. In 1963, when a large order of LSD and psilocybin reached Sandoz from the US (Timothy Leary ordered 100 grams of LSD and 25

28 Archiv IMG, N Hofmann 136: Korrespondenz mit Rudolf Gelpke (1961–1979): Brief von Albert Hofmann an Rudolf Gelpke, Bottmingen den 15. Dezember 1962.

29 Archiv IMG, N Hofmann 136: Korrespondenz mit Rudolf Gelpke (1961–1979): Brief von Albert Hofmann an Rudolf Gelpke, Bottmingen den 15. Dezember 1962.

30 FA Novartis, Sandoz, H 121.001, Protokoll der Geschäftsführungssitzung vom 20.3.63.

kilograms of psilocybin, which Sandoz ultimately declined),[31] LSD was at a crossroads: Either Sandoz officially stopped dispensing LSD in the US, or they immediately initiated a "New Drug Application to the FDA." Sandoz's management expressed the view that official registration with the FDA was the right way to go.[32]

But LSD did not only feel the headwind from the media, where certain publications stood out with particularly bizarre LSD fantasies. At least as fundamental for the ban were methodological changes in the approval of drugs due to the thalidomide scandal. Now, evidence from "double-blind" trials was demanded, especially by the FDA. Hallucinogenic substances had trouble fitting into this new methodology, which was considered "objective" and statistically evaluable. The well-known Canadian psychiatrist Humphry Osmond had already made rather condescending remarks about "some methodologists" to Albert Hofmann in 1962. These simply could not bear the thought that "their beloved 'double blind controlled experiments' don't necessarily work. I don't, of course, mean that they are useless or should never be done, but that they are one of a number of factors to take into account."[33] All the objectifying procedures introduced into LSD research up to that point, such as the Rorschach test, various writing procedures, drawing tests, writing samples, technical methods such as the EEG, or video recordings of the experiments, seemed flawed to the new regulatory requirements. Nor did it help that (following the elite theories) artists and authors were often chosen as test subjects because they were particularly skilled at introspection.[34]

Rudolf Gelpke described in a letter to Albert Hofmann how he perceived the statistical change. Some researchers, he conceded, had worked in a very "American" way. He himself "would never have had the idea that e.g. mystical experiences could be gradually recorded with a staff and translated into numbers on tables!"[35] Nevertheless, Gelpke could not avoid acknowledging: This path "is certainly the only correct and possible one with regard to the 'social integration' of these substances, their incorporation into the

31 See Tornay, *Zugriffe*, 234–37.

32 FA Novartis, Sandoz H 121.001, Protokoll der Geschäftsführungssitzung vom 19.2.1963.

33 Archiv IMG, N Hofmann 136: Einzel-Korrespondenz Nr. 2, Korrespondenz mit Humphry Osmond (1961–1973): Brief von Humphry Osmond an Albert Hofmann, 19.3.1962.

34 For the statistical turnaround, see Tornay, *Zugriffe*, 171–215.

35 Archiv IMG, N Hofmann 136: Korrespondenz mit Rudolf Gelpke (1961–1979): Brief von Rudolf Gelpke (Waldenburg) an Albert Hofmann, 29./30. Oktober 1964, 1.

public consciousness of our time."[36] To put it differently: It was not only the controversies surrounding the recreational use of LSD that stood in the way of its "social integration" in the 1960s and led to its illegalization, but also the difficulties in stabilizing their effects in experiments and in registering and licensing psychotropics as drugs.[37]

LSD as the Atomic Bomb for the Mind in the Cold War

During the Cold War, LSD and psilocybin migrated through a wide variety of social settings – including, last but not least, the dangers and potentials of warfare. In the event of a war, the focus would no longer have been on individuals but on population groups – and hence not micrograms but kilograms of warfare agents were deemed necessary. The narrative was less structured by risk than by danger.[38] Before and behind the Iron Curtain, psychotropic substances were traded as possible "truth serum." The potential use for "mind control" – in particular, the CIA's MK-ULTRA project, which was launched on a large scale in 1953 – has already been discussed in detail in the literature. Less well known is the potential use of psychotropic substances in a "humane war," as interpreted by the Swiss Army.

In 1961 a detailed report by Rolf Dolder, a captain in the Swiss Army, on the "Gas War in a New Perspective" was published in the *Neue Zürcher Zeitung*. Among the "modern chemical warfare agents" he distinguished the "silent" ones like LSD, and he wrote about a "humane" war, a hotly debated topic during this peak phase of the Cold War. While, according to Dolder, "conventional explosive weapon" and nuclear shells had both destroyed people and material and devastated countries, the nerve poisons had been taken a step further "in a rational way." In the light of a "quasi 'humane' warfare," in which "even the destruction of the enemy is completely renounced," "psychochemical warfare agents" such as LSD-25 and psilocybin seemed to open up completely unimagined possibilities. For these substances could

36 Archiv IMG, N Hofmann 136: Korrespondenz mit Rudolf Gelpke (1961–1979): Brief von Rudolf Gelpke (Waldenburg) an Albert Hofmann, 29./30. Oktober 1964, 2.

37 See Matthew Oram, "Efficacy and Enlightenment: LSD Psychotherapy and the Drug Amendments of 1962," *Journal of the History of Medicine and Allied Sciences* 69, no. 2 (2012): 221–50. For the methodology of LSD experiments see also Nancy D. Campbell and Laura Stark, "Making up 'Vulnerable' People: Human Subjects and the Subjective Experience of Medical Experiment," *Social History of Medicine* 28, no. 4 (2015): 825–48.

38 See Niklas Luhmann, "Risiko und Gefahr," in *Soziologische Aufklärung 5. Konstruktivistische Perspektiven*, 2nd ed. (Westdeutscher Verlag, 1993), 131–69.

temporarily turn those affected into "will-less ruins" without causing them "any lasting damage." In such a war there would be no more dead and no more injured – "only mentally raped and duped!" The industrial and labor potential of the subjugated would pass completely and undestroyed into the hands of the conqueror, who could then live effortlessly at the expense of the outwitted slaves. "The absurd perspectives are almost inconceivable."[39]

After Colonel H. Gessner, an ABC officer,[40] had contacted Albert Hofmann by telephone in 1962, he recorded the reason for his contact in a letter at his request. Since he considered it "very likely" that the large number of available atomic bombs would prevent "total nuclear war," Gessner feared that chemical weapons could be used instead. In addition to phosgene and prussic acid, he sensed potential new warfare agents in psychotropic drugs. He therefore wanted to receive detailed information about the production methods, costs, storage life, and possible forms of use of such substances. In his letter Gessner also mentioned the "problem of so-called 'humane warfare' (the term is of course nonsense in itself!)." Nevertheless, he asked Hofmann whether LSD could also be used in higher doses without "permanent damage." He concluded his request by asking whether Hofmann could give a lecture at the next ABC officers' course. He would oblige him to "sincere thanks in the name of the fatherland."[41]

When Hofmann finally gave some lectures about "LSD and psilocybin as potential warfare agents" in the 1960s in front of members of the Swiss army, he brought some LSD with him to give his audience a vivid impression of the tremendous effectiveness of this substance. He showed the audience a tube containing a whole gram of LSD and said that this quantity would be enough to incapacitate up to 20,000 humans for several hours of combat, provided you somehow managed to give each one their allotted dose of 0.05 mg, either in drinking water or as a spray. The extremely high effectiveness of LSD, Hofmann explained, had to do with the fact that it attacks a "very central regulation point" in the organism, the brain – the "highest command post." Hofmann continued making a war-metaphorical comparison: If one compared the "human organism" with the "complicated, differentiated organism of a modern army," then LSD would hit the general staff (the brain), leading to the disorganization of the entire army. "One grenade

39 Rolf Dolder, "Gaskrieg in neuer Sicht," *Neue Zürcher Zeitung*, November 10, 1961.

40 ABC stands for Atomic-, Biological- and Chemical-Officers.

41 FA Novartis, Sandoz, H. 124.006, Brief von Oberst Gessner (Abteilung für Sanität des Eidg. Militärdepartements) an Dr. K. Hoffmann [*sic*], Zürich, 15. März 1962, 3.

in the General Staff Headquarters has more catastrophic consequences than 10,000 grenades falling on the trenches at the front."[42]

On this occasion, Hofmann's closeness to the reactionary German writer Ernst Jünger, whom he deeply admired, becomes apparent.[43] In an elitist style, he called the brain the "highest command post," with LSD becoming the "grenade" hitting the top of the army. Hofmann had come into contact with Jünger's work in the officer school. "The Storm of Steel" had been "compulsory reading" in the late 1920s. Hofmann once described the relative effects of mescaline and LSD in similarly bellicose metaphors as Jünger's – probably precisely because Jünger, after his first LSD trip, had described it as a "domestic cat" compared to the "King Tiger Mescaline": Since LSD possessed a 5–10,000 times higher effect than mescaline, it deserved to be apostrophized the "atomic bomb" for the mind, according to Hofmann.[44] These martial analogies may be surprising until it is known that Hofmann was a former 'frontist' – a member of a Swiss pro-Nazi movement in the 1930s. When it came to LSD for the masses, he was more in line with the elitist disciple Jünger than with Timothy Leary.[45]

Hofmann's thoughts on psychotropic warfare agents were not quite as much in a vacuum as one might think. Psychotropics mobilized all kinds of fantasies and fitted in perfectly with the often phantasmatic patterns of perception and interpretation of the Cold War. There were further sandbox

42 Archiv IMG, N Hofmann 152, Mappe 152.7: Vortrag "LSD und Psilocybin als potentielle Kampfstoffe" gehalten vor den ABC-Offizieren Sektion Basel, 19.11.1964; N Hofmann 153, Mappe 153.1: "LSD und Psilocybin als potentielle Kampfstoffe" gehalten vor ABC-Offiziere in Dübendorf, 12.1.1965; Mappe 153.2: "LSD und Psilocybin als potentielle Kampfstoffe" gehalten vor ABC-Offiziere in Zürich und Umgebung, 25.3.1965, 10f.

43 See Deutsches Literaturarchiv Marbach, ed., *LSD. Albert Hofmann und Ernst Jünger. Der Briefwechsel 1947 bis 1997* (Offizin Scheufele Druck und Medien, 2013); Archiv IMG, N Hofmann 136: Einzel-Korrespondenz Nr. 2, Jünger, 1957 + 1970, Kopien; and Hofmann, *Sorgenkind*, chapter 11 ("Einstrahlung von Ernst Jünger"), 152–74.

44 "LSD ganz persönlich (Filmaufnahmen seines Vortrages bei der Tagung des Europäischen Collegium für Bewusstseinsstudien (ECBS)," Kongresshaus, Stadthalle Heidelberg, February 22–25, 1996 (here ca. mins. 9:58 and 25:35). For mescaline, see Mike Jay, *Mescaline: A Global History of the First Psychedelic* (Yale University Press, 2019).

45 This was recently uncovered in a Master's thesis at the University of Basel. The Front Movement, or Frontism, refers to heterogeneous movements in Switzerland in the 1920s, 30s, and 40s that were extreme right-wing, nationalist, fascist or National Socialist. Hofmann was a member of the "National Movement of Switzerland," the "Federal Collection" in Basel, and the Basel Palatinate until he left in 1942. See Tornay and Bächi, *Drogen*, 121.

games and evaluations of LSD as a possible weapon behind closed doors during the 1960s. Newly declassified files show that in spring 1963 a subgroup of the Swiss army was preparing a study on "the chemical weapon," wherein LSD and psilocybin played important roles. As far as the production of chemical warfare agents was concerned, the Swiss army was convinced that "our industry" would be technically capable of producing chemical warfare agents, "according to the same principles as insecticides." However, the army worried about the chemical industry raising concerns about the dangers of poisoning associated with large-scale production or refusing production on moral grounds. In the end, the decisive factor against such a program was the very high production cost of the substances "known to us (1 kg. LSD 25 around Fr. 100,000.-)."[46]

Outlook: From the Decline of the West to the Psychedelic Renaissance in the Era of the Brain

Today, LSD and psilocybin are experiencing a renaissance as micro-dosed fuels in the creative industries, Silicon Valley, and psychotherapy. Since the 2000s, and possibly influenced by the decade of the brain, there has also been renewed interest in neuroscientific and pharmacological hallucinogen research. While the counterculture of the sixties regarded them as a vehicle for escaping the meritocracy or for expanding consciousness, LSD, psilocybin, and MDMA are once again being used in a wide variety of therapeutic settings – whether as a remedy for depression, post-traumatic stress disorder, or trauma. In microdoses, they are used to increase creativity and performance or simply to provide a greater sense of well-being. When used in this way, psychedelic substances are all about self-optimization and working on the self. While the dose is reduced to the point where there is no longer any demonstrable effect, the established interpretative power of neuroscience is increasingly coming into play.[47]

Contrary to many popular accounts, this is in line with Hofmann's own thinking. In his view, LSD was a means to defend occidental against oriental values, which he saw connected to Hashish. Hence, in his mind, LSD functioned as a substance that did not threaten western culture (by the so-called counterculture), but that defended it against "oriental" ways of addressing the mind.

46 Schweizerisches Bundesarchiv Bern (BAR) E 5560 D, 2005/97, BD: 11, 244.1: Abteilung für Sanität EMD, ABC-Sektion: Studie über die chemische Waffe, Bern, den 3. April 1964 (Aktenexemplar, geheim, entklassifiziert 18. Feb. 2005), 13–15, 73.

47 See Tornay and Bächi, *Drogen*, 170–79.

To this point, a lecture from 1970 is quite illuminating. With regard to hallucinogenic drugs "as a contemporary problem and temptation," he stated that LSD and its "relatives" were not stimulants in the same sense as hashish, which encouraged repeated use. A single LSD experience generally causes effects for a long time, sometimes for a lifetime, which explains why the use of LSD, which had been widespread at American universities and colleges a few years ago, has declined sharply, while the consumption of hashish is constantly increasing there and also in Europe. In his opinion, the case of hashish was therefore less a "socio-medical" issue than a "cultural-political" one. For, Hofmann continued, the effects of hashish correspond to an "introverted philosophy of life," as it was native to the Eastern countries of origin of this drug, and were in contrast to "our Western world view, formed by antiquity and Christianity," in which active attention to the outside world and to one's fellow man constituted the meaning of life. It seemed questionable to him whether the continuity of Western culture, which was shaped by the "European spirit, could be maintained if the use of hashish, which originated in an Eastern culture, became generally accepted."[48] Here, the "objective element of the drug" is interwoven with cultural-political considerations and linked to the virulent discussions about the potential "downfall of the Occident" (Oswald Spengler) at the beginning of the twentieth century. It was probably precisely the "radiation" of Ernst Jünger that might have led Hofmann to these cultural pessimistic considerations. For Jünger, hashish was simply associated with "oriental tyranny."[49]

From Hofmann's point of view, LSD was both a risk and a promise for Western, European culture. For him, it was the social integration of this substance that mattered. If it was taken by profane people (the lower classes), it had the potential to jeopardize the dominant Western culture. If it was swallowed by elite, bourgeois bodies, it promised to inspire Western Christian culture to new heights. In this respect, LSD was a substance to protect the bourgeois, conservative elite from the mob – just as it seemingly had great potential in the Cold War to incapacitate the enemies of the West.

48 Archiv IMG, N Hofmann 154.7: Vortrag "Halluzinogene Rauschgifte als Problem und Versuchung der Gegenwart" gehalten anlässlich der Cusanus-Akademie, Brixen 2.4.1970, 20f.

49 Hofmann, *Sorgenkind*, 155.

Chapter Five

Hallucinations: 1960s Filmic Narratives of Subjective Lived Psychedelic Experiences and their Legal/Illegal Status

Christian Bonah

Risk and benefit are real but situational. In the context of medicines, they emerge from the interplay between pharmacological and social factors. These claims, made by the introduction to this book, require an addition. Risks and benefits of what? At the core of this narrative are psychotropic substances in the 1960s such as opium, hashish, psilocybin, mescaline or LSD (see Bächi in this volume). More precisely, it is not the substances per se, but rather the visions or hallucinations they produce that will be center stage. Self-experiments with new and old psychoactive substances by physicians and pharmaceutical company employees were part and parcel of the 1950s exploring and describing their effects (see Bächi in this volume). But how could these individual experiences be reported and mediated in a world of nascent controlled clinical trials and popularized psychedelic experiences?[1] How were drugs' psychic effects presented in (French) public space and the legal-illegal divide negotiated there?

Our entry point is a curious, industrial, short film *Images du monde visionnaire* (Images from the Visionary World, 1963–1964, 28 min/34 min) commissioned by the Swiss pharmaceutical company Sandoz, produced by the medical film maker Eric Duvivier and written and directed by the Belgian-born French poet, writer and painter Henri Michaux

1 Timothy Leary, Ralph Metzner, and Richard Alpert, *The Psychedelic Experience: A Manual Based on The Tibetan Book of the Dead* (University Books, 1964).

(1899–1984).[2] *Images from the Visionary World* is a two-part film showing "the visions presented to a subject with no special characteristics, subjected to two successive experiences. In the first, under the action of hallucinogen A (mescaline), he sees colored forms passing by, constantly changing, for no apparent reason, tremulous, a kind of structure of who-knows-what being, of who-knows-what matter, and moreover indefinitely on the way to becoming something else. In the second experiment with hallucinogen B (hashish), familiar objects and beings presented themselves to him, but distorted, singular, in enigmatic attitudes and situations. Impetuosity, overt or underlying brusqueness."[3]

Commenting, at the beginning of his film, the risks and benefits taken by producing such a first experimental film on drug induced hallucinations, Henri Michaux states: "When I was asked to make a film about mescaline visions, I declared and repeated and still repeat that it's undertaking the impossible. Whatever you do, this drug is beyond."[4] Despite his somewhat awkward disclaimer at the beginning of the film, and his evident frustration, Michaux did not block the film.

In contrast, a contemporary observer and reviewer highlights the benefits of this "film from within":

> As an explorer of the peaks and chasms of inner space, Henri Michaux has brought back for us, in the manner of a traveler, stories, drawings and even a film. The visions conjured up by hallucinogenic drugs are in a perpetual state of flux, and words and drawings are hard put to hold them back. At the outset of his vocation as a draughtsman, H. Michaux already noted his desire to "draw the flow of time," and all his painting seems to be an attempt not to immobilize the moment, but to restore movement itself. Thanks to the resources made available to him by a major laboratory (Sandoz), he was able to go one step further and make the first experimental film shot in the land of mescaline, then in the land of hashish ... Of course, this is not, nor does it claim to be, "mescaline, hashish as if you'd taken it," since the film cannot restore the visceral and emotional accompaniment first aroused by the drug, the importance of which is emphasized in all the accounts. But it is an exceptional success because, here as elsewhere,

2 Henri Michaux, *Œuvres complètes*, ed. Raymond Bellour with the collaboration of Ysé Tran (Gallimard/Pléiade), vol. 1 (1998); vol. 2 (2001); and vol. 3 (2004). Hereafter cited as *OC* with volume and page numbers.

3 Michaux, *OC* III, 221–62. See also Michaux, *OC* III, 1526–42.

4 *Images du monde visionnaire* (ScienceFilm, France, 1963/64), 00:39–03:00. The film is publicly available at: https://medfilm.unistra.fr/wiki/Images_du_monde_visionnaire.

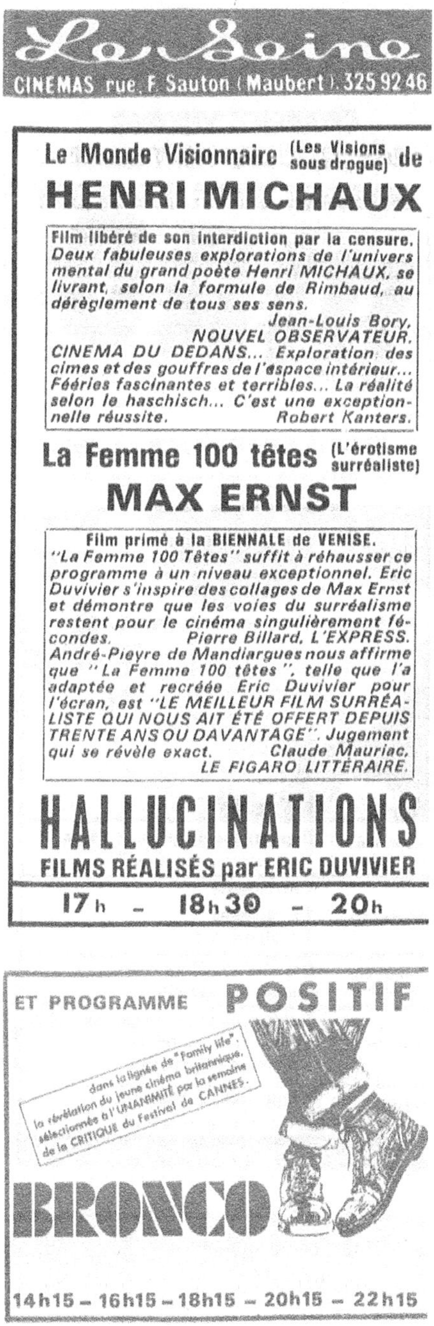
Le Seine
CINEMAS rue. F. Sauton (Maubert). 325 92 46
Le Monde Visionnaire (Les Visions sous drogue) de
HENRI MICHAUX
Film libéré de son interdiction par la censure.
Deux fabuleuses explorations de l'univers mental du grand poète Henri MICHAUX, se livrant, selon la formule de Rimbaud, au dérèglement de tous ses sens.
Jean-Louis Bory, NOUVEL OBSERVATEUR.
CINEMA DU DEDANS... Exploration des cimes et des gouffres de l'espace intérieur... Féeries fascinantes et terribles... La réalité selon le haschisch... C'est une exceptionnelle réussite.
Robert Kanters.
La Femme 100 têtes (L'érotisme surréaliste)
MAX ERNST
Film primé à la BIENNALE de VENISE.
"La Femme 100 Têtes" suffit à réhausser ce programme à un niveau exceptionnel. Eric Duvivier s'inspire des collages de Max Ernst et démontre que les voies du surréalisme restent pour le cinéma singulièrement fécondes.
Pierre Billard, L'EXPRESS.
André-Pieyre de Mandiargues nous affirme que "La Femme 100 têtes", telle que l'a adaptée et recréée Eric Duvivier pour l'écran, est "LE MEILLEUR FILM SURRÉALISTE QUI NOUS AIT ÉTÉ OFFERT DEPUIS TRENTE ANS OU DAVANTAGE". Jugement qui se révèle exact.
Claude Mauriac, LE FIGARO LITTÉRAIRE.
HALLUCINATIONS
FILMS RÉALISÉS par ERIC DUVIVIER
17h - 18h30 - 20h
ET PROGRAMME POSITIF
dans la lignée de "Family life", la révélation du jeune cinéma britannique, sélectionnée à l'UNANIMITÉ par la semaine de la CRITIQUE du Festival de CANNES.
BRONCO
14h15 - 16h15 - 18h15 - 20h15 - 22h15

Figure 1. Entrance ticket for the experimental surrealist short film program "Hallucinations" at the experimental movie theatre Le Seine in Paris in 1971.

> H. Michaux has succeeded in bringing together the psychological structures of a paramedical document and the structures of a work of art.[5]

In November 1968, the Parisian press announced widely the premiere of an experimental surrealist short film program entitled "Hallucinations" at the Le Ranelagh art gallery and movie theater in the capital's upper-class sixteenth arrondissement. Accompanied by a surrealist art exhibition (including works by Max Ernst, Henri Michaux, and Ferro), the film program featured *Images from the Visionary World*, *La femme 100 têtes* (The Woman One Hundred Heads, 1967, BW, 20 min, based on a 1929 graphic novel by Max Ernst) and *Concerto mécanique pour la folie* (*Mechanical Concerto for Insanity*, 1963, 25 min).

An hour prior to its opening, the 1968 art gallery screening of the "Hallucinations" film program was cancelled due to state film censorship of *Images from the Visionary World*. The French ministry of the interior and its film board considered that the public dissemination of colored visions and hallucinations experienced after mescaline and hashish intake were a risk to public order and an undue incitement to engage with psychoactive substances in and for recreational use. Nevertheless, the film had been screened several times between its 1964 release and the 1968 censorship.

What are the unexpected connections between surrealist artists, pharmaceutical industry and medical research? What are their expected benefits for producing an experimental film presenting drug induced hallucinatory visions "from within?" And who was concerned about potential risks presenting "visions conjured up by hallucinogenic drugs ... in a perpetual state of flux?" My contribution will first present the curious production triad (physicians – pharmaceutical industry – arts/film making) of *Images from the Visionary World*, analyzing in detail the benefits sought and risks taken by each one of the three stakeholders engaged in the film production. Then, in a second step I will portray the shifting perceptions of risks and benefits between the film's 1964 release and its 1968 ban trying to understand when and why the cinematographic expression of psychoactive drug induced visions changed its status from "experiments of great scientific value" [6] to reprimandable, subversive art and art shows.

5 Robert Kanters, "Cinéma du dedans," *L'Express*, January 16, 1964, 28. Archives Duvivier, Université de Strasbourg, DHVS, folder "Hallucinations. Coupures journaux, critiques, censure," n.p.

6 *Images du monde visionnaire*, 00:00–00:18.

Mobiles, Benefits and Risks of Producing an Industrial, Experimental Film

Strictly speaking, *Images from the Visionary World* is an industrial film, meaning here a film produced by or for use by an industrial corporation.[7] An early, longstanding, and little-studied sector of corporate film production concerns modern medicine-producing chemical-pharmaceutical industries in Europe and North America.[8] Emerging with the second industrial revolution in late nineteenth century and kin to business-merging and new techniques of public relations (PR), pharmaceutical companies engaged quickly, since the early 1920s, in industrial and medical filmmaking.[9] The advent of the so-called therapeutic revolution after 1945 that drastically multiplied drug research, development, promotion, and consumption,[10] increased investments in media communication practices by pharmaceutical giants even more so.

In 1958, and in the context of its marketing strategies, the Swiss pharmaceutical corporation Sandoz[11] initiated a pioneering medical film library

7 Vinzenz Hediger and Patrick Vonderau, eds., *Films That Work: Industrial Film and the Productivity of Media* (Amsterdam University Press, 2009); Yvonne Zimmermann, ed., *Schaufenster Schweiz: Dokumentarische Gebrauchsfilme 1896–1964* (Limmat, 2011); Yvonne Zimmermann, "Target Group Oriented Corporate Communication: Geigy Films," in *Corporate Diversity: Swiss Graphic Design and Advertising by Geigy 1940–1970*, ed. Museum für Gestaltung Zürich (Lars Müller Publishers, 2009), 48–57. Charles Acland and Haidee Wasson, eds., *Useful Cinema* (Duke University Press, 2011).

8 Gerard Leblanc, *Quand l'entreprise fait son cinéma: la médiathèque de Rhône-Poulenc (1972–1981)* (Cinéthique Presses Universitaires de Vincennes, 1983); Christian Bonah, "In the service of industry and human health. The Bayer Corporation, industrial film and promotional propaganda, 1934 –1942," in *Health Education and Film in the Twentieth Century*, ed. Christian Bonah, David Cantor, and Anja Laukötter (Rochester University Press, 2018), 85–142.

9 Stuart Ewen, *PR! A Social History of Spin* (Basic Books, 1996); Roland Marchand, *Creating the Corporate Soul. The Rise of Public Relations and Corporate Imagery in American Big Business* (University of California Press, 1998).

10 Jeremy A. Greene, Flurin Condrau, and Elizabeth Siegel Watkins, eds., *Therapeutic Revolutions: Pharmaceuticals and Social Change in the Twentieth Century* (University of Chicago Press, 2016). Nils Kessel, "Étudier les marchés du médicament : les entreprises pharmaceutiques et la transformation du marketing en Allemagne de l'Ouest (1960–1980)," in *Les marchés de la santé*, ed. Bruno Valat (Presses Universitaires du Midi, 2021), 175–99.

11 Anna Bálint, *Clariant Clareant. The Beginnings of a Specialty Chemicals Company* (Campus Verlag, 2012); Zimmermann, "Target Group Oriented Corporate Communication."

(*Cinémathèque*) used for promotion in medical and postgrad training.[12] The so-called medical film library was in fact a pharmaceutical corporation-based film distribution unit graciously renting out industry-commissioned medical films to professional audiences.[13] Contrary to what its name suggested, the film library was not just a place for the distribution of films with medical content; it was also the initiator of a new corporate film production strategy by Sandoz. It financed and distributed free copies of medical films produced by the pharmaceutical company for physicians. The *Cinémathèque* was therefore as much a film production agency as film distribution library.

Commissioned utility film led to the creation of film companies that produced exclusively industrial films for a large variety of different industrial medicines, producing sponsors. One of these film companies was run by the French professional industrial film maker Eric Duvivier (1928–2018)[14] who directed several production and distribution companies: Art & Science (1950–1960), ScienceFilm (1960–1979), and Films Art & Science (1979–1980).[15] Particularly active in Europe from the 1950s to the 1970s, the catalogue of Duvivier's film production company contains a list of approximately

12 "Cinémathèque," November 1981, 10, Firmenarchiv der Novartis AG, Vorarchiv, Service Audit Groupe Sandoz France. Zimmermann, "Target Group," 49.

13 Gerard Leblanc, "L'âge d'or du cinéma médical et l'aventure de *Médecine/Cinéma*: Entretien avec Gérard Leblanc," *Sociétés & représentations* 28, no. 2 (2009): 107–18; Leblanc, *Quand l'entreprise fait son cinéma.*

14 Thierry Lefebvre, "Les films d'Éric Duvivier: un cinema d'auteur," *MEDFILM*, Journée d'étude à l'Université Paris Diderot Grands Moulins, no. 2, September 21, 2012, https://medfilm.unistra.fr/wiki/Accueil:21_septembre_2012:https://medfilm-stream.u-strasbg.fr/36/duvivier_thierry_lefebvre/public.mp4. "Entretien avec le réalisateur Éric Duviver, présenté et animé par Thierry Lefebvre et Christian Bonah," *MEDFILM*, Journée d'étude à l'Université Paris Diderot Grands Moulins, no. 2, September 21, 2012. https://medfilm.unistra.fr/wiki/Accueil:21_septembre_2012:https://medfilm-stream.u-strasbg.fr/20/entretien_avec_ric_duvivier/public.mp4.

15 Christian Bonah, "'Réservé strictement au corps médical': les sociétés de production audiovisuelles d'Eric Duvivier, l'industrie pharmaceutique et leurs stratégies de co-production de films médicaux industriels, 1950-1980," *Cahiers d'histoire du CNAM*, special issue: "Le cinématographe pour l'industrie et dans les entreprises (1890–1970): histoire, acteurs, usages et configurations" (2020): 135–59. Christian Bonah, "Business and Art: Pharmaceutical Industries, Film Production and Circulation, and the French Film Production Company ScienceFilm, 1960–1980," in *Films that Work Harder. The Global Circulations of Industrial Cinema*, ed. Vinzenz Hediger, Florian Hoof, Yvonne Zimmermann, and Anthony Scott (Amsterdam University Press, 2023), 683–710.

seven hundred industrial films produced between 1950 and the 1990s.[16] In 1960, Duvivier's film production company ScienceFilm signed a series of ten contracts with Sandoz Laboratories in Basel to supply their new medical film library. In the list of films made for Sandoz, *Les embolies pulmonaires* (Pulmonary Embolisms), written by Professor Maurice and Doctor Scebat, rubbed shoulders with *Le grand problème des malformations congénitales* (The Great Problem with Congenital Malformations), written by Professor Lamy at the medical genetics clinic at the Hôpital des Enfants-Malades in Paris. From 1963 onwards, co-production agreements included sometimes several films in a single contract, as in the case of the three films *Les pathologies visuelles pathologiques* (Pathological Visual Pathologies), *Physiothérapie & Psychiatrie* (Psychotherapy and Psychiatry), and *Auto-Stop* in psychiatry.[17] By 1969, fifty-eight out of the 116 films sponsored by Sandoz were produced by ScienceFilm, i.e., fifty per cent of production.[18] Psychiatric films alone account for roughly one film out of five produced during the first ten years of the Cinémathèque's existence. In terms of numbers this is the most outstanding subject of films produced, a choice understandable since psychoactive substances were of particular interest to the company (see Bächi in this volume). Twelve of the twenty-six films listed under the "psychiatry" heading in the catalogue were creations of ScienceFilm and its director.[19]

Sandoz's rationale for financing industrial filmmaking, in line with commitments of many pharmaceutical companies,[20] was grounded in the fact that pharmaceutical markets were and are characterized by indirect consumption mediated by prescribing physicians. Accordingly, much of the PR in this sector was directed at professionals of medicine. In this context, pharmaceutical industry-sponsored films became boundary objects, where promotion was disguised to the point that their identity became almost

16 Art et Science, *596 films médicaux 16m/m couleurs sonores: Liste N° 17 référence des réalisations d'Éric Duvivier* (ScienceFilm, 1988).

17 Archives Duvivier, Université de Strasbourg, DHVS, Dossiers conventions, Laboratoires Sandoz, Conventions de coproduction *Les pathologies visuelles pathologiques*; *Physiothérapie & Psychiatrie*; *Auto-Stop en psychiatrie*, Convention collective, June 11, 1963.

18 *Films médico-scentifiques Sandoz: Edition 1969* (Sandoz, 1969).

19 For the corporate history of Sandoz, see Hans Fritz, *Industrielle Arzneimittelherstellung: Die pharmazeutische Industrie in Basel am Beispiel der Sandoz AG* (Wissenschaftliche Verlagsgesellschaft, 1992); Lukas Straumann and Daniel Wildmann, *Schweizer Chemieunternehmen im "Dritten Reich"* (Chronos Verlag, 2001); Christian Zeller, *Globalisierungsstrategien – Der Weg von Novartis* (Springer, 2001); Tobias Studer, "Die Geschichte der Sandoz im Lichte ihrer Diversifikationen" *Sandoz Bulletin* 22 (1986): 16–45.

20 Ewen, *PR!*; Marchand, *Creating the Corporate Soul.*

indistinguishable from educational medical films and sometimes from author documentary.[21] Manifold promotional practices including film, but as well specific journals such as Sandoz's *Médecine/Cinéma* and medical film libraries, catered to the social and cultural status of medical professionals. Sandoz's expected benefit from producing an experimental, artist-directed film on *Images from the Visionary World* consisted in creating a cultural event for physicians that specific promotional initiatives could be harnessed to. *Images from the Visionary World* excluded any form of product placement or direct promotional address. Medical professionals to whom corporate messages were addressed were often self-conscious about their status and self-image as a liberal profession, not businessmen with commercial interests. For many, this difference symbolized a deep divide between charlatanism and orthodox medical practice, and throughout the twentieth century physicians have generally been uncomfortable about being directly associated with commercial practices and advertising. Sandoz was well aware of medical etiquette and adapted its PR activities to it.

The première of *Images du monde visionnaire* took place on November 21, 1963, in the fashionable conference hall Salle Iéna in Paris. On invitation by Sandoz, "for professionals only,"[22] the event proposed a three-part film program, also including *Sur les traces de Marey* (In Marey's Footsteps, Sandoz/ScienceFilm, 1963) and *Le Poët et la Licorne* (The Poet and the Unicorn, a film by professor Müller from the Cery hospital in Lausanne, 1963). An observer, Jacques Brosse (1922–2008, naturalist and philosopher), whose very presence indicates a rather loose understanding of the "for physicians only" restriction, described the evening:

> Pharmacists with their ladies and kids, lots of pharmacists, physicians in compact groups ... a public that seems to come from a professional banquet, well-nourished and indulgent, the show is offered for free, but not at all prepared, oh no [a public] not prepared at all for what they were going to see.[23]

During social gatherings such as the one described, scientific films were accompanied by leaflets, hand-outs, and the like, including specific product-information messages not included in the films, and sales representatives could establish close and relaxed relationships with the physician-prescribers and pharmacists they were to visit in their office at some point or another. In

21 Devin Orgeron et al., eds., *Learning with the Lights Off: Educational Film in the United States* (Oxford University Press, 2012).

22 Films by Duvivier and Sandoz were usually premiered in this way, regularly stating "For physicians only" in the opening credits.

23 Michaux, *OC* III, 1538.

contrast to Michaux's above-stated skepticism, the film was effective and well received. Jacques Brosse concluded his description of the evening: "When the lights come back on, we look at ourselves, a little pale, a little embarrassed, deeply disturbed, with the feeling of having seen what we shouldn't see. Thanks to *Images du monde visionnaire*, we have touched the bottom of madness – provoked, experimental, ruthlessly observant madness." [24] Sandoz had obtained their goal, and the film screening became a memorable branding event.

The opening credits of the film projected at Salle Iéna conference hall placed the film under the patronage of Jean Delay, an opinion-leading Parisian psychiatrist directing clinical research with psychopharmaceuticals at the capital's St. Anne hospital. Securing medical patronage was a key element of Éric Duvivier's two-step film production strategy. This consisted in first ensuring the interest and collaboration of a high-profile medical expert whom Duvivier addressed as a disinterested artist-filmmaker. Acceptable to the physician from that third-party perspective, the proposal to produce a film allowed the physician public representation of himself or public display of his specific working topics and theories. Then the film director Duvivier, turning producer, used high-profile physicians as incentives for the industry to finance the production of "his" film. Sandoz might not have sponsored a film by Éric Duvivier, but would do so, and did, for a film "by" a medical professor such as Jean Delay or an artist like Henri Michaux. Leading physicians therefore engaged in film production with Duvivier as film professionals on medical subjects. Leaving financial aspects to the production company ScienceFilm, they apparently stayed clear of pharmaceutical advertising and promotion, a subject always potentially controversial to them. Identified as an opinion leader by the profession and the pharmaceutical industry, the mobilized medical expert's symbolic capital was then transformed by Duvivier into film-production budgets from the pharmaceutical industry. In terms of authorship, as ScienceFilm film production contracts show, this meant that the films were usually co-produced by the pharmaceutical company and ScienceFilm and they were co-authored or co-directed by ScienceFilm/Duvivier and a medical professional and sometimes an artist, as in the case of *Images from the Visionary World*. The outcome of such transactions of symbolic capital was gratifying to physician-authors or presenters. The opening of the film starts with the Sandoz logo, followed by a statement of the otherwise absent medical authority, Jean Delay:

> With extraordinary lucidity and incredible precision, Henri Michaux had succeeded in fixing in his memory such and such images of the visionary world as appeared under such and such a hallucinogenic substance. It was

24 Michaux, *OC* III, 1538.

> the great scientific value of these experiments that justified Éric Duvivier's initial medical interest in this achievement. … The analogy or identity of these experimental states, which can be produced and reduced in a few hours, with certain states of insanity, is at the origin of current research into the biochemical pathogenesis of psychoses.[25]

The benefit for the Parisian psychiatrist was the "great scientific value of these experiments," along with their transcription by artist Michaux and filmmaker Duvivier. The combination of artist and filmmaker represented an original qualitative recording device exploring hallucinations and, through them, psychosis and mental illness. The risk taken by Jean Delay as film instigator and presenter addressing "his" film to other physicians as his audience in a social evening setting of trustful physician talk consisted in pharmaceutical industries flattering individual physicians' egos, treating them as the pharmaceutical industry's little helpers in the guise of a corporate promotion. Through films like the one studied here, professional gatherings, postgraduate training, and conferences became arenas for scientific marketing and building influence. The practice was described and analyzed already in the 1970 as "promotional information" informing and educating practicing physicians, who in return offered opportunities of commercial profit through their prescriptions.[26] An opinion-leading physician, such as Jean Delay, played a central role in these indirect marketing strategies.

But how did artists like Henri Michaux become committed to participating in such social and scientific marketing set-ups? Why would they take the risk to compromise themselves with corporate marketing agendas and physicians' utilitarian requests? Henri Michaux was renowned for his highly original poetry and prose as well as for his art and drawings that obtained recognition in major shows of his work at the Parisian Museum of Modern Art and the Guggenheim Museum in New York in 1978. Between 1956 and 1966, he published a tetralogy – *Misérable Miracle (La mescaline)* (1956; *Miserable Miracle. Mescaline*, trans. Louise Varèse, 1963); *L'Infini turbulent* (1957; *Infinite Turbulence*, trans. Michael Fineberg, 1975); *Connaissance par les gouffres* (1961; *Light Through Darkness*, trans. Haakon Chevalier, 1963); and *Les Grandes Épreuves de l'esprit et les innombrables petites* (1966; *The Major Ordeals of the Mind*, trans. Richard Howard, 1974) – chronicling his psychedelic experiences with hallucinogens including LSD, mescaline, psilocybin, hashish, and cannabis.[27]

25 *Images du monde visionnaire*, 00:00–00:18.

26 P. Chantelou, "Information 'promotionnelle' par le film: Armour Montagu / La folie de Copp et la calcitonine," *Médecine/Cinéma* 13 (1972): 17.

27 Malcolm Bowie, *Henri Michaux: A Study of His Literary Works* (Clarendon Press, 1973). A fifth book could be added here: *Paix dans les brisements* (1959).

Michaux's acquaintance with hallucinogens started in 1953, at the age of fifty-four, informing himself about Peyotl.[28] Michaux engaged in a quest to explore the impact of induced hallucinations in his creative process and to elaborate a method how he could compose his work from bodily experiences, sensory perceptions, and hallucinations given to him by the toxic substances – from what Anne Brun designates as a "hallucinated body" (*le corps halluciné*).[29] In the summer of 1954 in an exchange of letters with his friend, writer and editor Jean Paulhan (1884–1968), Michaux states: "If you manage to find it [mescaline] I am your man. If you wish, your traveling companion and my apartment will be our take-off pad."[30] The experience was to include a third party, the writer Edith Boissonnas (1904–1989), and was to be conducted under the medical supervision of the French neurologist Théodore Alajouanine. The first ingestion can be dated to the of end 1954 or early 1955,[31] and a fourth administration of the toxic substance in June 1955 – actually an episode marred by a dosage error in which he ingested six times the advised dose[32] – swiftly led to the publication of *Miserable Miracle* in 1956.[33] The opening of the book states: "This is an exploration. By words, by signs, by drawings. Mescaline is explored." For Michaux the self-observation under influence comes at a price:

> I was not neutral either, for which I do not apologize. Mescaline and I were more often at odds with each other than together. I was shaken, broken, but I refused to be taken in by it. ... It was with *my* terrible buffetings that *it* put on its show. I was the fireworks that despise the pyrotechnist, even when it can be proved that it is itself the pyrotechnist. ... Should I speak of pleasure? It was unpleasant. Once the agony of the first hour is over (effect of the encounter with the poison), an agony so great that you wonder if you are not going to faint ... in my journal, during all those incredible hours, I find these words written more than fifty times, clumsily, and with difficulty: Intolerable, Unbearable. Such is the price of this paradise(!).[34]

28 Michaux, *OC* II, xxxii.

29 Anne Brun, *Henri Michaux ou le corps halluciné: Les empêcheurs de penser en rond* (Seuil, 1999).

30 Michaux, *OC* II, xxxvi.

31 Michaux, *OC* II, xxxvii.

32 Michaux, *OC* II, xxxvii; Michaux, *OC* II, 722.

33 Henri Michaux, *Miserable Miracle. Mescaline*, trans. Louise Varèse (City Lights Books, 1963). Hereafter, I cite from the 2002 reissue of this translation by the New York Review of Books.

34 Michaux, *Miserable Miracle*, 7–8. "Je n'étais pas neutre non plus, de quoi je ne me défends pas. La Mescaline et moi, nous étions souvent plus en lutte qu'ensemble. J'étais secoué, cassé, mais je ne marchais pas. ... C'est avec *mes* terribles secousses, qu'elle faisait son spectacle. J'étais le feu d'artifice, qui

Miserable miracle, chasm situations, aggressed by mescaline … the terms Michaux employed to describe his experiences after ingestion of what he termed hallucinogenic drugs or toxics were far from laudatory or seductive.[35] They were painful explorations rather than popular incitement.

Marie-Thérèse Wilhelm, a young Alsatian psychiatrist and author of a very recent medical thesis on a mescaline test for mental illness,[36] introduced Michaux to psychopathology, enabling him to communicate directly with her patients and sharing her medical observations with the him.[37] When Michaux published his second mescaline book, *L'Infini turbulent* the following year,[38] he acknowledged the Alsatian psychiatrist. His third book, exploring how (hallucinatory) drugs work, *Connaissance par les gouffres*[39] completed his reversal – only touched upon in *Infinite Turbulence* – from studying the drug and its effects to outlining the twelve "chasm-situations [*situations-gouffres*] defined as difficulties and problems encountered by the mentally deranged."[40] In *Infinite Turbulence*, Michaux considers his objective of an almost scientific description of mescaline experience, stating:

> Following several psychiatrists, I have employed repeatedly in *Miserable Miracle*, despite my suspicious hesitation, the term of experimental schizophrenia to characterize the state I was in after an overdose. It should not be called anything else than mescalinic madness. American psychiatrists have suggested "*experimental psychosis*" or "*model psychosis*" as terms characterizing the state after ingestion of L.S.D. 25.[41]

---

méprise l'artificier, si même on lui prouve qu'il est lui-même l'artificier. … Faut- il parler de plaisir? C'était déplaisant. Une fois l'angoisse de la première heure passée, résultat de la confrontation avec le poison, angoisse telle qu'on se demande si on ne va pas tomber évanoui … tout au long de ces heures inouïes, je trouve, dans mon journal, ces mots, écrits plus de cinquante fois, gauchement, difficilement: *Intolerable, Insupportable.* Tel est le prix de ce paradis (!)." Michaux, *OC* II, 620–21.

35 Henri Michaux, *Light Through Darkness*, trans. Haakon Chevalier (Orion Press, 1963), 139.

36 Marie-Thérèse Wilhelm, "L'intérêt de l'épreuve mescalinique dans les maladies mentales" (PhD dissertation, University of Strasbourg, 1955). Michaux, *OC* II, xlii, 828, 865.

37 Michaux, *OC* II, 1340.

38 Henri Michaux, *Infinite Turbulence*, trans. Michael Fineberg (Calder and Boyars, 1975).

39 Michaux, *Light Through Darkness.*

40 Michaux, *Light Through Darkness*, 129–90.

41 Michaux, *OC* II, 912.

This became the connecting point with the professionals of psychiatry, recurring to an artist as observer and translator of drug induced mental states considered by the physicians as "model psychosis."[42] In return, Michaux gained access to the substances desired, to patient narratives and drawings, and to medical supervision of his drug use. In his quest of the time to produce knowledge about the hallucinogenic drug-induced states, Michaux considered himself "a simple guinea pig, yet one that has the gift of writing [poetry]."[43] His benefits were literary as he stated while writing *Infinite Turbulence* in exchanges of letters with his editor Paulhan Michaux: "To pass from 'I' and from my narrative to 'it' and the other's experience (the mentally ill) is a profound *metamorphosis*. ... You will not regret your patience. It will be all of psychiatry re-digested that you will receive."[44]

Liaising in 1958 with Roger Heim, professor at the Muséum national d'histoire naturelle, who had just published a monograph on hallucinogenic mushrooms, Michaux was inducted into the "circle of experimenters"[45] so that he could participate on April 11, 1959, in his first experiment at St. Anne under the direction of Jean Delay's close collaborator professor Pierre Pichot and in presence of four physician observers.[46] At the time, psychiatrists at St. Anne were engaged in the idea to use artists as intermediary tools of observation of hallucinogenic drug induced experimental psychosis. But their observational presence disturbed Michaux in his interior exploration.[47] He set out his intention, against the physicians' resistance, to repeat the experience in his home as he had done with mescaline. It was this introduction into the "circle of experimenters" that, two years later, triggered the idea to produce a film where the "guinea pig with the gift of writing" could transpose his observations into a cinematic expression presenting the visual perceptions to a wider audience of physicians. The professional writer and painter thereby became a tool of transmission and communication.

His psychedelic writings and drawings in the late 1950s and early 1960s form the basis for the film *Images from the Visionary World*, produced between 1961 and 1963. Poetry and paintings were at once autonomous and complementary worlds for Michaux. And the moving image seemed

42 For a more recent approach, see Anne Brun. "Hallucinatoire et processus créateur: de l'œuvre d'H. Michaux aux enfants psychotiques," *Champ psychosomatique* 46, no. 2 (2007): 127–46.

43 Michaux, *OC* II, lii.

44 Michaux, *OC* II, liii.

45 Michaux, *OC* II, l.

46 Michaux, *OC* II, li.

47 In return, psychiatrists were not very satisfied with the outcome. Michaux, *OC* III, xi: "Les résultats ont été au moins dans l'expérience fait avec nous [docteur Pierre Pichot], assez décevants sous l'angle poétique."

to resonate with the rhythm, the instability and the mobility of Michaux's mescaline visions. Furthermore, Michaux was strongly attracted to cinema and especially documentary, be it scientific, medical, or anthropological. [48] His friend, the philosopher Emil Cioran (1911–1995), who accompanied him regularly going to the documentary movies, considered that it was Michaux's excessive quest for objectivity and rigor that grounded his fascination for these so scandalous impersonal scientific films.[49] Attracted to avant-garde cinema and surrealist poetry and having read *Connaissance par les gouffres* (1961), Eric Duvivier contacted Henri Michaux to make a film about the hallucinatory visions caused by hallucinogens.[50] Struggling with financial difficulties at the time, Michaux seized the opportunity to expand his universe of media to express his observations in the media he treasures but has not touched upon: film. Given his attraction to scientific documentary film and his style of writing sometimes referred to as "scientific," the fact that the proposal came from a scientific medical filmmaker and associated the psychiatrist Jean Delay with the pharmaceutical company producing LSD was enough to convince Michaux to "attempt the impossible," and to make a film on mescaline visions.[51] The condition *sine qua non*, stipulated in the production contract and unusual in comparison with similar ScienceFilm contracts, was that Michaux provided the scenario, had the artistic direction and, above all, "Michaux reserves his right to control by all necessary means the high fidelity of the illustrations [in the film] according to the descriptions he transmitted to Eric Duvivier, to take part in the shooting of some of the delicate scenes of the film, to assist at the work in progress projections and to control the film's dubbing and sonorization."[52] Indeed, Michaux dedicated much of his time between June 1961 and autumn 1963 to the project, as did Duvivier.

For Éric Duvivier, *Images from the Visionary World* was not a stand-alone film work. Addressing psychiatric and psycho-pathological themes regularly, Duvivier produced in 1961, sponsored by Sandoz and in collaboration with the psychiatrist Didier-Jacques Duché, *Le Monde du schizophrène* (The World of the Schizophrenic), a film that proposed in an "objective manner the

48 Michaux, *OC* III, 21–22.

49 Michaux, *OC* III, 22.

50 Anne Dymek and Vincent Lowy, "Toucher aux limites du filmique: Images du monde visionnaire (1963)," *Cahiers Louis-Lumière* 11, special issue: "Le cinéma face aux histoires du regard," ed. Laurent Jullier and Vincent Lowy (2018): 7070; Michaux, *OC* III, 1535.

51 Text read by Michaux at the beginning of the film. Michaux, *OC* III, 223.

52 Archives Duvivier, Université de Strasbourg, DHVS, Dossiers conventions, Laboratoires Sandoz, *Images du monde visionnaire*, Convention de coproduction, June 7, 1962.

subjective lived experiences of images and sound [experienced] by a schizophrenic patient."[53] The beginning of the film is very melancholy, turns strange and ends in an atmosphere of horror. No commentary accompanies the action; the camera follows the man, and the viewer is immersed in the atmosphere and directly confronted with the person's visions. Images of hallucinations and transformed perception start at 03:30, while the commentary is in the first person and repeated automatically. Objective and subjective vision alter from thereon in the film moving back and forth between the patient played by an actor and his hallucinatory visual and auditive perceptions. The film ends with a view of a wax statue of his face gradually melting, distorting and falling off. It marked a turning point in Duvivier's filmmaking. From here on, firstly, several of ScienceFilm's films resolutely adopted a patient-oriented perspective, which was in tune with *direct cinéma* in which directors attempted to completely immerse audiences in the world that was filmed.[54] Secondly, *Le Monde du schizophrène* engaged a much more experimental cinematic approach than prior productions. In his unpublished short manuscript on the history of medical film, Duvivier credits Duché with the exclamation that the film was "a considerable success, a film of a novel kind," which used complex and surreal tricks to recreate the visions presented.[55]

The same year, with *Phobie d'impulsion* (Impulsion Phobia, 1962), Professor Didier Jacques Duché and Éric Duvivier began a project they carried out together for Roche Products. The budget for this film was three times that of the previous year's *Activités électriques du cerveau* (Electrical Activities in the Brain).[56]. Illustrating impulsion phobia – in this case the

53 MedFilm database: *Le Monde du schizophrène* (France, 1961), https://medfilm.unistra.fr/wiki/Le_monde_du_schizophr%C3%A8ne, accessed August 21, 2023. Text cited from *Films médico-scientifiques Sandoz* (Sandoz, 1966), 136.

54 Christian Bonah and Joël Danet, "Le moment anthropologique du cinéma industriel pharmaceutique. Retour sur le film utilitaire médico-pharmaceutique francophone des années 1970," *Images du travail Travail des images* 4, special issue: "La relation soignants/soignés à l'épreuve de l'image," ed. Lucia Candelise, Sylvaine Conord, Nadine Michau, and Gilles Remillet (2017): http://09.edel.univ-poitiers.fr/imagesdutravail/index.php?id=1436. Christian Bonah, and Joël Danet, "Reglose Ödnis, erstickende Ödnis, betäubende Ödnis. Persönliche Geografien von Menschen mit Psychiatrie-Erfahrung im medizinischen Gebrauchsfilm der 1970er Jahre," in *Kopf/Kino. Psychische Erkrankungen und Film*, ed. Tobias Dietrich and Winfried Pauleit (Bertz&Fischer, 2022), 140–50.

55 Archives Duvivier, Université de Strasbourg, DHVS, Note "Petit historique du film medical," Éric Duvivier, n.d.

56 Archives Duvivier, Université de Strasbourg, DHVS, Dossiers conventions, Produits Roche, *Névrose d'angoisse*, Convention de coproduction, Novembre 20, 1961. Filmographie N° 172 sous le titre *Phobie d'impulsion*.

anxiety of a mother concerned about a possible death of her child – the camera follows a mother, played by Florence Guerfy, illustrating from her point of view situations where her phobia is triggered. Again, oscillating between the objective camera filming the mother and her child and subjective camera visions the film immerses the spectator in the interior world of the phobic mother. As the film progresses, the interior visions become more and more elaborate and strange.[57]

The artistic attempt to explore the unconscious was expanded by Duvivier the following year when in June 1962 Henri Michaux, Laboratoires Sandoz, and ScienceFilm signed a contract for a film based on a scenario by Henri Michaux. Sandoz produced a film directed by Eric Duvivier, in color, concerning "the visions produced in the course of experiments under administration of mescaline and hashish." The credits described it as "a film by Henri Michaux, directed by Eric Duvivier."[58] In this case, ScienceFilm's usual medical co-author was replaced by Michaux, and the Parisian professor of psychiatry Jean Delay was only visible as the presenter introducing the film. The production contract further specified that "any possible disposition has to be taken by ScienceFilm to enable Henri Michaux to control that illustrations are as accurate as possible to descriptions of the visions provided by Henri Michaux to Eric Duvivier." This time, it was not a patient, but a well-established artist returning to the voluntary use of hallucinogenic, mind-broadening substances, who would be the subject of the film and at the same time the author of the scenario. Exploring the unconscious from the subject's point of view therefore expanded into a collaboration with an artist who was collaborating with the psychiatrist Jean Delay to subjectively and experimentally explore visions produced by hallucinogens conceived as a form of experimental schizophrenia. Duvivier's benefits, working with Michaux and being financed by Sandoz, corresponded to his genuine business model. The original and complex dispositive of collaboration introducing a third party in the classical industrial film commission-production scenario – the opinion-leading physician alongside the film producer and film director and with Duvivier being part of both sides – co-producer and co-author provided ScienceFilm with considerable leway in terms of creative

57 Probably, given his intense engagement and work with Michaux and other contracts to honor, the production of *Phobie d'impulsion* was delayed. A situation that occurred several times in Duvivier's career as, e.g., with the high-profile film with Claude Vajda *Ces malades qui nous gouvernent* (These Ailments that Govern Us). *Phobie d'impulsion* was completed in 1967 and had visibly profited from Duvivier's work with Michaux.

58 Archives Duvivier, Université de Strasbourg, DHVS, Dossiers conventions, Laboratoires Sandoz, *Images du monde visionnaire*, Convention de coproduction, June 7, 1962. Filmographie N° 176.

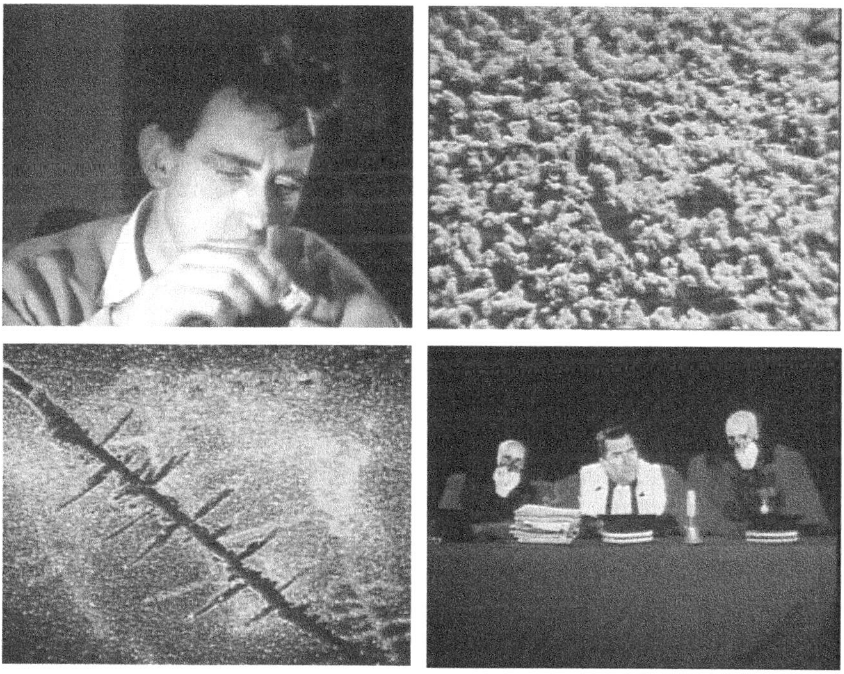

Figure 2. Film stills from Henri Michaux, *Images from the Visionary World*, 1963/64, 28'/34' (and its different versions).

liberty. Films produced by ScienceFilm opened with a company logo, e.g., "Sandoz presents," followed by the acknowledgment, e.g., "A film by Henri Michaux" (usually a physician here, and only in exceptional circumstances the artist), followed then by "directed by Eric Duvivier" and the further credits to camera, screen sets, and sound. Duvivier managed, given his production strategy, to avoid any product placement in his corporate medical films. The minimal recognition of the industrial sponsor/co-producer allowed for parallel lives and uses of these industrial films that were legally guaranteed by the production contracts. Beyond his creative freedom, the dispositive of collaboration also granted Duvivier considerable space for independent use of "his" films that included independent film screenings and programs as the 1968 "Hallucinations" event. For such occasions, the opening corporate logo – "Sandoz presents" in our case – was deleted from the screened film roll.

Screening "Hallucinations": Publics, Boundaries, and the Legal/Illegal Divide

The term "hallucinations" has several meanings: A sensory perception in the absence of an external stimulus; or an object or voice that has the qualities of a real perception. Initially, *alucinari* in Latin refers to misperception and erring in the mind. Medical theory adopted the term long ago, and in early nineteenth-century nascent modern psychiatry Esquirol defined hallucinations in the spectrum of mental disease symptoms.[59] Twentieth-century psychiatry included hallucinations in the standard definition of schizophrenia. A second medical meaning appears after World War II in the framework of the psychopharmacological revolution of the 1950s.[60] Non-intentional, drug-induced hallucinations became labeled as side effects of opioids, for example. And, as is so often the case in drug histories, unwanted secondary symptoms became attractive principal effects in differing contexts (See Greene and Gulino in this volume). Defined as hallucinogens, after 1945 drugs like mescaline, hashish, and lysergic acid diethylamide (LSD, discovered by Hofmann in 1943; see Bächi in this volume) stirred considerable interest in the 1950s for their potential use in psychotherapy and, in reverse, as tools to produce and explore psychosis experimentally. In the following, we will refer to this medical, utilitarian, and exploratory use as "psychodysleptic," using a term borrowed from contemporary medical writing. In the late 1950s, writers and artists including Michaux popularized these drugs for their mind-enhancing and -enlarging qualities. Their growing recreational use outside of medicine in the 1960s is referred to as psychedelic, again using a contemporary actor category and adjective. "Hallucinations" takes on yet a further and differing meaning in this contribution, referring to the November 1968 premiere of an experimental surrealist short film program entitled "Hallucinations" stagged at the Le Ranelagh art gallery and movie theatre in Paris upper class sixteenth arrondissement.

The 1968 art gallery screening of "Hallucinations" was cancelled due to state film censorship of *Images from the Visionary World.* Shifting the point of observation for our story about borderlands of medicines and illegal drugs, the focus of this contribution is not on a specific drug or a series of psychedelic drugs in the 1950s and 1960s, but rather the cinematographic

59 Jean-Etienne Esquirol, *Des maladies mentales considérées sous le rapport médical, hygiénique, et médico-légal*, 2 vols. (J.-B. Baillière, 1838).

60 Marvin E. Lickey and Barbara Gordon, *Drugs for Mental Illness: A Revolution in Psychiatry* (W. H. Freeman, 1983); David Healy, *The Creation of Psychopharmacology* (Harvard University Press, 2002). Joanna Moncrieff, (*The Myth of the Chemical Cure: A Critique of Psychiatric Drug Treatment* (Palgrave Macmillan, 2008).

presentation of their psychic effects in public space and how the legal/illegal divide was negotiated there in the 1960s. Evidently, the film censorship concerned the films as much as the substances that were used to produce the visions of these "hallucinated worlds."[61] Nevertheless, decentering from the substances to the projected visions of the visions they produce is the attempt to broaden the picture. It strives for an entangled history of substance use between art and science, understanding psychosis (better) and exploring literary and drawing drug induced creativity including attitudes towards drugs and the (promotional) presentation of their effects along a legal/illegal boundary setting. Shifting our focus from the product to the filmic representations of its effects transforms at the same time what the risk-benefit divide implies. Risks are no longer bodily impairments *per se* (even if they always remain the evidentiary endpoint), but rather the uncontrolled and multiplied circulation of projected visions outside of their medical control. The risk is thus that psychodysleptic, potentially harmful substances and the presentation of their visual effects get out of established medical control. Going psychedelic, meaning recreational here, hallucinogens transgressed regulation delegated to medical professionals and thus triggered state intervention.

Let us restart with the beginning of *Images from the Visionary World*'s public life in November 1963. Not all of the spectators in November 1963 in the Iéna hall were physicians or pharmacists. Press and art critics attended the event and reported on it over the following days and weeks. Robert Kanters, one of the most sensitive literary critics of Michaux, provided the film with a glowing review, cited above.[62] Despite such positive reviews in art circles, and given his disenchantment with the film, Michaux did nothing to promote "his" film. And the only screening directly associated with him consisted of two projections in February 1965 at the Cinémathèque Française in connection to the major retrospective of his work at the Musée National d'Art Moderne.[63]

The film's audience specific professional circulation with screenings and venues at medical conferences, postgraduate training sessions, and professional gatherings catering to forms of professional sociability including physician's dinners or receptions expanded in the following years and Eric Duvivier estimated that it was viewed by 150,000 spectators over the following years.[64]

Because they did not feature adverts for specific products, Duvivier's industrial films were also included in wider distribution circuits, including

61 "Hallucinated worlds" ("Mondes hallucinés") is the title of another film program organized around the "psychedelic films" produced in the 1960s by Eric Duvivier.

62 See above, page 000.

63 Michaux, *OC* III, 1539.

64 Michaux, *OC*, III, 1535.

those of the Ministry of Foreign Affairs, which in the early 1960s established the audiovisual catalogue of St. Antoine hospital, a catalogue made available to the cultural sections of French embassies throughout the world. Furthermore, they could be rented out, either by Sandoz or by ScienceFilm, to youth centers, trade unions, cultural associations, or film clubs. In April 1968, for example, *Bourdonnements*, the student journal of the prestigious Ecole Centrale in Paris, announced the screening of *Images du monde visionnaire* in the presence of Eric Duvivier, at their film club.

The film had been screened for five years in such parallel circuits, beyond Sandoz's professional screenings, when Eric Duvivier managed to make ends meet with one of the high-profile Parisian avant-garde movie theaters and art gallery Le Ranelagh. This time, it was ScienceFilm and Le Ranelagh that invited chosen spectators to what was termed "the first public presentation" of the film program "Hallucinations."

Whereas Sandoz announced the film in its 1969 film library catalogue as the attempt to present in "objective manner the subjective lived experiences of images and sound,"[65] the experimental surrealist short film program "Hallucinations" at La Ranelagh presented its film night program as follows:

> These four paramedical films united under the title "Hallucination – Hallucinated Worlds" explore the incredible domain of the unconscious in which surrealism after Freud and Lautreamont has found its source of poetic and revolutionary inspiration. It is this descent into hell and into the paradise of the imaginary that these films invite us to. A place where the marvelous, the erotic, and the strange compose a fantastic ballet of a surprising facture.[66]

Between the confidential Ecole Centrale screening and the highly publicized first public presentation at La Ranelagh, not only the audience addressed had changed. France had gone through the major student and worker revolt of May 1968. Antiauthoritarian in its essence, the social, political, and cultural revolt that paralyzed France for two months included, from the side of the youth, calls for greater self-determination, feminism, and sexual liberty and included questions about the rising recreational use of psychedelic drugs.

Widely announced in the press – *L'Information du spectacle*, *Une semaine de Paris*, *Elle*, *L'Officiel des spectacles*, *L'Humanité*, *Le Figaro*, *France Soir*,

65 *Films médico-scientifiques Sandoz* (Sandoz, 1969).

66 Archives Duvivier, Image Est/Centre Régional de l'Image Nancy, Box N° 21, N° 613–664. The later 1970 version of the *Hallucination* programme added *Perception et imaginaire* (Perception and the Imaginary, 1964, 25 min)

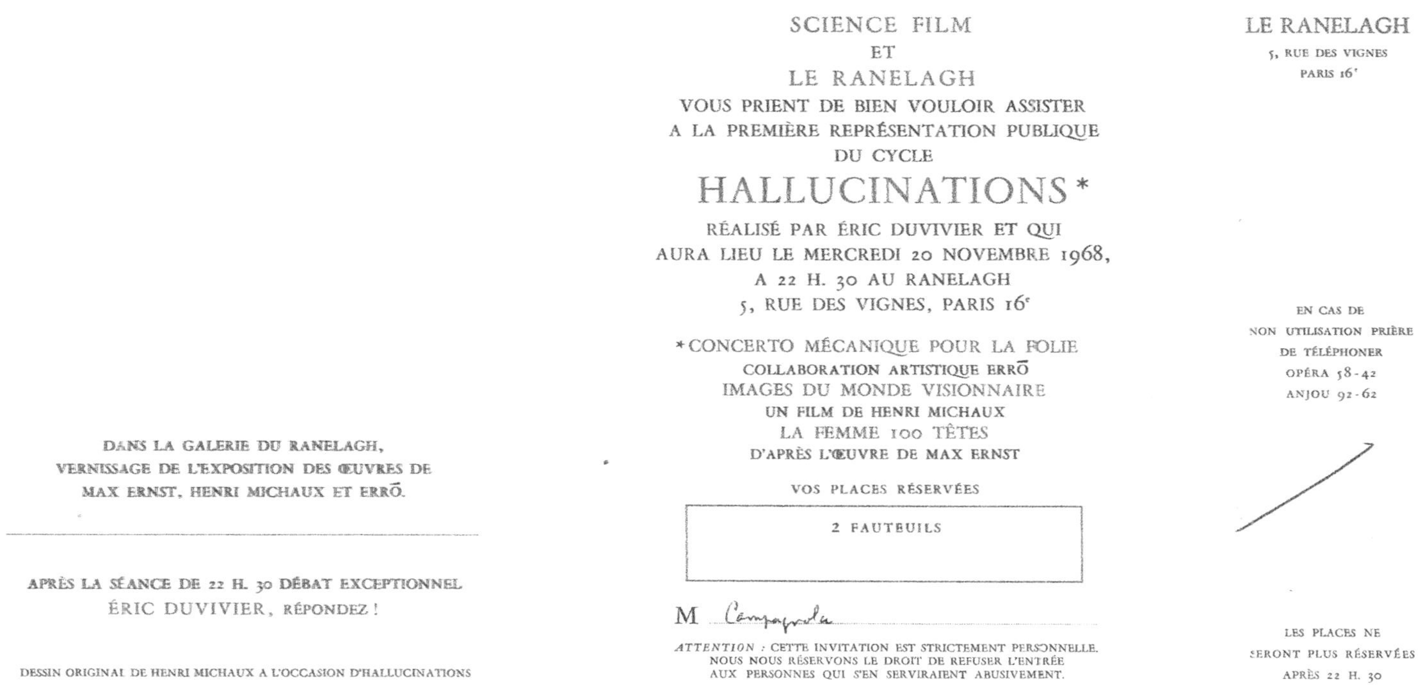

DANS LA GALERIE DU RANELAGH,
VERNISSAGE DE L'EXPOSITION DES ŒUVRES DE
MAX ERNST, HENRI MICHAUX ET ERRÕ.

APRÈS LA SÉANCE DE 22 H. 30 DÉBAT EXCEPTIONNEL
ÉRIC DUVIVIER, RÉPONDEZ !

DESSIN ORIGINAL DE HENRI MICHAUX A L'OCCASION D'HALLUCINATIONS

SCIENCE FILM
ET
LE RANELAGH
VOUS PRIENT DE BIEN VOULOIR ASSISTER
A LA PREMIÈRE REPRÉSENTATION PUBLIQUE
DU CYCLE

HALLUCINATIONS*

RÉALISÉ PAR ÉRIC DUVIVIER ET QUI
AURA LIEU LE MERCREDI 20 NOVEMBRE 1968,
A 22 H. 30 AU RANELAGH
5, RUE DES VIGNES, PARIS 16e

*CONCERTO MÉCANIQUE POUR LA FOLIE
COLLABORATION ARTISTIQUE ERRÕ
IMAGES DU MONDE VISIONNAIRE
UN FILM DE HENRI MICHAUX
LA FEMME 100 TÊTES
D'APRÈS L'ŒUVRE DE MAX ERNST

VOS PLACES RÉSERVÉES

2 FAUTEUILS

M Campagnola

ATTENTION : CETTE INVITATION EST STRICTEMENT PERSONNELLE.
NOUS NOUS RÉSERVONS LE DROIT DE REFUSER L'ENTRÉE
AUX PERSONNES QUI S'EN SERVIRAIENT ABUSIVEMENT.

LE RANELAGH
5, RUE DES VIGNES
PARIS 16e

EN CAS DE
NON UTILISATION PRIÈRE
DE TÉLÉPHONER
OPÉRA 58-42
ANJOU 92-62

LES PLACES NE
SERONT PLUS RÉSERVÉES
APRÈS 22 H. 30

Figure 3. Invitation card announcing the experimental surrealist short film program "Hallucinations" at the La Ranelagh art gallery and experimental movie theater Le Ranelagh in Paris, November 20, 1968.

etc.[67] – the projection of ***Images du Monde visionnaire*** was censured half an hour before the show and retrieved from the program under the whistles of the audience. In the following days, major newspapers commented on the event with headlines like "Le film ***Images du Monde visionnaire*** by Henri Michaux and Eric Duvivier banned" (*L'Humanité*) and "Duvivier banned but Pasolini acquitted..." (*Combat*).[68]

In a letter from the State Secretary of the Prime Minister in charge of information, dated from November 22, 1968, to the ScienceFilm Company, the Secretary Joël Le Theule informed Eric Duvivier that his film was banned. After two consecutive examinations the commission concluded: "notwithstanding the author's intentions or the audiences reactions, positive or negative, the film raises the issue of narcotics, and as such offers a real danger of suggesting or inciting practices that constitute the most serious of social evils."[69]

Le Monde came back to the issue in December 1968. Under the heading "Psychiatrists deplore the ban on ***Images du Monde Visionnaire***," the newspaper publicized their public letter to the Secretary of State Le Theule. It stressed that the film was "a scientific document of exceptional value," that to their mind the film "included neither image nor word that could be considered as in invitation to use mescaline or hashish," and that it was cinema's duty to address the question of narcotics."[70] The ban remained in place.

Material film history may provide a glimpse at how Duvivier tried to adapt to the risk of film censorship.[71] Camera materials and projection prints of the film *Images du Monde Visionnaire* exist in four versions that all show variations in length, image sequences, and color quality. The original camera

67 Archives Duvivier, Université de Strasbourg, DHVS, folder "Hallucinations. Coupures journaux, critiques, censure," n.p.

68 Newspaper clipping on censorship, Archives Duvivier, Université de Strasbourg, DHVS, folder "Hallucinations. Coupures journaux, critiques, censure," n.p.

69 Letter from the State Secretary of the Prime Minister in charge of information dated from November 22, 1968, to the ScienceFilm Company. Archives Duvivier, Université de Strasbourg, DHVS, folder "Hallucinations. Coupures journaux, critiques, censure," n.p.

70 "Des psychiatres déplorent l'interdiction d'Images du monde visionnaire," *Le Monde*, November 22, 1968.

71 Bregt Lameris, "Medical psychedelics. Eric Duvivier's *Mages du Monde Visionnaire*," in *Éric Duvivier, cinéaste medical*, ed. Christian Bonah and Joël Danet (Éditions Le Bord de l'Eau, forthcoming). Bregt Lameris, "Images du monde visionnaire. The representation of hallucinogenic vision in various ranges of color," in *Color mania: the material of color in photography and film*, ed. Barbara Flückiger, Eva Hielscher, and Nadine Wietlisbach (Lars Müller, 2020), 151–62.

LE SECRÉTAIRE D'ÉTAT
AUPRÈS DU PREMIER MINISTRE
CHARGÉ DE L'INFORMATION

Paris, le 22 NOV 1968

005375

1654

Messieurs,

Vous avez bien voulu me demander le visa d'exploitation et l'autorisation d'exportation, en faveur du film français de court métrage intitulé :

IMAGES DU MONDE VISIONNAIRE

J'ai l'honneur de vous faire connaître que la Commission de Contrôle des films cinématographiques, après avoir examiné cette production le 23 octobre en sous-commission et le 19 novembre en séance plénière, a émis un avis défavorable à son exploitation et à son exportation:

" la Commission consciente de ses responsabilités à
" l'égard du public dans son ensemble estime, à l'unanimité, que
" ce film, quelle que soit l'intention de son auteur et quelles
" que soient les réactions du spectateur dans un sens favorable
" ou défavorable, pose le problème des stupéfiants et que de ce
" fait, il offre un réel danger de suggestion ou d'incitation à
" des pratiques qui constituent le plus grave des fléaux sociaux.
"
" En conséquence, la Commission propose l'interdiction
" totale. "

Me rangeant à l'avis ainsi exprimé, j'ai décidé d'interdire totalement l'exploitation et l'exportation du film précité.

Je vous prie d'agréer, Messieurs, l'expression de mes sentiments distingués.

Société Sciencefilm
22, Boulevard Victor Hugo
92 - Clichy

J. Le Theule

Joël LE THEULE

Figure 4. Letter from the State Secretary of the Prime Minister in charge of Information, dated November 22, 1968, to ScienceFilm, banning *Images du Monde Visionnaire*.

material (Kodakchrome II Type A) corresponds to the film described so far. One duplicate (V2: Eastman Reversal Color Print) is missing the Sandoz logo and the Delay introduction at the beginning suggesting that it is one of the copies used for non-medical projections. In a third print (V4 patchwork of Kodakchrome, Eastman, and Gevachrome) the titles cards "Mescaline" and "Hashish" introducing the two parts are replaced by "Substance A/B." Bregt Lameris conjectures that this may correspond to an adapted version after the ban bargaining for public release.[72] In the context of this analysis this element from material film history shows that "the film" is not one fixed object and that Duvivier's first strategy to counter censorship was to accommodate some of the "packaging" of his and Michaux's visions of hallucinogenic visions to keep his experimental film on the "market." As V2 indicates, this was already a practice employed when transferring the film to avant-garde experimental film circuits (clearing out Sandoz and Delay), and was extended here to diffuse censor's apprehension about "inciting practices" deleting drug's names. Be it these arrangements, or changes in French social, moral, and political life in the aftermath of May 68, the film ban was lifted by July 1969.[73]

Eventually, with the progressive end of French state paternalist film censorship, art house movie theaters like Le Seine (which in its name exchanged the usual female article "La" of the Paris river for the male "Le"), Le Racine or Gït-le-Coeur successfully screened the four short experimental cinema films of the "Hallucinations" program, including *Images du monde Visionnaire*, for the general public.[74] Income tax declarations from the Gït-le-Coeur movie theater for the week of April 7–13, 1971, for example, indicate that there were 3,694 paying spectators that week.[75]

Conclusion

In the English language, "drugs" is an ambiguous term that suggests both medicines and their potential, diverging reemployment for non-therapeutic use. Hallucinations produced by psychoactive substances analyzed in this

72 Lameris, "Medical psychedelics. Eric Duvivier's *Mages du Monde Visionnaire*". See also Dymek and Lowy, "Toucher aux limites du filmique," 78.

73 Newspaper clippings in Archives Duvivier indicate that the ban on the film was lifted in July 1969, when the movie theater Le Racine presented it as "finally authorized." Archives Duvivier, Université de Strasbourg, DHVS, folder "Hallucinations. Coupures journaux, critiques, censure," n.p.

74 Laurent Garreau, *Archives secrètes du cinéma français, 1945–1975* (PUF, 2009), 245.

75 Archives Duvivier, Université de Strasbourg, DHVS, folder "Hallucinations. Coupures journaux, critiques, censure," n.p.

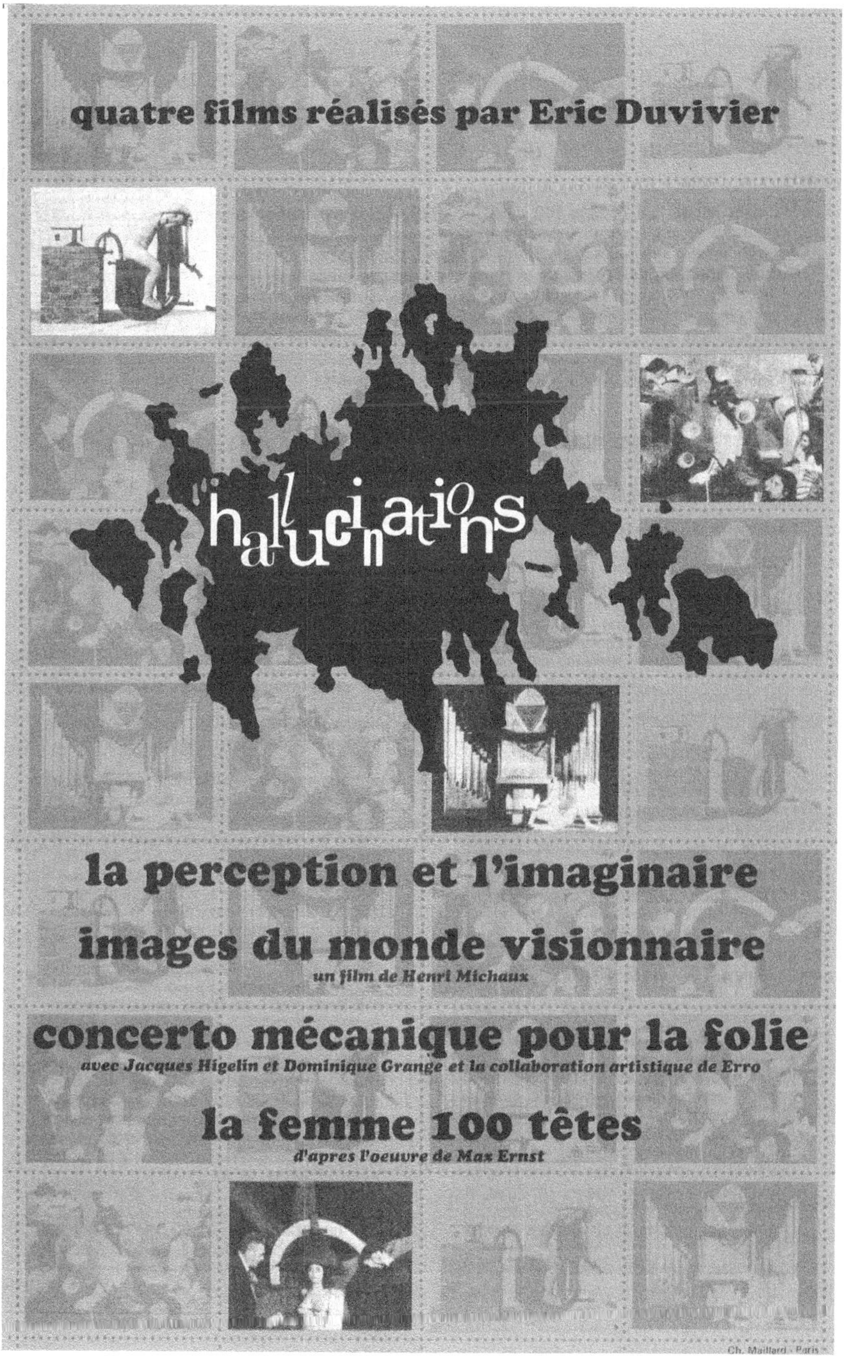
quatre films réalisés par Eric Duvivier
hallucinations
la perception et l'imaginaire
images du monde visionnaire
un film de Henri Michaux
concerto mécanique pour la folie
avec Jacques Higelin et Dominique Grange et la collaboration artistique de Erro
la femme 100 têtes
d'apres l'oeuvre de Max Ernst

Figure 5. Poster announcing the experimental surrealist short film program "Hallucinations" at the experimental movie theater Le Seine in early 1970.

contribution are alternately sensory perceptions in the absence of an external stimulus, mental disease symptoms, drug induced effects or side-effects used in psychotherapy and as tools for the experimental exploration of psychosis, and eventually the title of an experimental surrealist art and short film program. Asking how these drugs' psychic effects were presented in (French) public space and the legal/illegal divide negotiated there, my chapter has investigated how hallucinogenic drugs were relabeled, moving from medical to public space and from psychodysleptic to psychedelic.

These drugs were psychodysleptic when they served medical, utilitarian exploration of psychosis, controlled by physicians as Jean Delay at St Anne hospital and elsewhere. Cinematographic transcriptions and translations of lived experiences and visions could be publicly screened. But they remained under social control as film screenings were restricted to "physicians only," even if that was a decoy, as many spectators in fact were not physicians at all. Control of drug-induced hallucinatory visions was delegated by the state, as for medicines on prescription, to the medical profession supposed capable of arbitrating between use and misuse.

Such substances became psychedelic in the early 1960s, as writers and artists including Henri Michaux popularized them, and the visions they produced, as enhancing and enlarging one's mind. Their growing recreational use outside of medicine, their psychedelic status using here an actor category, sparked concerns about their societal diffusion. The 1968 French ban of *Images from the Visionary World* was a first step towards state intervention when delegated medical control seemed to be falling short of effectively arbitrating use and misuse. When cinematographic hallucinations and their film moved from "physicians-only nights" to a surrealist film manifesto attracting trendy youths, a turning point was reached. Benefit and risk were situational and their evaluation squarely changed: the same film and the same drug-induced images were reframed as illegal; their distribution and screening banned. Delegation of control to the medical corporation stopped when *Images from the Visionary World* entered the wider public sphere of 1968 France. Thereby, the French 1968 film ban foreshadowed what happened to the drugs themselves: their legal prohibition in most Western countries in the 1970s, supposedly due to a lack of safety for use outside of medical supervision, and their high potential for what was now framed as abuse.

Through analyzing projected cinematographic visions of drug-induced hallucinatory visions, I have attempted to broaden our sense of a history of drug use and alternative reemployment, of socially endorsed use, and publicly decried misuse, or who defined what was, when and where, legal or illegal about psychodysleptic-psychedelic substance presentations in public space. And in doing so, I have argued that films are relevant in a history of the risks and benefits of drugs.

My analysis of *Images from the Visionary World* and its public screenings started with the uncanny production and distribution triangle of an experimental movie aligning benefits and risks of a pharmaceutical company, a psychiatrist studying psychodysleptic drug effects, a medical filmmaker, and an established poet and painter. In the end, and after four years of semi-public screenings of the experimental film "from within," a specific post-1968 triangle emerges in which hallucinogenic drugs and the public display of the visions they produce became a dangerous matter, perceived as dangerous enough to enforce legal prohibition. Film was a media used for mobilization and activism, it appealed particularly to students and youth, and the film program "Hallucinations" presented a substance that could enhance the mind and, in consequence, open up new possibilities of perceiving, understanding, and potentially changing the world. The fact that the film was banned in November 1968 indicates that battles over control not only concerned the substances per se, but just as much imagined risks of drug-induced visions only shown on screen. "Of course," to quote Robert Kanters once again, the film "is not, nor does it claim to be, 'mescaline, hashish as if you'd taken it,' since the film cannot restore the visceral and emotional accompaniment first aroused by the drug"; but silver screen images from a visionary world were perceived as a situated risk by themselves, testifying to the power of film that contemporaries associated with this media and to the socially constructed nature of risks.

Chapter Six

Proscribing and Prescribing: Drug Education in 1980s Britain[1]

Alex Mold

In April 1985, a series of advertisements warning young people against heroin use appeared in English media outlets. The "Heroin Screws You Up" campaign consisted of two short TV films, press and magazine advertisements, a poster, and a leaflet for parents. The advertisements featured a mixture of male and female protagonists, all were young, and all were white. Each was presented in a state of distress, caused, so the text accompanying the images suggested, by their use of heroin. The viewer was told: "If a friend offers you heroin, you know what to say. HEROIN SCREWS YOU UP." The "Heroin Screws You Up" campaign was one of the first major anti-drug education programs ever launched in England. Health educators and drug use experts alike had long warned against such efforts for fear that these would backfire, that telling young people about drugs would encourage them to start using illegal substances. However, the apparent dramatic increase in the number of "known heroin addicts" (heroin users who came to the notice of doctors and were reported to the Home Office) over the course of the 1980s prompted a change in tack. Politicians and policymakers felt compelled to act, and in the absence of effective measures to curb heroin use, opted for an anti-drug use education message. From the 1960s

1 This chapter is based on research conducted as part of a Wellcome Trust Medical Humanities Investigator Award, grant number WT 100586/Z/12/Z. I would like to thank David Herzberg, Nils Kessel, and Joseph M. Gabriel for their feedback on the chapter, and the audience members at the "Governing Uncertainty in Drugs and Medicines" workshop for their questions and comments.

onwards, there had been many campaigns that addressed smoking, and a handful focused on alcohol, but anti-illegal drug use campaigns were practically non-existent. As drug use began to increase in the 1980s, this started to change, with the UK following the example of other countries, like the US, in launching efforts to encourage young people to "Just Say No."

Although the "Heroin Screws You Up" campaign was a novel departure with respect to dealing with illegal drugs in Britain, it was not the first attempt to persuade the public to think carefully about their consumption of drugs of any kind. Since at least the 1960s, health officials had tried to deliver a message that not every visit to the doctor would result in a prescription for medication. One campaign, which pre-dated "Heroin Screws You Up" by just a few years, asserted that "[t]he doctor may not give you a prescription. His [*sic*] advice may be all you need." Another, which ran during the 1980s, stated: "You don't need a pill for every ill." Of course, unlike "Heroin Screws You Up," such campaigns were not against substance use per se, but rather concerned with the correct use of prescription drugs under medical guidance as well as the management of patient demands and the promotion of healthy living. Indeed, there were many differences between anti-illegal drug campaigns and efforts to prompt the more rational consumption of prescription drugs. Nonetheless, considering these initiatives alongside one another provides some useful insights. The ways in which messages about drugs and drug taking, both illegal and legal, were delivered and the motives that lay behind these reveal some distinctions, but also important similarities. This chapter considers the imagery and reception of the "Heroin Screws You Up" campaign, drawing out issues relating to risk, responsibility, and individual behavior. The "You don't need a pill for every ill" efforts offer a point of contrast, serving to demonstrate not only what was peculiar to narratives about illegal drugs, but also areas of overlap with the framing of prescription drugs. These commonalities and distinctions were underpinned by a deeper set of issues around notions of risk, the construction of drugs and drug users, as well as the proscription and prescription of certain substances and behaviors. Notions of benefit figure more obliquely in these campaigns. On one level, the supposed benefits were the opposite of the supposed risks: the benefit of better and collective individual health the inverse of the risk of damaging these. Yet, on another level, there were a set of "shadow benefits": aspects of continuing proscribed behaviors that individuals prioritized over avoiding risks. For illegal drug users, this may have meant getting high or avoiding withdrawal; for those ignoring healthy lifestyle messages this meant continuing to enjoy "unhealthy" behaviors like eating too much. These "shadow benefits" were left out of any discussions about why individuals behaved the way that they did and helped to contribute towards the campaigns failing to achieve their goals.

To explore these issues, this chapter will begin by setting the campaigns in context. The recent history of illegal drug policy in the UK, the development of health education, and the importance of the concept of risk within what became known as the "new public health" all help explain the "Heroin Screws You Up" campaign and the reaction to it. Visual analysis of some of the campaign materials highlights the importance of narratives of risk in the presentation of heroin and its users. An assessment of the response to "Heroin Screws You Up" points to numerous problems with how the campaign was received, problems which were rooted in wider issues connected to the use of risk in health education messages. Taking a brief look at roughly contemporary campaigns to encourage the public not to demand a prescription at every consultation with their doctor underscores similarities and differences in the framing of illegal and legal drugs and those that used them. The chapter concludes by reflecting on the prescription and proscription not only of certain substances, but also particular behaviors. These behaviors were out of line with an individualized framing of risk but also prioritized a different set of benefits that sat uneasily with the elevation of individual and collective health above other goals.

Risk, Health Education, and Drugs

The narratives of risk on display in anti-drug campaigns like "Heroin Screws You Up" need to be understood with reference to a larger debate about the place of risk in modern society and in the philosophy and practice of public health. In the post-war period, a series of epidemiological studies in the US, the UK, and other parts of Europe identified specific factors that appeared to increase the likelihood of individuals developing certain kinds of diseases.[2] For instance, high cholesterol and elevated blood pressure were linked to heart disease, and cigarette smoking to lung cancer. These characteristics

2 Gerald M Oppenheimer, "Profiling Risk: The Emergence of Coronary Heart Disease Epidemiology in the United States (1947–70)," *International Journal of Epidemiology* 35, no. 3 (2006): 720–30; Luc Berlivet, "'Association or Causation?' The Debate on the Scientific Status of Risk Factor Epidemiology, 1947–c.1965," in *Making Health Policy: Networks in Research and Policy after 1945*, ed. Virginia Berridge (Rodopi, 2005), 39–74; Carsten Timmermann, "Appropriating Risk Factors: The Reception of an American Approach to Chronic Disease in the Two German States, c. 1950–1990," *Social History of Medicine* 25, no. 1 (2012): 157–74; Virginia Berridge, "Disease, Risk, Harm and Safety: Trends in Post-War British Alcohol Policy," in *Images of Disease: Science, Public Policy and Health in Post War Europe*, ed. Illana Lowy and John Krige (Office for Official Publications of the EU, 2001), 41–52.

and the behaviors associated with them were described as "risk factors."[3] By the 1960s, risk-factor epidemiology was a key part of public health research, and it quickly filtered into public health practice, with multiple efforts made to identify and address risk factors within the population.[4]

Intersecting with this specific sense of risk was a broader conceptualization of risk and its place in modern society. Ulrich Beck, in *The Risk Society*, argued that new technologies posed risks to individuals and societies on an unprecedented scale.[5] Anthony Giddens suggested that there were two kinds of risks: "external risks" which could strike individuals unexpectedly from the outside, but were predictable enough to be insurable. The second kind of risk was "manufactured risk," risks that were created by progress, and especially science and technology. "Manufactured risk" was thus a feature of late/post-modern societies.[6] Responding to such risks became a key task for government in its many domains. In public health, this can be seen in the centrality of risk to what has been described as the "new public health." The "new public health" incorporated the findings of risk factor epidemiology and the broader discussions about risk, individual behavior, and the environment to arrive at a specific formulation of the public, its health and what should be done about it.[7] This emphasized individual responsibility for dealing with and avoiding health risks.[8] Health risks were something for the "entrepreneurial self" to manage, especially through behavior change such as giving up smoking or reducing alcohol consumption.[9]

3 Élodie Giroux, "The Framingham Study and the Constitution of a Restrictive Concept of Risk Factor," *Social History of Medicine* 26, no. 1 (2013): 94–112; William G. Rothstein, *Public Health and the Risk Factor: A History of an Uneven Medical Revolution* (University of Rochester Press, 2003).

4 George Weisz, *Chronic Disease in the Twentieth Century: A History* (Johns Hopkins University Press, 2014).

5 Ulrich Beck, *Risk Society: Towards a New Modernity* (Sage Publications, 1992).

6 Anthony Giddens, "Risk and Responsibility," *The Modern Law Review* 62, no. 1 (1999): 1–10.

7 Alan Petersen and Deborah Lupton, *The New Public Health: Health and Self in the Age of Risk* (Sage Publications, 1996).

8 Nike Ayo, "Understanding Health Promotion in a Neoliberal Climate and the Making of Health Conscious Citizens," *Critical Public Health* 22, no. 1 (2012): 99–105; David Armstrong, "Origins of the Problem of Health-Related Behaviours A Genealogical Study," *Social Studies of Science* 39, no. 6 (2009): 909–26; R. Crawford, "Healthism and the Medicalization of Everyday Life," *International Journal of Health Services: Planning, Administration, Evaluation* 10, no. 3 (1980): 365–88.

9 Alan Petersen, "Risk, Governance and the New Public Health," in *Foucault, Health and Medicine*, ed. Alan Petersen and Bryan Turner (Routledge, 1997), 189–206.

One of the principal methods of attempting to provoke behavior change was health education. From the 1960s onwards, greater emphasis was placed on educating the public about the risks certain kinds of behaviors posed to their health. Informing people about dangers to health had long been part of public health practice, but this took on a new level of importance in the second half of the twentieth century.[10] As chronic disease linked to lifestyle became the leading cause of morbidity and mortality, emphasis was placed on telling people about health risks and persuading them to change their behavior. Mass media health education campaigns were increasingly common from the 1960s onwards. In 1964, the Cohen committee on health education recommended that greater use be made of the mass media not only to provide health information, but also to change behavior.[11] In the wake of the Cohen committee the Health Education Council (HEC) was set up in 1968 in England and Wales, and the Scottish Health Education Group (SHEG) in Scotland. Numerous campaigns on various issues were launched by these groups, on topics including obesity, alcohol and the dangers posed by smoking.[12] By the early 1980s, however, doubts about the ability of such campaigns to change behavior and reduce harmful outcomes were beginning to arise. An editorial published in the *British Medical Journal* in 1982 argued that the HEC had achieved little.[13] A didactic approach was increasingly regarded as unlikely to lead to lasting behavior change. Some health educators stressed the importance of social context and rejected a sole focus

10 David Serlin, ed., *Imagining Illness: Public Health and Visual Culture* (University of Minnesota Press, 2010); Christian Bonah, David Cantor, and Anja Laukötter, eds., *Health Education Films in the Twentieth Century* (University of Rochester Press, 2018).

11 Ministry of Health, *Health Education: Report of a Joint Committee of the Central and Scottish Health Services Councils* (HMSO, 1964).

12 Virginia Berridge, *Marketing Health: Smoking and the Discourse of Public Health in Britain, 1945–2000* (Oxford University Press, 2007); Virginia Berridge and Kelly Loughlin, "Smoking and the New Health Education in Britain 1950s–1970s," *American Journal of Public Health* 95, no. 6 (2005): 956–64; Jane Hand, "'Look after Yourself': Visualising Obesity as a Public Health Concern in 1970s and 1980s Britain," in *Balancing the Self: Medicine, Politics and the Regulation of Health in the Twentieth Century*, ed. Mark Jackson and Martin Moore (Manchester University Press, 2020), 95–124; Alex Mold, "'Everybody Likes a Drink. Nobody Likes a Drunk.' Alcohol, Health Education and the Public in 1970s Britain," *Social History of Medicine* 30, no. 3 (2017): 612–36.

13 "New Thoughts for the Health Education Council," *British Medical Journal (Clinical Research Edition)* 285, no. 6357 (1982): 1761–62.

on individual behavior change.[14] In the UK and at the global level, a wider focus on "health promotion," rather than simply "health education," was put forward.[15] This encompassed the environmental, social, and economic determinants of health and advocated for a set of policies that went beyond health education in order to improve public health.

In addition to questions about the overall effectiveness of health education campaigns, there were specific reasons why anti-drug use campaigns had not been attempted in Britain. Paul Manning argues that the lack of drug education campaigns prior to the 1980s was influenced by the British approach to drugs which was primarily medical, unlike the US, which framed drug use in moral terms.[16] But there were more prosaic elements at work too. Although cannabis and LSD use increased in Britain during the 1960s and 1970s, the use of "hard" drugs like heroin and cocaine was relatively rare. The number of what were called "known heroin addicts" (those who were notified to the Home Office) did not exceed 2,000 until the end of the 1970s.[17] There was also considerable professional opposition to the utilization of drug education campaigns, from both health educators and drug use experts alike. A leaflet on young people and drugs produced by the HEC and the Institute for the Study of Drug Dependence (ISDD) in 1975 was a rare exception, and even this was aimed primarily at parents. The leaflet stated that "We know it is not any use talking at young people, nor trying to scare them by depicting horrific consequences."[18] Indeed, there was some evidence of substance awareness campaigns in the US leading to a rise in drug use, the so-called "boomerang effect."[19] In the UK, in 1979, the

14 Sue Rodmell and Alison Watt, eds., *The Politics of Health Education: Raising the Issues* (Routledge and Kegan Paul, 1986).

15 Peter Duncan, "Failing to Professionalise, Struggling to Specialise: The Rise and Fall of Health Promotion as a Putative Specialism in England, 1980–2000," *Medical History* 57, no. 3 (2013): 377–96; Ilona Kickbusch, "The Contribution of the World Health Organization to a New Public Health and Health Promotion," *American Journal of Public Health* 93, no. 3 (2003): 383–88.

16 Paul Manning, "'No Reefer Madness Please – We're British': Accounting for the Remarkable Absence of Mediated Drugs Education in Post-War Britain 1945–1985," *Media History* 19, no. 4 (2013): 479–95.

17 Advisory Council on the Misuse of Drugs, *Treatment and Rehabilitation* (HMSO, 1983).

18 Institute for the Study of Drug Dependence and Health Education Council, "Young People and Drugs: How We Can Help" (HEC, 1975).

19 Jack B. Haskins, "Evaluating the Effect of a One-Day Drug Education Program on High School Journalists," *Journal of Drug Education* 9, no. 3 (1979): 263–71; John D. Swisher et al., "Drug Education: Pushing or Preventing?," *Peabody Journal of Education* 49, no. 1 (1971): 68–75.

Central Office of Information (COI) echoed such fears warning that an "ill-advised approach by feeding interest in drugs in the wrong way, may actually encourage experimentation."[20]

However, when heroin use started to increase, the value of drug education was re-evaluated. In 1977, there were 2,016 "known heroin addicts"; by 1982 there were 4,371.[21] In 1984, the government's expert body on drugs, the Advisory Council on the Misuse of Drugs (ACMD), examined the issue of health education campaigns. They asserted that "education aimed specifically at preventing drug misuse is not yet common because of the fear that it will promote experimentation."[22] The ACMD warned against "shock and horror" tactics, noting that campaigns "based on such measures on their own are likely to be ineffective or, at worst, positively harmful."[23] The Council also raised questions about the whole premise of drug education, noting that "we do not accept that educational programmes based only on the provision of accurate factual information about drugs and their potential dangers are sufficient to prevent drug misuse. It is now generally accepted that knowledge of itself does not usually change attitudes, far less alter behaviour."[24] Instead, the ACMD argued that drug education was better placed within a broader program of health education messaging aimed at promoting a healthy lifestyle – taking exercise, not smoking, eating a good diet, and so on.

By the early 1980s, the rising number of people using heroin, and a growing moral and media panic around heroin use, made a health education campaign politically expedient, even if it was not well-supported amongst experts. In 1983 there were 5,079 "known heroin addicts"; by 1987 there were 10,389, with many thousands more going undetected. At the same time, social and economic conditions facilitated the development of problematic drug use and heightened the sense of fear that surrounded this. Mass unemployment, particularly amongst young people, and high levels of deprivation were linked to rising levels of drug use, especially in urban areas.[25] Popular and media presentations of young people tended to portray them as either vulnerable or violent, perceptions that were strongly influenced by

20 Central Office of Information, "The Prevention and Treatment of Drug Misuse in Britain" (HMSO, 1979), 17.

21 ACMD, *Treatment and Rehabilitation.*

22 Advisory Council on the Misuse of Drugs, *Prevention: Report of the Advisory Council on the Misuse of Drugs* (HMSO, 1984), 20.

23 ACMD, *Prevention*, 35–36.

24 ACMD, *Prevention*, 36.

25 Susanne MacGregor, ed., *Drugs and British Society: Responses to a Social Problem in the 1980s* (Routledge, 1989).

notions of race, ethnicity and class.[26] Increasing drug use amongst young people was one of a number of social problems that demanded political and practical attention.

The "Heroin Screws You Up" Campaign

Given this context, it is unsurprising that the impetus for the "Heroin Screws You Up" campaign came from government ministers. The Department of Health and Social Security (DHSS) initially asked the HEC if they would run an anti-heroin campaign. The HEC were reluctant, as a specific education campaign to tackle drug use went against the advice of health educators and drug experts. The HEC also wanted time to gather information and to develop materials, as well as additional resources, but the government demanded swift action.[27] Instead, the DHSS turned to the COI, the government's official communications body, to run the campaign. The COI commissioned the advertising agency Yellowhammer to develop the campaign, where it was designed by Sammy Harai, who went on to produce the famous AIDS education campaign featuring a tombstone and the voice of actor John Hurt a few years later.

In the absence of a full archival record, the strategy behind "Heroin Screws You Up" can be gleaned from what was said about it at the time and from the materials themselves. A report on the campaign stated that it was intended to "prevent further increases in the prevalence of drug misuse, and ultimately to reduce its incidence, especially where heroin is concerned."[28] According to the Conservative party health minister Ray Whitney, the aim of the campaign was to influence and inform young people deemed to be "most at risk."[29] These were defined as: young people who had been involved in the "misuse of other drugs but not heroin"; or who were "living in areas where heroin use prevailed"; where there were "adverse social and economic

26 Kieran Connell, *Black Handsworth: Race in 1980s Britain* (University of California Press, 2019); Simon Peplow, *Race and Riots in Thatcher's Britain* (Manchester University Press, 2019).

27 House of Commons Social Services Select Committee, *Misuse of Drugs with Special Reference to the Treatment and Rehabilitation of Misusers of Hard Drugs. Evidence given by the Health Education Council, 6 March 1985*, Session 1984–85 (1985).

28 Research Bureau International, *Heroin Misuse Campaign Evaluation: Report of Findings* (Research Bureau International, 1986).

29 Ray Whitney, "Drugs Campaign: A View from the Department," *The Health Service Journal*, March 27, 1986, 427.

circumstances"; or they had "friends using heroin."[30] The identification of the target audience was thus related to a particular construction of the population "at risk" that was rooted in wider social and economic issues. But the mitigation of such risks was a task for the individual, not for government. As with other health education campaigns at the time, this was intended to make those thought to be at risk or engaging in risky behaviors responsible for dealing with these.[31]

The "Heroin Screws You Up" campaign included two TV films, a series of press and magazine advertisements, a poster, and a leaflet for parents. It ran from April 1985 to March 1986, and it cost £2 million. The magazine and newspaper advertisements were mostly black and white. This meant that they were cheaper to reproduce, but also the monotone coloring exaggerated the dark message of the advertisements and the dangerousness of heroin. The advertisements featured a mixture of male and female protagonists, all of whom were young, and all of whom were white. Each one of the different images had a similar look, but a slightly different emphasis, presumably designed to reach slightly different audiences. For instance, the advertisement titled "Skin Care by Heroin" (Figure 1) featured in teenage magazines targeted at girls, such as *Just Seventeen*. This image was reminiscent of the cosmetic and skin care advertisements common in this type of publication. The placing of the advertisements within the magazine was also interesting – these were often situated next to the problem page where readers wrote in to the magazine's Agony Aunt. The suggestion was that this might be a section where someone with an incipient heroin problem would be looking for advice, and so they might come across the "Heroin Screws You Up" advertisement.

Scrutinizing some of the material produced by the campaign in more depth illustrates the extent to which narratives of risk prevailed. Many of the images focused on the physical and mental consequences of heroin use. In "Your mind isn't the only thing heroin damages," the viewer is confronted with a black and white image of a young man seated in a hunched over position. He appears to be pale, sweaty, and dirty and has spots on his skin. Superimposed on top of the image are seven text labels. These catalogue the physical effects of injecting drug use and addiction to heroin, including skin infections, blood diseases, liver complaints, and "mental problems." The text underneath the image elaborates on these side effects and emphasizes

30 Andrew Irving Associates, "Anti-Heroin Misuse Campaign: Qualitative Evaluation Report" (1986).

31 Deborah Lupton, *The Imperative of Health: Public Health and the Regulated Body* (Sage Publications, 1995).

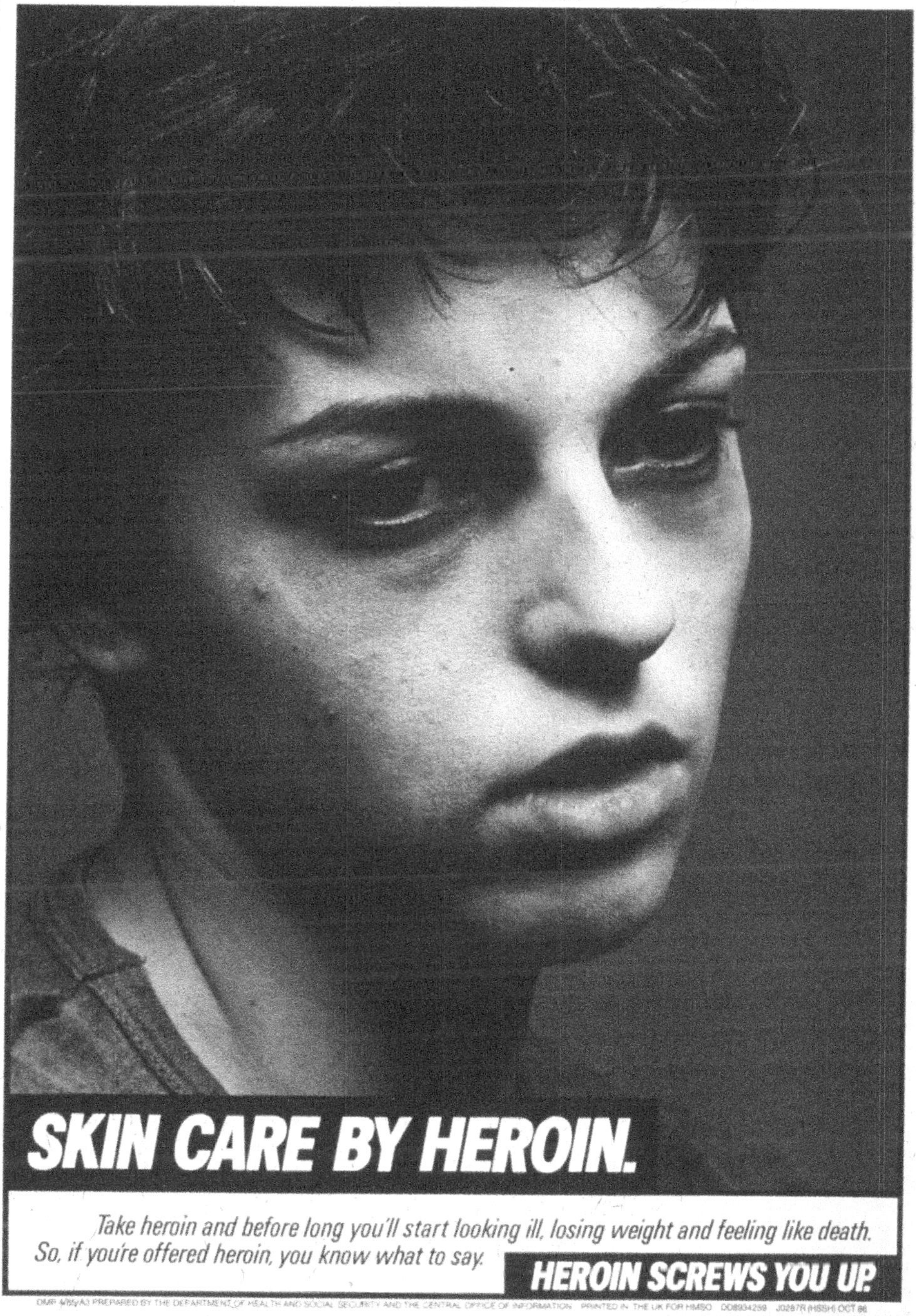

Figure 1. Skin Care by Heroin. Central Office of Information, Heroin Screws You Up campaign, 1985–86.

how these began before addiction occurs. The text offers a narrative of progressive decline and loss of control, from use to sickness and addiction.

Similar tropes were at work in other images from the campaign. In "At first he was sure he'd never become a heroin addict. Now he's not sure he'll ever be anything else" (Figure 2), we find another pale and gaunt young man, this time seated on a chair with his hand on his head in a seemingly distraught manner. The text underneath states: "Take heroin and before long you'll start looking ill, losing weight and feeling like death. So if you're offered heroin, you know what to say. HEROIN SCREWS YOU UP." This message emphasizes the apparent inevitability of addiction, even for those who are sure they can "handle it."

The theme of loss of control and progressive decline loomed especially large in "How much is heroin likely to cost you." The advertisement features a succession of images of the same young woman, moving from left to right across the page. In the first image she appears healthy and confident, with her hand on her hip and looking directly into the camera. In the second image, she is standing but looking downwards. In the third image, the woman is seated on a chair; her hair appears to be greasy and she has dark circles around her eyes. In the final image, she is seated on the floor, hunched over with a hand pulling at her hair. Superimposed on top of each image is a short text label indicating what heroin will cost the user: "It'll cost you your friends," "Your looks," "Your possessions," and "Your health." The text underneath the image echoes the narrative of progressive decline, but also emphasizes the price of heroin use in relation to the loss of possessions, as well as the danger to health.

"How much will heroin cost you" and "Skin care by heroin" were clearly targeted at young women, as denoted by both the images of women and the fact that unlike the ones aimed at young men, these advertisements placed greater emphasis on the risk heroin use posed to physical appearance, a trope presumably thought to be of more appeal to women. The gendered dimensions of this campaign also sat alongside emphasis on the effect heroin might have on a teenagers' possessions and their ability to acquire new ones. Such tactics were representative of the place of the teenager (itself a relatively new construction) in a burgeoning consumer society. Risk in some ways was equated with cost, and this was conceptualized as both cost to the health of the individual, but also economic and social cost. There was no acknowledgment of any benefit heroin use might bring. This was, of course, unsurprising in an anti-drug campaign, but ignoring the reasons why people might take drugs helped to distance the message from some members of its audience. Few could miss the assertion that heroin, and by extension those that used it, was "bad." This tactic, however, backfired as reaction to the campaign demonstrated.

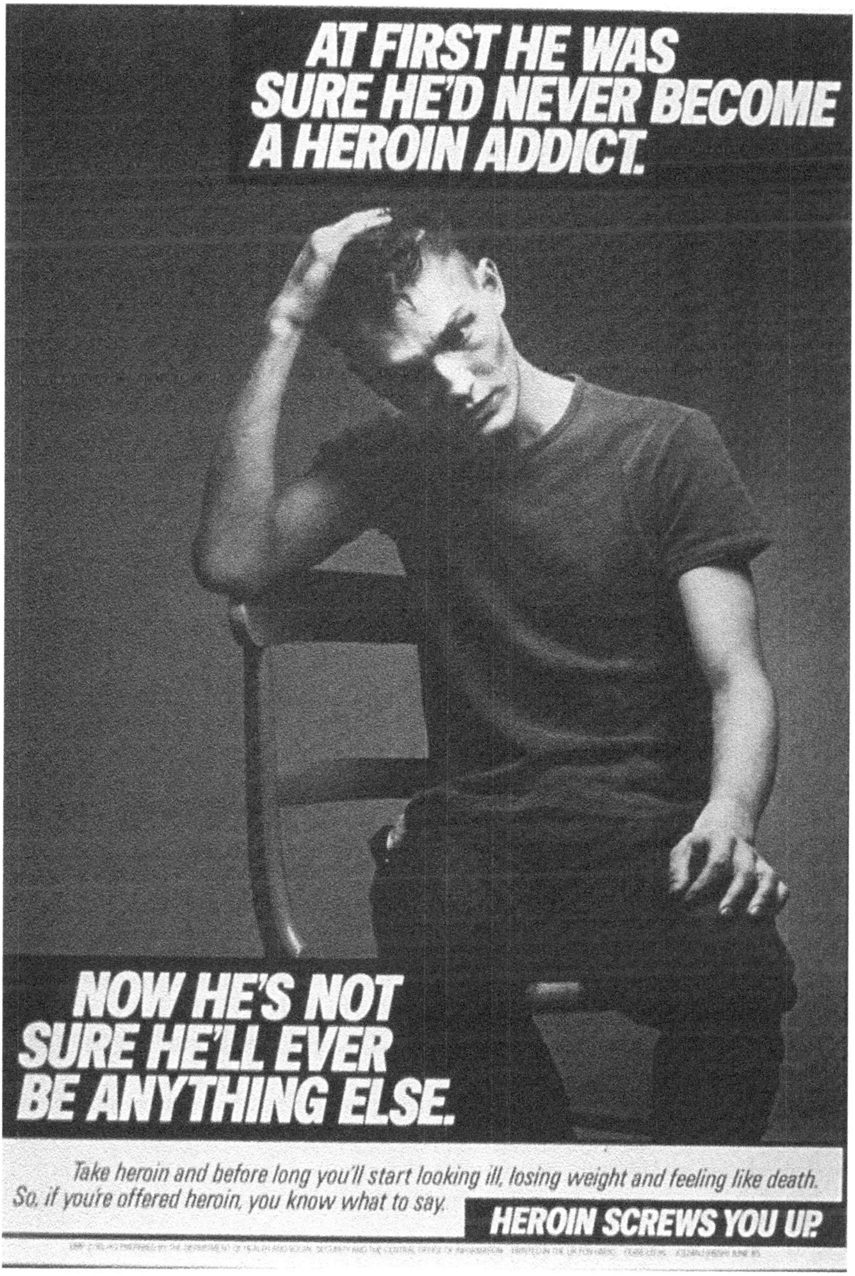

Figure 2. "At first he was sure he'd never become a heroin addict. Now he's not sure he'll ever be anything else." Central Office of Information, Heroin Screws You Up campaign, 1985–86.

The Response to "Heroin Screws You Up"

There were a series of different responses to the campaign including formal evaluations, critiques by drug experts, and those from young people themselves. The campaign was evaluated for the DHSS and the COI by two commercial market research companies. One agency carried out a quantitative study. They surveyed 700 young people aged between thirteen and twenty, both before and after the campaign. The agency found that: 95% of respondents had heard of the campaign; 80% had seen the TV advertisements; 64% the posters; and 56% the newspaper advertisements. Moreover, the survey suggested that there had been significant change before and after the campaign in relation to awareness about the health risks associated with heroin use. Respondents also reported being less likely to take heroin if offered it by a friend after having seen the campaign. However, the survey noted an increased belief that death was an inevitable consequence of heroin usage.[32] This was obviously an erroneous view, but it was perhaps not surprising that respondents held this, given the tone of the campaign.

A qualitative study, based on focus groups and in-depth interviews, dug more deeply into the attitudes, beliefs, and behaviors of the target audience. This also found high levels of recall of the campaign amongst those who had seen it, and that the overall message appeared to have registered, especially with those thought to be most "at risk" from using heroin. The evaluators asserted that the campaign had fostered and reinforced negative attitudes and beliefs about heroin "misuse" across the sample. They also pointed to an apparent increased confidence amongst what the report called heroin "rejectors" by providing them with information about the downsides of using the drug. However, the report did sound some notes of caution. Although "[t]he campaign has achieved in many ways its initial objectives of alerting young people to the risks of trials of heroin," the report's authors felt that "the current commercials and press advertisements show signs of wear out: if young people become bored with the executions, they may begin to become more resistant to and react against the message." The effects of the campaign, the report cautioned, were likely to be short-term, and "long-term effects might be less favourable unless future activity is handled with care and is both sensitive and responsive to the changing attitudes amongst young people."[33]

Notwithstanding these warnings, the campaign's paymasters appear to have been moderately happy with the results. Health minister Whitney pointed to the high levels of recall amongst respondents and the suggestion

32 Research Bureau International, *Heroin Misuse Campaign Evaluation.*

33 Andrew Irving Associates, *Anti-Heroin Misuse Campaign: Qualitative Evaluation Report* (1986).

that attitudes towards heroin were more cautious after the campaign as a sign of its success. He asserted that although unrealistic claims for the effect of the campaign should not be made, the results were "encouraging."[34] Yet the campaign came in for widespread criticism from those working in the drugs field, the wider media, and even an internal DHSS review. The methods used in the evaluation of the campaign were questioned. Critics pointed to the small sample size, and therefore the lack of confidence one could put in their findings. This mattered especially in relation to the assertion that a change in attitudes had occurred after the campaign.[35] But it was the campaign itself that provoked the most ire. Some detractors saw the use of fear tactics to scare young people into not using drugs as increasing the stigmatization around drugs and drug users, but also worried that such images would not be credible to those more familiar with drugs.[36] For individuals who had used drugs, the potential harms seemed exaggerated and did not outweigh the benefits they derived from taking drugs. These benefits included the pleasurable experience of drug use, self-medication for other conditions, or the relief of withdrawal symptoms. There is a long history of ignoring pleasure in the response to substance use, and this was certainly not on the agenda in Britain during the 1980s.[37] However, by ignoring the "shadow benefits" associated with drug use, the campaign distanced itself from those it most hoped to reach. Worse still, from a prevention standpoint, scare tactics might actually have encouraged young people to use drugs as an act of rebellion.[38] Other critics pointed out that the campaigns were too broadly targeted, unlikely to achieve behavior or attitude change, that attitudes towards drugs were influenced by a range of other media, and embedded within broader cultural and social structures and values.[39]

34 Whitney, "Drugs campaign," 427.

35 LSHTM archive, GB 0809 Berridge/6/1/1, Drug misuse campaign evaluation, partial review for Homelessness and Addictions Research Liaison Group, DHSS, no date.

36 Tim Rhodes, "The Politics of Anti-Drugs Campaigns," *Druglink*, May/June 1990, 16–18.

37 David Moore, "Erasing Pleasure from Public Discourse on Illicit Drugs: On the Creation and Reproduction of an Absence," *International Journal of Drug Policy* 19, no. 5 (2008): 353–58; Pat O'Malley and Mariana Valverde, "Pleasure, Freedom and Drugs: The Uses of 'Pleasure' in Liberal Governance of Drug and Alcohol Consumption," *Sociology* 38, no. 1 (2004): 25–42.

38 Jane Falk-Whynes, "Drug Issues in Health Education: Demand Reduction or Public Panacea?," in *Policing and Prescribing: The British System of Drug Control*, ed. David Whynes and Philip Bean (Macmillan, 1991), 217–44.

39 A. Hansen, "Will the Government's Mass Media Campaign on Drugs Work?," *British Medical Journal (Clinical Research Edition)* 290, no. 6474 (1985):

Indeed, looking at the public response to the campaign, there were signs that it did more than miss the mark. There were reports that young people deliberately appropriated the campaign and its imagery. There were numerous accounts of teenagers taking the poster or the magazine and newspaper advertisements and putting them up on their bedroom walls, not in support of the message, but in an ironic commentary on it.[40] In 1989, Barry Sheerman (Labour MP for Huddersfield East) told the House of Commons that "[t]he rather effete young man in the heroin posters became a pin-up for some young girls." Health Minister David Mellor responded that this was an allegation that had never been proven, and it probably is hard to say for certain whether this happened.[41] But, irrespective of the truth or otherwise of this, the campaign clearly did nothing to reverse the upward trend in heroin use. Moreover, the imagery the campaign featured was open to wider cultural appropriation or re-appropriation. This is an example of what media studies theorists describe as the "polysemic" nature of "texts": that these are open to multiple interpretations and readings, some of which may be in direct opposition to that which the creators intended.[42] This went beyond the immediate context of the campaign. In the mid-1990s, a "look" became popular within the fashion world known as "heroin chic." Models displaying heroin chic had emaciated features with pale skin, dark circles underneath the eyes, and were often androgynous.[43] Visually, this look was like that portrayed in the "Heroin Screws You Up" campaign. Of course, the campaign did not lead directly to the creation of heroin chic. There were a whole host of other elements to this, but the similarity between the visuals, at least on the surface, speaks to the way in which imagery created for one purpose in one context is not owned by any one group or fit for one purpose. Just as the "Heroin Screws You Up" campaign drew on stereotypical images of drug users to try and sell an anti-drug message, the fashion industry could

---

1054–55; Ruth Woodcock, "Would This Make You Stop and Think Twice?," *Health and Social Service Journal*, February 20, 1986, 248–49; Robert Power, "Drugs and the Media: Prevention Campaigns and Television," in *Drugs and British Society*, ed. MacGregor, 129–42.

40 Robert Ashton, *This Is Heroin* (Sanctuary House, 2002), 137.

41 House of Commons Debate, December 8, 1989.

42 David Miller et al., eds., *The Circuit of Mass Communication: Media Strategies, Representation and Audience Reception in the AIDS Crisis* (SAGE, 1998), 210–11.

43 Rebecca Arnold, "Heroin Chic," *Fashion Theory* 3, no. 3 (1999): 279–95; Christine L. Harold, "Tracking Heroin Chic: The Abject Body Reconfigures the Rational Argument," *Argumentation and Advocacy* 36, no. 2 (1999): 65–76; Timothy A. Hickman, "Heroin Chic: The Visual Culture of Narcotic Addiction," *Third Text* 16, no. 2 (2002): 119–36.

use similar visual tactics to sell clothes and a particular body image. The multiple readings and mobilization of images was hardly unique to the 1980s, or to public health campaigns, but the enmeshing of drug-related motifs with commercial products illustrates the extent to which these efforts and a particular notion of risk had become embedded within the consumer society.

Problematizing Narratives of Risk and Benefit

Around the same time as the "Heroin Screws You Up" campaign, research was being conducted on other health education efforts that began to raise concerns about the usefulness, purpose, and efficacy of these, and especially the presentation of risk. Although there had been much optimism about the value of health education in the 1960s, by the 1970s, doubts were beginning to set in. A landmark government report on prevention and health published in 1976 advocated more education as one of the chief ways of improving public health, but a number of groups and individuals pointed out the limitations of such a strategy.[44] The public were often well aware of the dangers to health posed by things like smoking, poor diet, and lack of exercise, but they seemed reluctant to abandon such practices, presumably because they derived some benefit from them.[45] There was considerable skepticism about the ability of health education to change behavior, even amongst health educators themselves. The HEC ran a series of campaigns on alcohol use from the late 1970s onwards, but they were quick to argue that the success of these should not be judged by their ability to reduce alcohol consumption.[46] Other critics pointed to structural factors that served to undermine health education. Commercial interests, such as the tobacco and alcohol industries, worked against changing behaviors that were – for them – extremely profitable.[47] Socioeconomic inequalities and environmental factors also played a significant part in both determining health and shaping the capacity of the individual to change their behavior and make healthy "choices."[48] A broader

44 Department of Health and Social Security, *Prevention and Health: Everybody's Business. A Reassessment of Public and Personal Health* (HMSO, 1976).

45 Peder Clark, "'Problems of Today and Tomorrow': Prevention and the National Health Service in the 1970s," *Social History of Medicine* 33, no. 3 (2020): 981–1000.

46 Mold, "'Everybody Likes a Drink.'"

47 Wendy Farrant and Jill Russell, *Health Education Council Publications: A Case Study in the Production, Distribution and Use of Health Information* (University of London, 1985).

48 Hilary Graham, "Women's Smoking and Family Health," *Social Science & Medicine* 25, no. 1 (1987): 47–56.

attack on lifestyle public health and its focus on individual behavior as both the cause and remedy of ill health was underway.[49] Viewed through this lens, campaigns like "Heroin Screws You Up" were not only futile and potentially damaging, but also served to disguise larger issues.

A key strand of such critiques of health education centered on the mobilization of notions of risk. Shortly after the "Heroin Screws You Up" campaign took place, a piece of research was conducted on another contemporaneous health education campaign. "Heartbeat Wales" was designed to educate the public in South Wales about the risk factors for developing heart disease. A team of researchers, including epidemiologists and an anthropologist, interviewed people who had seen the campaign. They found that respondents constructed their beliefs about heart disease and risk through a combination of official pronouncements, the lived experiences of friends and family and depictions in the mass media. These beliefs, which the researchers termed "lay epidemiology" could work against official presentations of the risk factors for heart disease.[50] Many respondents spoke of an aged and healthy friend, acquaintance, or relative – an "Uncle Norman" – who has smoked heavily for years, eats a diet rich in cream cakes and chips, and/or drinks "like a fish." Despite his behavior, "Uncle Norman" lived to a ripe old age. The researchers asserted that "A single Uncle Norman, it seems, may be worth an entire volume of medical statistics and several million pounds of official advertising."[51] As with the "Heroin Screws You Up" campaign, relying on risk as a way to communicate a health education message was a flawed and potentially damaging technique as it failed to take into account the pre-existing beliefs and lived experiences of those who received it.

"You Don't Need a Pill for Every Ill"

Despite such difficulties, the language of risk proliferated throughout a range of health education efforts. Risk came to occupy a role in attempts to manage legal drug use partly through the dissuasion of the public from demanding a prescription at every consultation with their doctor. The cost

49 Rodmell and Watt, *The Politics of Health Education.*

50 S. Frankel, C. Davison, and G. D. Smith, "Lay Epidemiology and the Rationality of Responses to Health Education," *The British Journal of General Practice* 41, no. 351 (1991): 428–30; Charlie Davison, George Davey Smith, and Stephen Frankel, "Lay Epidemiology and the Prevention Paradox: The Implications of Coronary Candidacy for Health Education," *Sociology of Health & Illness* 13, no. 1 (1991): 1–19.

51 Charlie Davison, "Eggs and Sceptical Eater," *New Scientist* 1655 (1989): 45–49.

of prescription drugs and the management of patient demand had long been an issue. From at least the 1950s, health officials were concerned about the cost of prescription drugs to Britain's National Health Service (NHS). Although prescription medication was initially provided to patients for free, a flat-rate prescription charge was introduced in 1952 to help offset the rising drugs bill. This was followed by a series of attempts to control NHS expenditure on medicines, without much success.[52] By the mid-1980s, spending on prescribing made up almost half of the primary care budget, and costs were increasing by 5% a year.[53] To get drug spending under control, the Conservative government attempted to introduce restrictions on what General Practitioners (GPs) could prescribe, encouraging them to prescribe cheaper, generic, and older drugs. Alongside such initiatives, there were also efforts to reduce demand by persuading patients that a prescription for medication was not always necessary. In 1977, a survey of patients' views of general practice conducted by social researchers Ann Cartwright and Robert Anderson found that 41% of patients said that they went to an appointment with their doctor expecting a prescription. This was lower than the two thirds of patients who were given a prescription after a consultation. The vast majority of patients (89%) thought that their doctor was "reasonable" about giving out prescriptions, and just 4% of respondents believed that their doctor was "rather reluctant to give a prescription."[54]

Nonetheless, there was a perception amongst health officials and some doctors that patients demanded prescriptions inappropriately, pressurizing doctors into over-prescribing medication. In 1978, the HEC, at the request of the DHSS and the British Medical Association, produced a campaign with the aim of cutting the cost of medicines and reducing pressure on doctors to over-prescribe. This campaign also had the "complementary" objective of promoting "acceptance by patients that not all consultations with their general practitioners should end with a prescription; and hence to embark on the formidable process of weaning the public off their dependence on others for the discharge of a responsibility which, at least in principle, the great majority can and should carry for themselves."[55] The campaign poster told patients: "Be prepared to leave this surgery empty-handed. The doctor may

52 J. P. Griffin, "An Historical Survey of UK Government Measures to Control the NHS Medicines Expenditure from 1948 to 1996," *PharmacoEconomics* 10, no. 3 (1996): 210–24.

53 Rudolf Klein, *The New Politics of the NHS: From Creation to Reinvention*, 5th ed. (Radcliffe Publishing, 2006), 131.

54 Ann Cartwright and Robert Anderson, *General Practice Revisited: A Second Study of Patients and Their Doctors* (Tavistock Publications, 1981), 51, 49.

55 Health Education Council, *Health Education Council Annual Report, 1979* (Health Education Council, 1979), 14.

not give you a prescription. His [*sic*] advice may be all you need! You can be sure that if you really need one – you'll get one." Such a message obviously reinforced medical authority over both the patient and the decision about if a prescription was needed. But the campaign was also intended to get the public to take "responsibility," although it was not made explicit what they should take responsibility for or how this was to be achieved.

Exactly what the public should do instead of demanding a prescription was made clearer in the "You don't need a pill for every ill" campaign. Little is known about the campaign, although it appears to be from England during the 1980s. There is no archival record detailing the campaign's design or production, but images of the posters have been preserved in the National Library of Medicine's digital history of medicine collection.[56] It consisted of a series of posters featuring cartoons of patients visiting a GP's surgery. In one, an overweight man eating a chocolate bar, with various snack foods falling out of his trouser pocket, demands: "Doctor, doctor – my stomach's bad, can I have a prescription?" (See Figure 3).

In another poster, a different man, also overweight, is depicted walking away from his visit with the doctor reading his "prescription." A speech bubble coming out of his mouth says "What kind of prescription is this? Five miles walk a day and keep off the beer and cigs!" (See Figure 4).

Both posters feature a strap line at the bottom that states: "You don't need a pill for every ill. Let the doctor decide." These images and the messages they delivered were not, therefore, just about reducing demand for prescription drugs, but also about encouraging patients to make lifestyle changes that would reduce their risk of developing various chronic diseases. The campaign was thus underpinned by risk factor epidemiology, but also a broader shift to place the responsibility for reducing the risk of ill health on the individual. This approach, characteristic of the "new public health," can be found in health education campaigns in Britain from the late 1970s onwards. Individuals were told to stop smoking, reduce their consumption of alcohol, change their diets, and take regular exercise to lower their risk of ill-health.[57] The "You don't need a pill for every ill" campaign is an illustration not just of the extent to which notions of risk had permeated approaches to drugs, both legal and illegal, but also public health policy and practice more broadly. As with the "Heroin Screws You Up" campaign, there was no acknowledgment of the benefits that individuals may have derived from their supposedly

56 "National Library of Medicine Digital Collections," n.d., https://collections.nlm.nih.gov.

57 Mold, "'Everybody Likes a Drink'" ; Hand, "'Look after Yourself'"; Berridge and Loughlin, "Smoking and the New Health Education"; Alex Mold, "Alcohol, Health Education and Changing Notions of Risk in Britain, 1980–1990," *Drugs: Education, Prevention and Policy* 28, no. 1 (2020): 48–58.

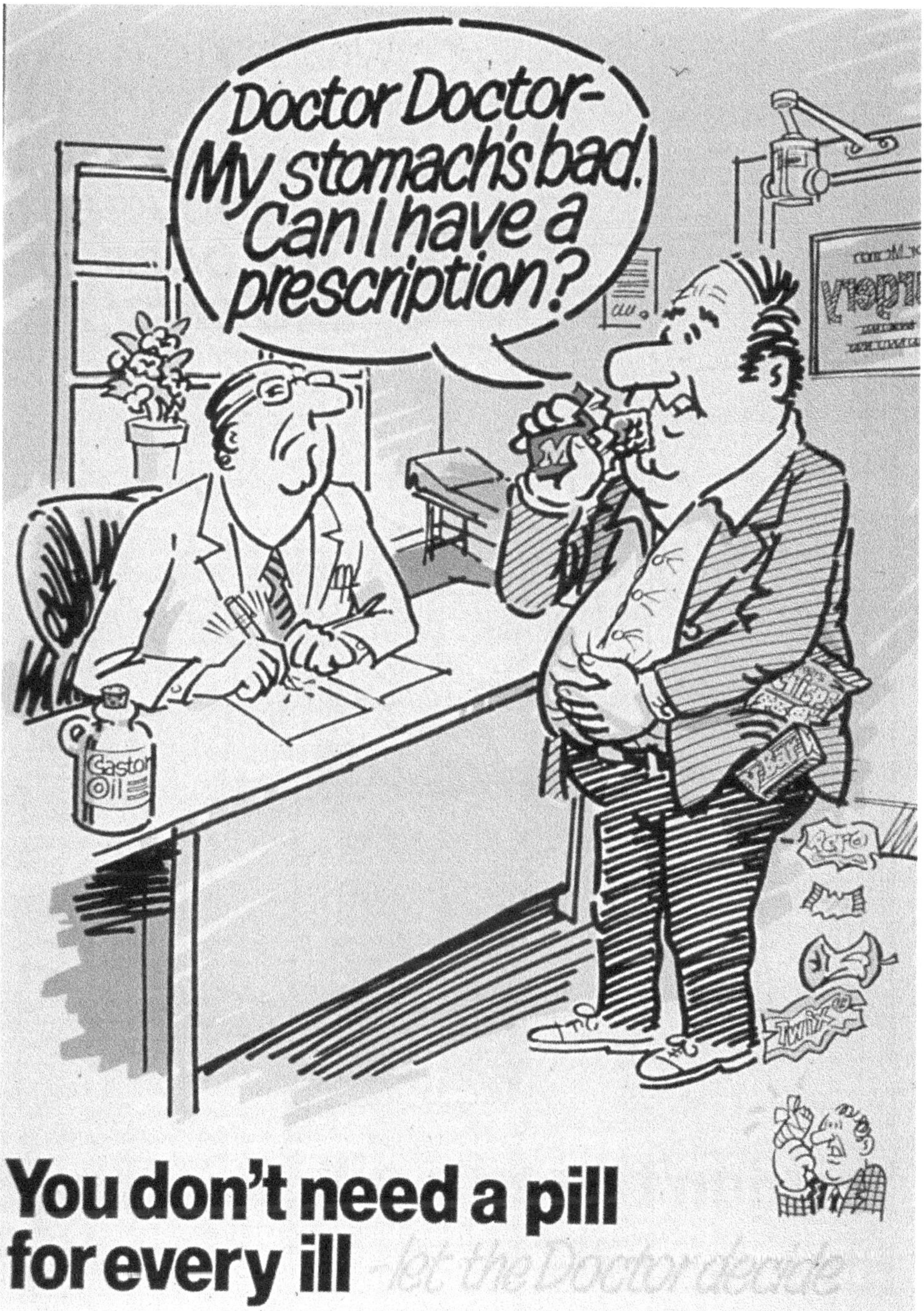

Figure 3. "You don't need a pill for every ill." "Doctor, doctor – my stomach's bad." England, c. 1980s.

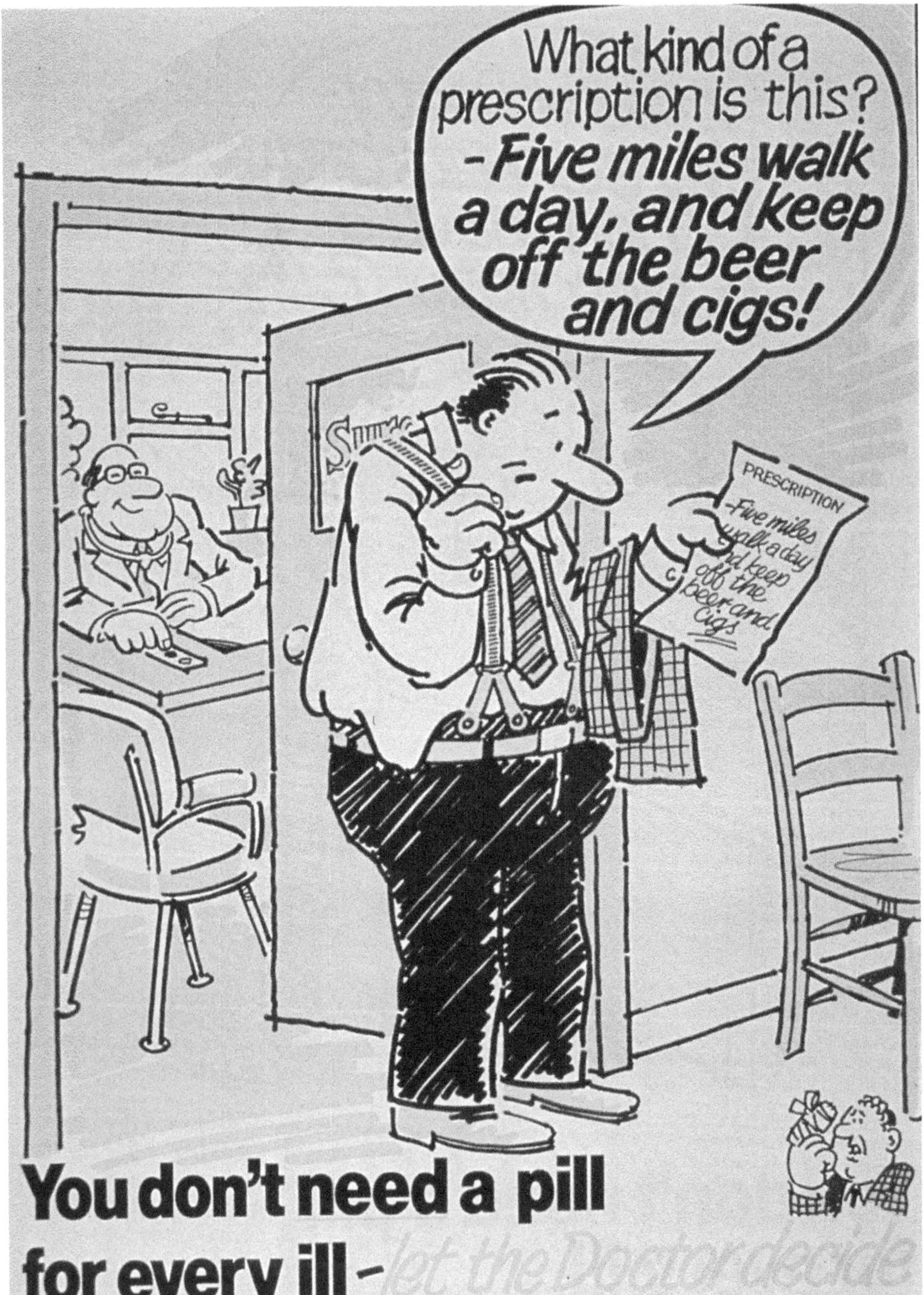
What kind of a prescription is this?
-Five miles walk a day, and keep off the beer and cigs!
PRESCRIPTION
You don't need a pill for every ill - let the Doctor decide

Figure 4. "You don't need a pill for every ill." "What kind of prescription is this?" England, c. 1980s.

"risky" behavior, or any consideration of the role structure, socioeconomic and environmental, may have played in driving and maintaining this.

Conclusion: Proscribing and Prescribing

Considering the similarities and differences between anti-illegal drug use campaigns like "Heroin Screws You Up" and efforts to discourage the public from demanding prescription drugs serves to highlight some important areas of overlap and disjuncture. Notions of risk, whether overtly or beneath the surface, were fundamental to the framing and approach to both issues, albeit in slightly different ways. In the "Heroin Screws You Up" campaign, concern was directed towards individuals thought to be "at risk" from starting to use drugs, and the putative risks of heroin use featured prominently in the materials themselves. In campaigns like "You don't need a pill for every ill," discussion of risk was less overt, but it was present as these were aimed at encouraging individual behavior change as an alternative to the prescription of pharmaceutical drugs and to reduce the risk of chronic disease. Beyond the pervasiveness of risk-based approaches to improving public health, these campaigns had other commonalities. Both aimed to reaffirm medical authority over drugs and drug users, whether legal or illegal. Despite the more consumerist context of Britain in the 1980s, there were limits to the power of consumer demand in medical settings.[58] Both campaigns sought to proscribe certain kinds of behavior (taking illegal drugs, demanding a prescription) and prescribe others (taking exercise, eating a healthy diet). But there were also areas of divergence. Campaigns designed to reduce patient demand for prescriptions were not intended to stop people taking drugs altogether, but rather appeal for more "sensible" use. In this way, they paralleled campaigns around alcohol that sought not to dissuade people from drinking entirely, but to do so "sensibly." In the case of illegal drugs, however, "sensible" use was beyond the pale. If prescription drug demand reduction campaigns were predicated on a notion of a consumer who could be persuaded to act rationally, this was not afforded to those taking illegal drugs. In part this could be attributed to the relative youth of the target audience of "Heroin Screws You Up," but this was also reflective of the status of illegal drugs and their users. Illegal drug use was thought to pose wider risks to society and morality and so could not be dealt with in the same way as demands for prescription drugs, no matter how inappropriate these were thought to be.

58 Alex Mold, *Making the Patient-Consumer: Patient Organisations and Health Consumerism in Britain* (Manchester University Press, 2015).

The centrality of notions of risk to public health messaging around drugs, both legal and illegal, and all sorts of other kinds of substances and activities, could, as this chapter has suggested, have unexpected and undesired consequences. The complexities associated with the public's understanding of risk in a vast array of spheres, from health to financial services and the environment, is now well known. In health, health educators and promoters speak about the need to improve "health literacy" so that members of the public are better able to "read" the messages they are presented with.[59] No matter how well intentioned, such efforts ignore two important problems with focusing on risk in health. Firstly, by conceptualizing risk as something that individuals encounter and must manage, the wider structural determinants governing the production of these risks are ignored. Whether these be socioeconomic or environmental, risk is not evenly distributed, with poorer people facing more risks and having less capacity to address these. Secondly, focusing only on the risks certain behaviors pose fails to acknowledge the powerful reasons why people behave in these ways to begin with. Smoking, drinking, taking illegal drugs, and eating calorie-dense food all come with benefits, most often in the form of pleasure or relief from pain of one sort or another. Failing to acknowledge structural factors and the "shadow benefits" derived from "risky" behavior meant that health education campaigns were divorced from the reality that many of their audiences lived with. Notions of risk continue to form a cornerstone of public health approaches to a range of issues, including drug use. But, as this chapter has shown, such a strategy itself carries risks. Drugs, drug use, and drugs users all present risks, but by focusing on these too heavily there is a risk that not only will such tactics miss their target, but that they may do more harm than good.

59 Don Nutbeam, "Health Literacy as a Public Health Goal: A Challenge for Contemporary Health Education and Communication Strategies into the 21st Century," *Health Promotion International* 15, no. 3 (2000): 259–67.

Part Three

Crises of Risk and Benefit

Chapter Seven

Depo-Provera and Medical Controversies in Britain, 1970s–1980s[1]

Caroline Rusterholz

In 1976, the licensing authority authorized the three-month injectable drug Depo-Provera (DP), produced by the manufacturer Upjohn Company, for short-term use in Britain. In Britain, marketing authorization for a drug depended on the licensing authority, who took their decision based on the recommendation of the Committee on Safety of Medicines. Under section 6 of the Medicines Act 1968, the licensing authority "was the authority responsible for the grant, renewal, variation, suspension and revocation of licenses and certificates. It was made up of a body of Ministers consisting of the Secretary of State for Health and Social Services, the Secretary of State for Scotland, the Secretary of State for Wales, the Minister of Health and Social Services for Northern Ireland, the Minister of Agriculture, Fisheries and Food and the Minister of Agriculture in Northern Ireland."[2] Initially, DP was approved for two specific contraceptive reasons only: for women who had been immunized against rubella to provide contraceptive cover during the active period of the virus; and for those whose partners had had

1 I am grateful to the Swiss National Science Foundation for funding this research through the grant PCEFP1_203399. I would like to thank Nils Kessel, David Herzberg, and Joseph M. Gabriel for their comments and their editing work. I would also like to thank Laura Kelly who provided comments on an earlier version of this chapter.

2 John P. Griffin, "History of drug regulation in the UK," in *The Textbook for Pharmaceutical Medicine*, ed. John P. Griffin, 6th ed. (Wiley-Blackwell, 2009), 424.

a vasectomy but whose sperm count was not yet negative. The rubella vaccine could engender birth damage or birth defects for women who received it while pregnant. To limit the risk of birth defects, women who were vaccinated were given DP, and very often without their informed consent. However, despite the licensing authority's recommendation not to prescribe DP for contraception more generally, several doctors in Britain used it off-label as a contraceptive, either for short-term or long-term use. In 1982, the Committee on Safety of Medicines (CSM) recommended the marketing of DP as a long-term contraceptive. This recommendation was not followed by the licensing authority, which rejected the CSM's advice due to safety concerns. This marked the first instance in which a CSM recommendation was not followed. This decision provoked strong condemnation from the medical community and Upjohn submitted an appeal. Consequently, a public inquiry was held in 1983, at which doctors extensively debated the potential authorization of DP for long-term use. Following this hearing, the panel recommended that DP should be licensed in Britain for long-term contraceptive use only when other forms of contraception were unsuitable and only when patients understood and accepted the risk of side effects and possible delay in return to fertility.

The debate surrounding DP in Britain during this period involved conflicting views; the drug was presented both as a potential new medicine with individual and collective benefits – since it avoided unwanted pregnancies for women who requested it or in the case when other forms of contraception were not suitable and birth defects – and as a dangerous drug with long-lasting side effects, with its health risks outweighing the benefits of preventing pregnancies. Analyzing the medical debate around DP provides valuable insights into the way new drugs with potential side effects were assessed through the risk and benefit framework. It highlights the roles of doctors and activists in this process in Britain, who resorted to these situated categories,[3] and to borrow from the introduction of this edited collection, who "characterized risk and benefit in different ways."

While recent literature has primarily focused on the battle to authorize DP in the US and its use in the Global South, notable contributions have been made in understanding the drug's evaluation process. William Green has shown how the idea of risk and benefit was invoked by the Food and Drug Administration (FDA) to keep clinical trials of the method running, even in the face of concerns around its carcinogenic risk.[4] Wendy Kline's

3 For an overview of how risks and benefits are situated categories see the introduction to this volume.

4 William Green, *Contraceptive Risk: The FDA, Depo-Provera, and the Politics of Experimental Medicine* (New York University Press, 2017).

analysis of the 1983 Congressional Board of Inquiry on DP in the US sheds light on the inquiry's role in exposing scientific flaws in US clinical trials.[5] Emily Callaci has argued that the campaign against DP in the Global South helped to create a shared sense of solidarity, fostering close ties between activists.[6] In Britain, a recent article by Caitlin Lambert has explored the role of the Women's Liberation Movement in condemning the use of DP outside of the recommended guidelines.[7] With Laura Kelly, we have also explored the role of domiciliary family planning services, the fact that family planning advice and methods were given by medical staff to women in their home, in the prescription of DP in Glasgow and Haringey, London. Our work reveals that the doctors in these domiciliary services were influenced by classist and racist biases and prescribed DP for long-term use prior to the 1983 panel recommendation.[8] Research on DP is also part of a broader body of academic work on contraceptive technologies, their risks and benefits, and their stratified use to control population, as well as the ways women fought back to assert their individual choices[9]. For instance, Elizabeth Siegel Watkins has shown how lawmakers and judges welcomed Norplant as a technological fix for (Black) women on benefits and teenage Black girls in the 1990s. Yet, women were not passive victims of the method. Women using or likely to use the method grew increasingly dissatisfied with it, especially given its side effects and the difficulty in removing the device. As a result, large numbers abandoned the method.[10]

5 Wendy Kline, "Bodies of evidence: activists, patients, and the FDA regulation of Depo-Provera," *Journal of Women's History* 22, no. 3 (2010): 64–87.

6 Emily Callaci, "'Injectable development': Depo-Provera and creation of the Global South," *Radical History Review* 131 (2018): 82–104.

7 Caitlin Lambert, "'The objectionable injectable': recovering the lost history of the WLM through the Campaign Against Depo-Provera." *Women's History Review* 29, no. 3 (2020): 520–39.

8 Caroline Rusterholz and Laura Kelly, "Depo-Provera, Class, Race, and the Domiciliary Family Planning Services in Glasgow and Haringey, 1970–1983," *The Historical Journal* 68, no. 1 (2025): 216–38.

9 Johanna Schoen, *Choice & Coercion: Birth Control, Sterilization, and Abortion in Public Health and Welfare* (University of North Carolina Press, 2005); Chikako Takeshita, *The Global Biopolitics of the IUD: How Science Constructs Contraceptive Users and Women's Bodies* (MIT Press, 2011); Dorothy Roberts, *Killing the Black Body: Race, Reproduction, and the Meaning of Liberty* (Vintage, 2014).

10 Elizabeth Siegel Watkins, "From breakthrough to bust: the brief life of Norplant, the contraceptive implant," *Journal of Women's History* 22, no. 3 (2010): 88–111.

This chapter builds upon these works and explores the medical debates that occurred prior to and during the hearings in Britain. It first provides historical and contextual information about the drug's development before delving into an analysis of the debates through the risk and benefit framework. The chapter initially focuses on doctors prescribing the drug outside of its license parameters, then proceeds to examine the arguments presented by the supporters and opponents of DP. In looking at the controversies for the British case, we learn how the perceptions of risk and benefit varied depending on who was assessing the drug. This illustrates how the marketing and acceptance of a new drug were shaped by those whose voices were heard and considered legitimate.

Depo-Provera: Origin and International Use

DP was (and still is) a three-month contraceptive injection made of medroxyprogesterone acetate. It suppresses the hormones that trigger ovulation. Developed by the US company Upjohn, it was approved by the FDA in 1959 to treat amenorrhea, irregular uterine bleeding, and endometriosis.[11] Its contraceptive properties were also noted; clinical trials to assess DP as a contraceptive were implemented in Chile, Mexico, Thailand, America, Australia, and New Zealand. In 1967, the FDA refused to grant Upjohn a license to commercialize DP as a contraceptive because of fears around side effects and safety, but encouraged the company to carry out further preclinical trials with animals. The results of the first trials with beagles hinted towards an increased risk of breast cancer. In 1973, the link between DP and cervical cancer was made clear; however, the FDA did not consider these studies as definitive evidence and planned to authorize the use of DP under specific conditions. Following widespread protest from diverse health agencies and media coverage of the link between the drug and cervical cancer, the FDA postponed its authorization.

In 1978, the FDA officially announced its rejection of DP as a contraceptive in America. The grounds for this rejection were based on the risk and benefit framework. The FDA decided that the possible benefits did not outweigh the potential risks to US women. In other words, the FDA concluded that the risk-benefit ratio of DP was unfavorable for American women.[12] This risk-benefit ratio refers to the comparison of good results when using a drug versus the potential harm that might come from using it. Effectiveness

11 Green, *Contraceptive Risk*.

12 WL, SA/FPA/C/F/1/2/3, "IPPF Factsheet, November 1978, Depo Provera and its use: The current legal controversy."

(lower fertility), side effects, and financial cost were key factors in determining this ratio. However, the ratio was said to differ between countries. The commissioner of the FDA, Donald Kennedy, expressed this view in a letter to the International Planned Parenthood Federation (IPPF): "we wish to emphasize that the benefit-risk judgement made for the US is not necessarily appropriate for other countries and the FDA disapproval of a drug does not necessarily signify that it is unsafe for contraceptive use in other countries."[13] This assertion should be understood in a context in which DP was being used in the setting out of international development and population policies in more than eighty countries. Since the Second World War, fears had grown about overpopulation and the risk it posed to democratic societies. Population growth was said to increase the risks of severe resource shortages and political instability, which population experts deemed fertile ground for communism.[14] One solution proposed to tackle this issue was spreading the ideal of the small nuclear family through the dissemination of contraceptive information and devices. DP was therefore perceived as a technological fix to curb overpopulation, especially in geographical contexts where infant and maternal mortality rates were high. In these circumstances, international organization experts argued, DP's risks were outweighed by its benefits. As argued in an IPPF factsheet on DP, entitled "Depo-Provera: the current legal controversy," "one country's drug regulations are not necessarily appropriate for another and should in no way be imposed either through withholding supplies or by exerting other influences on national programmes."[15] The factsheet went on to argue that "countries have the right to determine for themselves the acceptability, safety and effectiveness of methods of contraception, acknowledging the needs and choices of their own people." Moreover, the IPPF reaffirmed the position of its Central Medical Committee, who downplayed the "alleged risk of carcinoma" by arguing that this risk was not supported by "all available evidence." The committee added that DP was particularly well-suited for women in the postpartum period, since it did not have a detrimental effect on lactation. While they did recognize a delay in return to fertility in comparison with other contraceptive methods, they emphasized that this delay was not permanent, and that "by 24 months

13 "IPPF Factsheet, November 1978."

14 Matthew Connelly, *Fatal Misconception: The Struggle to Control World Population* (Harvard University Press, 2010); Emily Klancher Merchant, *Building the Population Bomb* (Oxford University Press, 2021); Alison Bashford, *Global Population: History, Geopolitics, and Life on Earth* (Columbia University Press, 2014); Simon Szreter, "The Idea of Demographic Transition and the Study of Fertility Change. A Critical Intellectual History," *Population and Development Review* 19, no. 4 (1993): 659–701.

15 "IPPF Factsheet, November 1978."

fertility had returned in most users." Therefore, they concluded that DP "represented a most dependable and useful method of family planning" and that "the injectable may therefore be used in all women who qualify for them." However, they also encouraged the monitoring of the injection in collaboration with the International Fertility Research Programme and urged users to report back at periodic intervals so as to gather more knowledge of "use-effectiveness, occurrence of known and expected side-effects and the early detection of unforeseen ones."[16]

Depo-Provera in Britain up to 1982

In Britain, DP received marketing licenses for treatment of endometriosis (1973), for use as a short-term contraception for wives of men undergoing vasectomy and for women being immunized against rubella (1976), and for treatment of endometrial, renal, and breast cancer (1981). However, the prescription of DP proved problematic and did not follow the guidelines set by the Committee on Safety of Medicines. Several cases of abuse of medical power, where the drug had been prescribed without the informed consent of the patient and outside of the licensing authority's recommendations, were uncovered in the years preceding the 1983 hearing, shedding light on how DP prescription was stratified along lines of class and race. These cases of abuse came to light as a result of the campaigning activities of the Campaign Against Depo-Provera (CADP), a group established in 1978 whose main aims were to ban the drug, document instances of abuse, and raise awareness about DP's detrimental side effects. The group was headed by Janet Hadley, a committed feminist whose entry into radical politics, however, came from her experiences of the Black Power movement in the late 1960s and early 1970s, following her relationship with a Caribbean man. Hadley recounts meeting prominent activist C. L. R. James and she cites these experiences as having provided her with a framework for understanding forms of oppression;[17] she also collaborated with Black women health activists, such as Stella Dadzie. The group collected a significant amount of evidence of abuse through calls for testimonies placed in local newspapers and via the spread of their findings in the press and on TV.

First, it appeared that DP was being administered alongside the rubella vaccine without full consent. For instance, in a letter sent to CADP, a woman from Bristol explained that she had given birth to her first daughter in 1978. Just after the birth, she was immunized against rubella and given

16 "IPPF Factsheet, November 1978."

17 Lambert, "'The objectionable injectable.'"

DP at the same time. The woman explained that she had limited knowledge of the drug apart from the fact that it was a hormonal drug. No other information was given to her and she was not offered the option of "whether to have it or not."[18] When she asked about the side effects, the doctor replied: "well we hope it will stop you getting pregnant." The woman added that she felt "very angry that I wasn't given any choice in the matter and that nothing was explained fully to me, especially as it is given at a time when one is feeling particularly acquiescent, in the couple of days after the birth of a baby in hospital."

In addition, while DP had been authorized alongside the rubella vaccine, there was no recommendation that made it the go-to contraceptive; other forms of efficient contraception would also have worked. Some hospitals seemed to have instigated a policy making DP the only contraceptive available alongside the rubella vaccine, taking contraceptive freedom away from women. It seems that doctors and nurses had decided that the risks of pregnancy, more specifically birth defects and damage linked to the rubella vaccine, were too high and that some women could not be trusted to use efficient methods of birth control. For instance, in west London, a junior doctor questioned the hospital's policy of automatically prescribing DP alongside the vaccine without providing adequate information.[19] He explained that in 1982, on the post-natal ward, he had been told that a woman could only receive the rubella vaccine if she was also given DP. If the woman refused, the vaccine instead had to be administered by her GP. The junior doctor asked the consultant to offer a choice of methods; initially, the consultant agreed, but went back on his decision a few days later, maintaining there was no issue with DP. The following week, the consultant reproached the junior doctor for providing too much information about the side effects of the injectable and for offering information about the cap. The consultant then warned the junior doctor to seek training elsewhere if the policy of the hospital was not followed. The junior doctor sought further help, turning to a woman consultant; this consultant shared the first consultant's view, explaining in derogatory language that "women around here were so stupid they could forget to take the pill." The junior doctor ended up writing to the Chief Medical Officer of the borough to complain about

18 WL, SA/FPA/C/F/1/2/3, "Letter dated February 1983, Bristol," in "Appendix 5 Reports of Women Given Depo-Provera Without Their Knowledge or Consent, The Co-ordinating Group on Depo-Provera Evidence Submitted to Public Enquiry, March 1983."

19 WL, SA/FPA/C/F/1/2/3, "Letter from London Junior Doctor, March 1983" in "Appendix 4 Women Who Were Pressured or Coerced into Accepting DP, The Co-ordinating Group on Depo-Provera Evidence Submitted to Public Enquiry, March 1983."

the policy. This example shows that DP was being prescribed to women who were deemed "stupid" and were believed to behave "irresponsibly" by forgetting their pill. In this instance, the benefit of the drug was calculated through social factors and specifically social hierarchies of class and ability.

Another doctor went even as far as refusing to perform an abortion in the hypothetical case where a woman who had received the rubella vaccine but had refused DP found herself pregnant. This doctor justified the systematic use of DP alongside the rubella vaccine in a letter sent to the District Community Physician, who seemed to have raised an objection to the prescription of DP without the provision of adequate information on its side effects. The consultant gynecologist wrote: "As you know it is essential that mothers given rubella vaccine in the puerperium take adequate measures to avoid conception, for at least eight weeks after the injection. Whilst the risk of pregnancy during this time is small, instances have occurred when the mother had been left to make her own contraceptive arrangements with the results that there has been a subsequent request for termination of pregnancy."[20] He then went on to explain, signifying that the District Community Physician might have suggested the provision of a leaflet listing the side-effects of DP to potential patients: "If however you feel that some form of written explanation would be desirable I can see no objection to this, but I should, however, like to make it plain that if a woman conceives as a result of inadequate contraception after this explanation I should not be able to terminate her pregnancy here."[21] This last statement sheds considerable light on the reluctance of doctors to provide adequate information to women about the risks of birth defect linked to the vaccine in the first twelve weeks after injection, but also on the potential side effects of DP preventing them from making an informed choice. It illustrates the fear that if women were to receive information about the side effects of the drug, they would no longer want to receive it. It also shows that doctors tended to believe that they were in a better position than women to assess the risk-benefit ratio of the drug, ultimately deciding what was best for the patient. This therefore problematizes the notion of informed consent and demonstrates the patronizing view held by many doctors about women's lack of ability to decide. Moreover, some women did not even speak English, showing that seeking informed consent was not standard procedure. In all, this points to a "eugenic rationale," whereby doctors decided to prevent potential birth

20 WL, SA/FPA/C/F/1/2/3, "Letter from a consultant gynaecologist in reply to his District Community Physician, dated 1979 in Submission to the Public Hearing on Depo-Provera."

21 "Letter from a consultant gynaecologist."

defects and birth damages and their social costs, such as care costs, by prescribing DP without giving any information to the recipients.

Even more problematic than prescribing the drug alongside the rubella vaccine without explaining the potential risks of birth defects from the vaccines, as well as side effects of DP, is the fact that, according to the evidence, the drug was also disproportionally given to ethnic minority women as a short-term and sometimes long-term contraceptive, outside of the Department of Health and Social Security's recommendation. In 1978, the gynecologist Wendy Savage published an article in *Fertility and Contraception*, documenting abuse around lack of informed consent in an East London hospital. Asian women were disproportionally being given DP for short-term contraceptive use without being given the information about its side effects.[22] Similarly, Brent Health Council put out a call for witnesses in order to shed light on several instances in which the drug had been prescribed to Black and Asian women in higher proportions and without their consent; the council argued that "there is no doubt that DP is far more readily given to black and Asian women in Brent."[23] In addition, this report also showed that women were not being given information about alternative methods of birth control such as the cap or diaphragm; according to one of the consultants, Asian women "did not know where their vaginas were." Another case was reported by a health education officer who worked in West London between 1979 and 1981, promoting sex education in the community with youth workers and social workers. He expressed his concern that many of his colleagues had found that DP was prescribed "quite frequently for their clients, who included many black and working-class women, and many young women (16–18)";[24] these women were not being given sufficient information and were suffering unpleasant side effects such as constant heavy bleeding, weight gain, and bad leg pain.

The drug was also prescribed to women who had just undergone an abortion without their informed consent. A famous case was that of a fourteen-year-old Caribbean girl who had been given DP after an abortion and who was considered to be "ESN," i.e., "educationally subnormal." The young girl, who was in the care system, testified in an ITV documentary on DP, broadcast in June 1979. Before the procedure, she was asked which type of contraceptive she would use in the future and opted for a coil; however, on

22 Wendy Savage, "The use of Depo-Provera in East London," *Fertility and Contraception* 2, no. 3 (1978): 41.

23 WL, SA/FPA/C/F/1/2/3, "Depo-Provera in the Brent Health District, Observations by Brent Community Health Council February 1983, Submission to the Public Hearing on Depo-Provera."

24 WL, SA/FPA/C/F/1/2/3, "Charmian Kenner, 'My experience of Depo-Provera Use in West London' in Submission to the Public Hearing on Depo-Provera."

coming round from the general anesthetic, she found herself being injected in the leg. She struggled against the injection and only discovered the following day that the coil had not been fitted: instead, she had been given a three-month dose of DP, without her consent and against her will. Justifying the provision of DP without the patient's knowledge, the consultant interviewed on ITV replied: "well she was certainly not the sort of person with whom you could discuss the chemical complications of hormone contraceptive treatment."[25] Challenged by the journalist about the circumstances under which patients were given DP, the consultant replied: "Well, I'd like to know both the political and moral inclinations, because to me it was a straightforward decision." He explained that he had made the decision as a "medical man, parent and citizen of the UK" and expressed his shock at having to do "a termination on a 14-year-old girl." These remarks clearly indicate that the surgeon evaluated the benefits of DP through the lens of class, race and age – specifically, in this case, referencing a young Black teenager described as "educationally subnormal" who had undergone an abortion.

DP was also being prescribed off-label by several doctors and agencies to working-class and ethnic minority patients. Dr. Elphis Christopher from Haringey and Dr. Elizabeth Wilson from Glasgow had used it through their domiciliary family planning services. In these instances, the drug was used to prevent some women from becoming pregnant. In particular, as my own research conducted with Laura Kelly has revealed, in Glasgow DP was regarded as particularly well suited for "promiscuous girls," "psychiatric patients," and "retarded patients."[26] Dr. Wilson started to prescribe the drug in 1973, before it was given the green light by the Committee on Safety of Medicines; she prescribed it as a routine contraceptive for many women in her domiciliary family planning service. Consent was not systematically sought; in particular, for patients with learning difficulties the extent to which they were in a position to understand the side effects was questionable. Moreover, patients were given little information about the drug's side effects. In Haringey, more than half of the patients using DP were from the Caribbean Islands, raising the question of a racist use of the drug. Elphis Christopher stated that she only prescribed the drug to women who had asked for it and when other methods had not been acceptable.[27] However,

25 WL, SA/FPA/C/F/1/2/3, "Interview London Program, LWT, Script dated May 1979, in Submission to the Public Hearing on Depo-Provera."

26 Rusterholz and Kelly, "Depo-Provera, Class, Race, and the Domiciliary Family Planning Services"; Elizabeth Wilson, "Use of long-acting depot progestogen in domiciliary family planning," *British Medical Journal* 2, no. 6049 (1976): 1435.

27 WL, SA/FPA/C/G/8/3, "Elphis Christopher, 'Depo Provera,' January 1980."

the extent to which her patients understood or were informed about the side effects could be questioned, in view of the statement she made in the 1979 ITV documentary: "I think that the amount that you tell a woman has to be graded with what you feel her level of understanding might be. I mean you can worry people very much by going into all the list of side effects and that puts them off completely and they can't evaluate the risks."[28] What is interesting in this quotation is that Dr. Christopher refers to the risk and benefit framework, according to which withholding information was presented as a way of ensuring that women were in a position to make an informed choice; this was based on the belief that if women had knowledge about the side effects, it would cloud their judgement and, obviously, lead them to decide against the drug.

The prescription of DP within domiciliary family planning services was recognized as falling outside of the recommendation of the Department of Health and Social Security, but was said to be useful by Michael Smith, honorary chief medical officer of the Family Planning Association (FPA). In two articles, in 1977 and 1978, he defended the utility of DP for "domiciliary patients, mentally retarded and psychiatric patients." He went on to emphasize the risk-benefit ratio in order to justify the use of the drug: "the Family Planning Association is fully aware of the short-term and the possible long-term hazards of injectable contraceptives, but these need to be weighed up against the benefits to the individual patient, to her family and to society as a whole." Based on this, the FPA felt that "the present restrictions on the use of Depo-Provera prevent a considerable number of women, particularly many who are most in need of contraceptive protection, from regulating their fertility and would welcome a change in the product licence which would allow Depo-Provera to be prescribed more freely." As a result, the FPA sent a request for the lifting of the prescription restrictions to the Committee on Safety of Medicines in 1977.[29] Similarly, in 1978, Smith explained that while DP had not received a license for long-term contraceptive use, its use could be justified "in women who are unable or unwilling to adopt alternative methods of contraception, particularly domiciliary patients, but the responsibility for the use of the product to this group of patients rests with the individual doctor in charge."[30]

28 "Interview London Program."

29 Michael Smith, "Injectable Contraceptives," *Fertility and Contraception* 1, no. 2 (1977): 32.

30 Michael Smith, "Depo Provera injectable contraceptive – a review," *Scottish Medical Journal* 23, no. 3 (1978): 225.

Regulations and Medical Opposition

Lack of informed consent played a key role in the assessment of the risks and benefits of using Depo-Provera. In 1982, the Committee on Safety of Medicines recommended that a product license should be granted for the long-term use of DP as a contraceptive only in "women for whom other contraceptives were contraindicated or had caused unacceptable side effects or were unsatisfactory."[31] In addition, the CSM asked Upjohn to add four warnings to the drug's data sheet (which was sent out to doctors who were considering prescribing the drug): (1) Madroxyprogesterone and it its metabolites are secreted in the breast milk; (2) Doctors are advised that they should check whether patients are pregnant before initial injection and also if any of the subsequent injections are overdue in their administration; (3) Tumors have developed in monkeys given fifty times the human dose, but the relevance of this to humans has not been established; and (4) A few cases of breast cancer have been reported in women taking DP, but no causal relationship has been established.

However, Kenneth Clarke, the Minister for Health and a member of the licensing authority, overturned the CSM's recommendation. His argument was based on the consideration of risks and benefits; this framework proved essential in assessing the utility and safety of DP. He stated that the CSM was "very guarded" in its approval,[32] recommending the drug as a last resort when all other contraceptives were considered unsatisfactory. The licensing authority[33] was of the view that "in these circumstances the risk of using DP appears to outweigh the benefit from such use. It considers that it is particularly important that, in a case such as this, the risk-benefit ratio should be clearly favourable." Clarke argued that there was no way to ensure DP was used "only as a drug of last resort." In addition, the CSM had also advised that the drug should be restricted to a group of women of whom many would have difficulty in giving informed consent to their treatment, such as the "mentally ill or handicapped." In addition, Clarke stated: "some

31 "CMS advice to licensing authority, 1982," in *Depo-Provera, Hearing Under Section 21 Medicines Act 1968, Preliminary Statement* (1983–84).

32 "Social service Depo-Provera," in "Parliamentary Questions and populations references," *Hansard*, May 12, 1982, vol. 23, no. 114, col. 273 REF H:3194.

33 Under section 6 of the Medicines Act 1968, the Licensing Authority (LA) was the authority responsible for the grant, renewal, variation, suspension and revocation of licenses and certificates. It was made up of a body of ministers consisting of the Secretary of State for Social Services, the Secretary of State for Scotland, the Secretary of State for Wales, the Minister of Health and Social Services for Northern Ireland, the Minister of Agriculture, Fisheries and Food, and the Minister of Agriculture in Northern Ireland.

say it should be used on promiscuous women who keep having abortions. I do not think that would be very popular."[34] The licensing authority therefore proposed refusing the license application.[35] Clarke's reservation about informed consent was most likely informed by the non-consensual use of DP that had occurred in Britain; these had hit the headlines in the preceding years due to the dedication of several women's groups set up to protest against the use of the drug.

Doctors were quick to condemn the interference of the Government in the CSM's recommendation. An editorial published in the *British Medical Journal*, entitled "Rejecting scientific advice," presented Clarke's decision as "another example of Government rejection of the considered judgement of its scientific advisory bodies."[36] The editorial went on to argue that Clarke's rejection amounted to saying that "doctors cannot be trusted to exercise competent clinical judgement in the use of a second-line drug." Moreover, in an article published in 1982 in the magazine *Doctor*, the journalist Charles Christian accused the Government of "undermin[ing] what confidence people have in the committee by turning down one of its recommendations."[37] He attributed this interference to "pressures from a motley collection of women's groups." He further explained that these groups "have been campaigning against the drug for some time, claiming that it has been given without proper consent to socially deprived women, the mentally handicapped and to Asian women with a poor understanding of English, without explaining the drug's sometimes unpleasant side-effects." Christian then quoted Wendy Savage, who had denounced the use of DP in Asian women without their informed consent in an East London Hospital: "the way to protect women who are incapable of giving informed consent is not to refuse to license the drug but to ensure that doctors use it in a responsible way."

Alongside their public stances in journal articles, Wendy Savage, Dr. Elphis Christopher, and Dr. Elizabeth Wilson, the latter two of whom had both used Depo-Provera in their domiciliary family planning services in Haringey and Glasgow, respectively, wrote to Kenneth Clarke to protest the government's decision. The three doctors stated that singling out DP due to concern that it may be given to "mentally handicapped women" without their consent was "unreasonable," since the same issue could apply to

34 Rodney Deitch, "Minister Declines to Approve Injectable Contraceptives," *The Lancet*, May 15, 1982, 1134.

35 "Depo-Provera risks outweigh the benefits," *The Times*, May 13, 1982.

36 "Rejecting scientific advice," *British Medical Journal (Clinical Research Edition)* 284, no. 6327 (1982): 1426.

37 Charles Christian, "Women sink Depo-Provera," *Doctor*, June 3, 1982.

various other treatments. They argued for the availability of the drug "as an extra option for women able to choose and for the minority who were unable to use other methods."[38] In addition, Dr. Michael Smith, the honorary chief medical officer of the FPA, criticized Clarke's decision and lamented that "the decision will deprive thousands of women of a valuable form of contraception."[39] The National Association of Family Planning doctors also shared their disappointment in Clarke's decision and encouraged him to follow the CSM's recommendation.[40]

The 1983 Public Hearing

The manufacturer of Depo-Provera, Upjohn, decided to appeal against the decision under section 21 of the Medicine Act; they requested a hearing in public to consider their representation. Such an appeal procedure had never been invoked before. As soon as Upjohn decided to appeal the decision, they made contact with potential witnesses and supporters of DP within medical circles. They wrote to Michael Smith, who replied that he "could appear at a public hearing as a spokesman for the FPA."[41] Upjohn planned to call independent witnesses to support their claims around the safety, effectiveness, and value of DP within the community.[42]

In April 1983, a public hearing took place in front of a panel. The panel was comprised of five professors: Prof. Rosalinde Hurley, chairman and Professor of Medical Microbiology, University of London; Prof. A. W. Asscher, Professor of Renal Medicine, Welsh National School of Medicine; Prof. I. Kennedy, Director, Centre of Law and Ethics, King's College London; Prof. H. S. Jacob, Middlesex Hospital Medical School; and Prof. Langley, Emeritus Professor of Obstetrics and Gynaecology at Manchester University. Twenty-four witnesses were called to support the use of DP. All were scientific experts holding prestigious medical positions. Among them were Dame Josephine Barnes, Dr. Elphis Christopher, Dr. Elizabeth Wilson, Michael Smith, and Prof. Colin Dollery of the Royal Postgraduate Medical School. According to these experts, DP should be given a long-term license for two reasons: because it was safe; and because doctors could use their clinical judgement.

38 "Depo-Provera restriction criticised," May 12, 1982.

39 "Drug advice rejected by health ministers," *The Times*, April 30, 1982.

40 WL, SA/FPA/C/G/8/3, "Letter from the National Association of family planning doctors to Kenneth Clarke."

41 WL, SA/FPA/C/G/8/3, "Letter from Michael Smith to Upjohn, 31 August 1982."

42 "Contraceptive makers to appeal over ban," *The Times*, May 20, 1982.

The safety of DP was presented through references to international organizations that had carried out literature reviews and assessed the drug's safety. For instance, Dame Josephine Barnes – whose numerous prestigious titles and scientific credentials were given[43] – insisted that she was familiar with the IPPF and WHO document that had reviewed the safety aspects of DP; based on these documents, she said, she was convinced "that it has been established that Depo-Provera is a safe drug."[44] She later emphasized that the committees of these organizations were made up of leading experts in the field; for instance, the Committee on Safety of Medicines "comprise doctors who are extremely well qualified, have a great deal of experience and are leading experts in their field. It is an extremely responsible and conservative body." These references to international and national scientific expertise served as an opposing point against the lack of medical qualifications held by Clarke, who she referred to as a "civil servant" and an opponent of scientific recommendation. In addition, international experts were called to testify to support the safety of the drug; these included Dr. Pramilla Senanayake, Medical Director of the IPPF, who stated that "while there was no ideal contraceptive, Depo-Provera was a safe and effective contraceptive option," and Dr. Elof Johannson, Professor of Obstetrics and Gynecology at Uppsala University (where DP had received a long-term license), who presented the drug as "highly effective and safe."[45]

The witnesses also emphasized doctors' freedom of clinical judgement, meaning that doctors were free to assess and decide on the risk-benefit ratio. For instance, Dr. Elphis Christopher stressed that the ruling of the CSM was not mandatory; the "responsibility then rests with the doctor to use the drug with due care." She added: "the authorities must trust the doctor to advise patients on what is in the patient's best interests in individual circumstances. Doctors are an educated profession and are quite aware of the responsibility for individual prescription which is placed upon them."[46] Dame Josephine

43 These titles included Fellow of the Royal College of Physicians, Fellow of the Royal College of Obstetricians and Gynaecologists, Fellow of the Royal College of Surgeons, President of the National Association of Family Planning Doctors, and a member of the 1982 review group set up by the World Health Organization to undertake a special assessment of the Special Programme of Research, Development and Research Training in Human Reproduction.

44 WL, SA/FPA/C/G/8/3, "Depo-Provera Statement to the Panel by Dame Josephine Barnes," in "Public Hearing on Depo-Provera, 25–29 April 1983."

45 WL, SA/FPA/C/G/8/3, "International medical experts recount extensive safety data on Depo-Provera, 27 April 1983."

46 WL, SA/FPA/C/G/8/3, "Depo-Provera Statement to the Panel by Dr Elphis Christopher," in "Public Hearing on Depo-Provera, 25–29 April 1983."

Barnes also attacked Clarke for implying that doctors could not be trusted to prescribe the drug properly: "It is tantamount to saying that doctors in this country are unreliable and act unethically: that they pay no attention to the need for obtaining an informed consent: that they do not explain potential risks and unpleasant side-effects; that they treat patients in a total arbitrary and uncaring fashion. These sorts of accusations are unworthy of any intelligent person."[47] However, with regards to informed consent, Barnes's comments show again the difficulty of ensuring that doctors provided enough information about side effects. She stated: "when a woman consults a doctor for advice on contraception, she has gone a long way toward giving an implied consent to many of the consequences, such as vaginal inspection, IUD insertion, the taking of a blood sample or an injection."[48]

The procedure of the hearing was criticized in the panel report because it only allowed Upjohn to present witnesses. Panel members recommended amending section 21(5) of the Medicine Act 1968 to allow some "direct participation in future hearings of representatives of interested parties other than the application company."[49] This remark referred to the protest made by members of the Coordinating Group on Depo-Provera (CGDP), who had provided written information to the panel but had not been allowed to express their views publicly. The CGDP had been created in 1982 by Marge Berer, at that time a campaign worker in the National Abortion Campaign; Jill Rakusen, a community worker and founding member of the Women's Health Information Centre; and Jean Robinson, a lay member of the General Medical Council. Their aim was to gather documentation and testimonies to present to the jury in the hope that the latter would ban DP. While this group collected a substantial amount of evidence, it was, however, banned from taking a stance publicly, limiting its intervention to background knowledge. In 1983, the CADP was dissolved; the materials they had gathered were passed on to the coordinating group and served as a basis for the 400 pages of written documentation provided to the panel. This documentation included more than eighty cases of women reporting bad experiences with the method, either in terms of side effects, such as migraines, weight gain, nausea, dizziness, loss of libido, anxiety, and depression, or in terms of lack of consent and information about the prescription of the drug. The attorney representing Upjohn dismissed these eighty-eight testimonies as anecdotal and irrelevant.

47 WL, SA/FPA/C/G/8/3, "Depo-Provera Statement to the Panel by Dame Josephine Barnes," in "Public Hearing on Depo-Provera, 25–29 April 1983."

48 "Depo-Provera Statement to the Panel by Dame Josephine Barnes."

49 "Report of the panel of persons appointed by the licensing authority to hear the application by Upjohn LTD for a product licence to market the drug Depo-Provera as a long term contraceptive" (Department of Health and Social Security, 1984).

The group submitted a wide range of evidence that, in addition to providing experiential expertise, used the language of risk and benefit. For instance, in one submitted report, entitled "Information, choice and informed consent," Marge Berer referred to the risk-benefit ratio invoked by doctors, notably Dr. Christopher, to justify the withholding of information. Berer used a similar reasoning to argue that women should be presented with all the information about the benefits and risks of DP: "the possibility of getting a particular adverse effect – however common – may be unacceptable for some women according to their own benefit-risk ratio. No doctor can be expected to know what the personal risk-benefit ratio is."[50]

In addition, the evidence revealed a disturbing difference between the significance of the risks of DP acknowledged by researchers and the adverse effects and non-medical problems revealed by the testimonies. In particular, the group called for close monitoring of side effects such as weight gain, heavy bleeding, depression, loss of libido, headache, and pain in the legs.

The group also submitted a pamphlet on DP that connected the evidence at national and international levels. In the pamphlet, the fate of women in the third world who had been prescribed DP was compared to that of women in Britain and the US. The pamphlet concluded: "the side-effects of women are the same wherever Depo-Provera is given – the risks of cancer are the same. We cannot call for Depo-Provera to be banned in Britain and condone its use in Asia, Africa and Latin America. If a drug is too risky to be used it is *too risky* – there can be no question of double standard."[51]

The hearing provided the opportunity to discuss the risk-benefit framework of the drug in depth, but it failed to allow activists to voice their position. However, the panel questions were informed by the concerns raised in the evidence presented by the group, notably around issues of informed consent and potential for abuse.

Conclusion

Depo-Provera provides a fascinating case study, enabling us to understand better how different experts clashed in the assessment of a new drug. This chapter has argued that both opponents and supporters of the drug invoked the concept of risk and benefit when advocating for or opposing its

50 WL, SA/FPA/C/F/1/2/3, "Marge Berer, 'Information, choice and informed consent,' March 1983," in "Submission to the Public Hearing on Depo-Provera."

51 "Depo-Provera: A Report by the Campaign Against Depo-Provera" (CADP, ca. 1983), 39.

long-term licensing. By examining how doctors used the concept of risk and benefit to evaluate the efficacy of the drug, this chapter has put forth four key arguments. First, it has demonstrated the ambiguous legal status of DP. Although officially authorized on restricted grounds only, the drug appears to have been widely prescribed by certain doctors with the intention of managing unwanted pregnancies and occasionally reducing the fertility of vulnerable populations, i.e., women from socially deprived backgrounds and of minority ethnicities. As in the case of the US, this example seems to be part of a bigger story of reproductive control.[52] In their groundbreaking book, the *Heart of the Race: Black Women's Lives in Britain*, Beverley Bryan, Stella Dadzie, and Suzanne Scafe emphasize doctors' will to "exercise control over [their] fertility in the interests of (white) society. The consequences of this are evident in the numerous cases of Black women who receive unwanted sterilisations or terminations, or the damaging long-term contraceptive DP (Depo Provera), all in the interests of controlling the numbers of 'unwanted' Black babies."[53]

Secondly, the chapter has argued that the application of the risk-benefit framework varied according to local circumstances and was stratified along lines of class and race. Doctors used DP with the rubella vaccines to prevent the risks of birth defects but without informing their patients about these risks and the side-effects of DP. In addition, doctors justified the prescription of DP outside of the recommendations of the CSM by invoking their freedom of judgement. They perceived vulnerable women as being at risk of additional pregnancies; this risk was deemed higher than that of the side effects. For opponents of the drug, the risk-benefit ratio was too high to allow the contraceptive to be prescribed, both in light with the abuses committed by doctors and because the drug was mainly prescribed to vulnerable women and often non-consenting women. In addition, the opponents highlighted a wide range of side effects that they believed had not been investigated properly.

Thirdly, the chapter has illustrated the influence of international debates surrounding DP on the prevailing framework. Doctors who prescribed the drug often referenced the policies of international organizations, which regarded DP as a valuable contraceptive with benefits that outweighed its potential risks. Conversely, activists who denounced the use of DP referred

52 For reproductive control see Alexandra Minna Stern, "Sterilized in the name of public health: race, immigration, and reproductive control in modern California," *American Journal of Public Health* 95, no. 7 (2005): 1128–38.

53 Beverley Bryan, Stella Dadzie, and Suzanne Scafe, *Heart of the Race: Black Women's Life in Britain* (Verso, 2018), 133.

to international discussions on its side effects and instances of coercion in order to campaign for the drug's prohibition.

Finally, the influence of activists' work on the panel recommendation has been highlighted. This fear that informed consent would prove problematic led the panel to recommend that DP should be approved for long-term contraception only as a last resort when other methods were unacceptable and only when patients understood both the side effects and the delay in return to fertility. Based on this guideline, Kenneth Clarke authorized DP for long-term use in 1984. Consequently, Upjohn had to comply with several rules; they had to publish a leaflet about the side effects of the drug that was translated into different languages. General practitioners were to receive a letter informing them that they should only prescribe DP if other methods had proven inadequate and only after a long period of counselling with the patient. Informed consent was presented as paramount. Finally, Upjohn was asked to carry out follow-up surveys documenting the side effects of the drug. These strict conditions were implemented in order to ensure that patients could make an informed decision, knowing the risks and benefits of the drug.

Chapter Eight

Trivializing an Extra-ordinary Analgesic: The Example of Tramadol in General Practice

Joséphine Eberhart

Topalgic, Ixprim, Zaldiar, Contramal, Zamudol, … In France, these are the brand names of painkillers that contain tramadol, either alone or in combination with acetaminophen. In the "three-step analgesic ladder" created in 1987 by the World Health Organization (WHO),[1] tramadol is considered as a "weak opioid" – the second step of this WHO classification, on par with codeine and opium powder. Unlike non-opioid analgesics – or Step I analgesics – like aspirin or acetaminophen, Step II analgesics are only available on prescription, because their active principles are similar to morphine, which is a Step III analgesic or "strong" opioid. However, although both Step II and Step III analgesics are opioids that affect the central nervous system, Step II painkillers have a lower analgesic efficacy. As a result, weak opioid analgesics are easier to prescribe[2] than strong opioids whose prescription and delivery is more regulated and marginal in France.

However, in the weak opioid analgesics market, tramadol stands out for its spectacular prescription trajectory. Authorized in France since 1997, tramadol has rapidly become a cornerstone of the painkiller market and is now one of the most prescribed analgesics, far ahead of opium powder and codeine, even though these two painkillers have been in use for more than a century and are therefore better known and understood. In France, tramadol

1 World Health Organization, "Cancer pain relief" (WHO, 1986).

2 Until March 2025, they could not be prescribed using a standard prescription form, and instead required the use of the special secured forms reserved for narcotics.

accounts for 48% of the total weak opioid consumption,[3] which makes it the most common analgesic in this category.

This success can seem surprising for several reasons. First, tramadol-based products have specific characteristics making them atypical analgesics that are not easily manageable in routine clinical use. Second, tramadol was introduced to the French market in the early 2000s, when another pain medication, combining dextropropoxyphene (DXP) and acetaminophen, and marketed under the name Di-Antalvic, was the most prescribed painkiller by far before being withdrawn from the European market in 2011. So how did tramadol come to be prescribed so routinely that it became the first "weak" opioid painkiller used in France in the early 2010s, doubling the famous Di-Antalvic despite characteristics that make it anything but an ordinary painkiller?

The aim of this chapter is to show how, despite tramadol's unfavorable pharmacological risk/benefit profile, pharmaceutical marketers successfully leveraged an alternative evaluative framework – the WHO's influential three-step painkiller ladder – to promote the drug to physicians in a way that emphasized its benefits while downplaying its risks. This chapter examines the different stages of tramadol's trajectory, drawing on multiple sources. It is based on interviews with around thirty general practitioners working in both urban and rural settings, an analysis of pharmaceutical advertisements from a medical newspaper widely read by general practitioners (*Le Quotidien du Médecin*) and a review of scientific, regulatory, and academic literature on tramadol. Although access to internal pharmaceutical company records was denied, the combination of these materials allows for a partial reconstruction of industry strategies and sheds light on how tramadol has been framed in medical practice and discourse. Advertisements are a particularly interesting source, not only because they serve as tools of promotion, but also because they reveal the rhetorical strategies that may be mobilized across other promotional formats used by the pharmaceutical industry, such as training sessions, symposia, or meetings with sales representatives. These ads are specifically designed to "speak" to physicians and to them alone, since in France, direct-to-consumer advertising for prescription drugs is strictly prohibited.

The chapter begins by reviewing the elements that make tramadol an atypical analgesic and explains why its success in general medicine can be described as paradoxical. Then, it examines the role played by the

3 K.Hider-Mlynarz, P. Cavalié, and P. Maison, "Trends in Analgesic Consumption in France over the Last 10 Years and Comparison of Patterns across Europe," *British Journal of Clinical Pharmacology* 84, no. 6 (2018): 1324–34.

pharmaceutical industry to market this unusual molecule as an everyday painkiller. The chapter finally studies the consequences of these strategies on prescribers by showing how the risks inherent in prescribing a painkiller presented as mainstream have been made invisible or, on the contrary, integrated into doctors' prescribing practices.

Tramadol as an Atypical Pain Reliever: Unusual Side Effects in Everyday Clinical Practice

Tramadol is an atypical pain reliever because of its molecular structure. Although it is pharmacologically similar to an opioid, tramadol also shares part of its molecular structure with MAOIs (MonoAmine Oxidase Inhibitors), a particular class of antidepressants. This particular molecular structure is the reason why tramadol causes unusual side effects, even more so because its particular molecular structure allows it to interact with a wide range of medications: this is particularly true for several antidepressants, but also for migraine medications (triptans), some antibiotics (such as linezolid), and some mood stabilizers (such as lithium).

First, the short-term risks of tramadol use are unusual because of their particularly high number and frequency. The label of a codeine-based product has a much smaller number of side effects than the label of a tramadol-based product, which carries greater risk because of its mixed molecular structure. Then, these side effects are also unusual in that physicians are used to dealing with the "classic" side effects of opioids (constipation, nausea, drowsiness) when they prescribe analgesics but they are less likely to have to manage effects such as those of tramadol (confusion, vomiting, euphoria, hallucinations, anxiety, dizziness), especially when such adverse effects seem to be very frequent.[4]

In addition, these side effects seriously affect compliance with other ongoing treatments, as this practitioner explains:

> The problem with tramadol is that in the elderly, it's extremely confusing and, more importantly, it goes through the liver, so for people who already have a lot of medications ... [...] And then when it hurts their liver, they feel queasy, and when they're queasy, they don't take the medication ... But when they get confused with the medication ... In the elderly, it's very common. And then, because they don't realize it, they don't remember it and they keep taking it and it gets worse and worse. *Interview with CV, 55/60-year-old woman, GP in a group practice in the Paris region.*

4 The appendix reproduces the "side effects" section from the leaflets of two medications, one containing codeine and the other tramadol, each combined with acetaminophen.

Finally, the side effects of tramadol are unusual in the sense that they seem particularly unpredictable. Several practitioners described them as "on-off": for some patients everything goes well, while for others the treatment is very poorly tolerated – and this is noticeable from the very first pill. In that case, intolerance is described as "dramatic" or "violent," as this practitioner testifies:

> I prescribe more codeine, maybe because I find tramadol a bit on-off, not when it comes to the quality of the analgesic effect but in terms of side effects. With tramadol, either you can take it or you can't. I mean, from what I've seen in my experience, I've seen it even with young people – not only with the elderly who may become confused or something – but in a twenty-five-year-old. I've seen people who can take it without a hitch and others who come back after two hours and say "I'm vomiting, I'm not feeling well." Oh yeah, yeah, there are some who are not well at all! You can really get knocked down by the side effects of tramadol. *Interview with GB, a 30/35-year-old man, GP in a group practice in Burgundy.*

Here, the fact that the intolerance affects "young people" and not just "elderly people" – who are generally regarded as more vulnerable and therefore seen as more sensitive to the effects of the drug – is what seems to alert the practitioner.

"*Primum non nocere*": The Imperatives of Contemporary General Medicine

Given the short- and long-term risks associated with the use of tramadol-based analgesics, the drug's success is all the more surprising, especially if we consider the contemporary trends in general medicine. Indeed, due to the aging of the population,[5] the shift to ambulatory care,[6] and the increasing prevalence of chronic diseases,[7] practitioners must care for patients who have ever longer prescriptions and who need to begin treatment earlier in their lives. Prescriptions are written by various specialists and are based on a fragile balance of treatments. The general practitioner's role is to ensure that the whole prescription remains consistent when it is renewed or when a problem arises (e.g., error in medication use, missed doses, intercurrent illness). It is

5 L. Auvray and C. Sermet, "Consommations et prescriptions pharmaceutiques chez les personnes âgées. Un état des lieux," *Gérontologie et société* 4, no. 103 (2002): 13–27.

6 M. Bungener, L. Demagny, K. Holtedahl, and A. Letourmy, "La prise en charge du cancer: quel partage des rôles entre médecine générale et médecine spécialisée?," *Pratiques et Organisation des Soins* 40, no. 3 (2009): 191–96.

7 J. Dumit, "Illnesses You Have to Fight to Get: Facts as Forces in Uncertain, Emergent Illnesses," *Social Science & Medicine* 62, no. 3 (2006): 577–90.

also the general practitioner's responsibility to manage medication-related risks, which are more likely to occur as the size of the prescription increases.

The prescription of analgesics is no exception, since all the doctors interviewed indicated that the issue of side effects is central to their choice of medication: a "good" painkiller is, above all, one that causes no or few adverse effects. This is especially true for analgesics, which are perceived as "palliative" drugs intended to act on the symptoms of a condition and therefore increase well-being by alleviating pain. While the short-term risks of "cure" drugs – i.e., those that act on the cause of the condition like antibiotics, for example – can be minimized or ignored by physicians as they represent a "necessary evil,"[8] such effects are considered unacceptable in the case of analgesics precisely because they should not replace pain with other symptoms that could cause more discomfort or functional impairment. As a result, the (apparent) absence of side effects is seen by physicians as one of the advantages of Di-Antalvic – an advantage that tramadol obviously cannot match, to the extent that almost all respondents spontaneously expressed regret at the withdrawal of Di-Antalvic:

> Well, that's when we wonder why we stopped using Di-Antalvic! We didn't have that with Di-Antalvic. Di-Antalvic didn't do that at all, or very rarely! Intolerance to Di-Antalvic is rare. But it is common with tramadol. Side effects are not rare, they're frequent. *Interview with EV, 55/60-year-old woman, GP in a single practice in Burgundy.*

These words could have been uttered by almost all the respondents, as they all compared Di-Antalvic with tramadol during the interview, and they praised Di-Antalvic's safety and efficacy compared to tramadol's frequent side effects.

Tramadol Scrutinized by Health Authorities Over Addiction Risk

Beyond these short-term risks, tramadol's addictive effects are also a cause for concern, which is why it began to be monitored only a few years after its market launch. Since 2009, the French drug agency AFSSAPS[9] has conducted numerous studies on tramadol. In October 2010, the reviewer of

8 A. Vega, "Positivisme et dépendance: les usages socioculturels du médicament chez les médecins généralistes français," *Sciences sociales et santé* 30, no. 3 (2012): 71–102.

9 Agence Française de Sécurité Sanitaire des Produits de Santé (French Agency for the Safety of Health Products), which became the ANSM (Agence

these studies advised that "the prescription of tramadol should not be trivialized." This caution was based on data from the US, Germany, the UK, and Sweden which show that tramadol can be misused and abused because of its psychiatric effects (euphoria, hallucinations, and a heightened sense of of well-being). In addition, the report also indicated that it causes dependence, even at therapeutic doses, and that tramadol withdrawal is particularly difficult to achieve. As a result, AFSSAPS requested that the summary of product characteristics for tramadol include "the risk of misuse, dependence, abuse, and occurrence of a withdrawal syndrome on discontinuation of treatment" and called for "the removal of the qualifier 'low' regarding tramadol's abuse potential," describing the adjective as "falsely reassuring for prescribers."[10] Consequently, the monitoring of tramadol misuse and dependence was strengthened: the conditions for its renewal have become more restrictive and the number of tablets per box as well as the duration of treatment have both been reduced. Since March 2025, tramadol – like other weak opioids – can only be prescribed using "secure prescriptions," a format previously reserved for strong opioids and other controlled substances.

The relatively short period of time between the initial marketing of tramadol and the beginning of its monitoring, as well as the magnitude of the long-term risks identified as warranting surveillance, make it a very different analgesic from codeine-based products, for which such level of risks has not been identified. More significantly, during the European re-evaluation of Di-Antalvic, the French Medicines Agency actively fought to keep dextropropoxyphene on the market – while the UK agency was advocating for its withdrawal due to the risks associated with a drug that was rarely used in their country. The French agency argued that Di-Antalvic was a widely prescribed and well-tolerated analgesic, and therefore safe in clinical practice. One of the main arguments it put forward at the time was that withdrawing Di-Antalvic would likely lead to substitution with tramadol – a newer drug already associated with twice as many adverse events as other weak opioids. In that sense, the French agency's defense of Di-Antalvic was motivated by the desire to limit the public health risks posed by the increasing use of tramadol.

Beyond the positions taken by regulatory agencies, our review of the literature – covering all articles on tramadol indexed in PubMed since the 1980s – shows that tramadol dependence is also becoming a public health issue for countries in North Africa and the Middle East. Indeed, since the 2010s, more

Nationale de Sécurité du Médicament et des Produits de Santé or National Agency for the Safety of Medicines and Health Products) in 2011.

10 Commission Nationale des Stupéfiants et des Psychotropes de l'Afssaps, "Compte rendu de la 89ième réunion du 22 octobre 2010. Adopté le 17 décembre 2010" (AFSSAPS, 2010), 6.

and more papers have highlighted the fact that tramadol has become widely available in these societies. This widespread availability can be explained by the fact that these countries have historically been zones of production and/or transit of opioid substances (especially opium), but also because these are countries with a Muslim tradition and where for many, repression towards psychoactive substances (particularly alcohol) is very strong. The use of a medical substance like tramadol is more socially and legally acceptable and its misuse has multiplied to the point that this drug now represents an important gateway to addiction. Authors from Nigeria,[11] Yemen,[12] the United Arab Emirates,[13] and especially Egypt[14] all discuss the addiction problems caused by tramadol, which one article describes as the substance behind the "African opioid crisis."[15] The common feature of this public health issue in all of these countries is the fact that tramadol addiction particularly affects young urban men. However, this common category masks major social differences in the ways tramadol is used: students (over-)use tramadol for its psychoactive effects to improve both their academic

11 A. Idowu, t A. O. Aremu, A. Olumide, and A. O. Ogunlaja, "Substance abuse among students in selected secondary schools of an urban community of Oyo-state, South West Nigeria: implication for policy action," *African Health Sciences* 18, no. 3 (2018): 776–85.

12 E. A. Abood, J. Scott, and M. Wazaify, "User Experiences of Prescription and Over-The-Counter Drug Abuse in Aden City, Yemen," *Pharmacy: Journal of Pharmacy Education and Practice* 6, no. 3 (2018): 99.

13 H. Alblooshi, G. K. Hulse, A. El Kashef et al., "The pattern of substance use disorder in the United Arab Emirates in 2015: results of a National Rehabilitation Centre cohort study," *Substance Abuse Treatment, Prevention, and Policy* 11, no. 1 (2016): 19.

14 M. Bassiony, G. M. Salah El-Deen, U. Yousef et al., "Adolescent Tramadol Use and Abuse in Egypt," *The American Journal of Drug and Alcohol Abuse* 41, no. 3 (2015): 206–11; M. Bassiony, M. Abdelghani, G. Salah El-Deen, M. Hassan, H. El-Gohari, and U. Youssef, "Opioid Use Disorders Attributed to Tramadol Among Egyptian University Students," *Journal of Addiction Medicine* 12, no. 2 (2018): 150–55; M. Bassiony, U. M. Youssif, R. A. Hussein, and M. Saeed, "Psychiatric Comorbidity Among Egyptian Patients With Opioid Use Disorders Attributed to Tramadol," *Journal of Addiction Medicine* 10, no. 4 (2016): 262–68; I. El-Safty, E. Eltamany, A. Shouman, O. El-Gamel, A. Nada, and W. Ali, "Effect of tramadol addiction alone and its co-abuse with cannabis on urinary excretion of Copper, Zinc, and Calcium among Egyptian addicts," *African Health Sciences* 18, no. 3 (2018): 767–75; C. A. Loffredo, D. N. K. Boulos, Doa'a A. Saleh et al., "Substance Use by Egyptian Youth: Current Patterns and Potential Avenues for Prevention," *Substance Use & Misuse* 50, no 5 (2015): 609–18.

15 L. Salm-Reifferscheidt, "Tramadol: Africa's Opioid Crisis," *Lancet* 391, no. 10134 (2018): 1982–83.

and sexual performances (because tramadol can have an effect on the duration of erection), while poor workers use it to calm the pain, anxiety, and depression caused by their hard working conditions and the absence of social protection.

The focus on the risks of tramadol dependence has been increasingly visible in package inserts. As early as 2006, tramadol dependence issues were included in the list of warnings in the user recommendation for some tramadol-containing medications. Similarly, the list of side effects related to tramadol dependence has become longer and more specific. Since 2015, for Ixprim and Zaldiar, a new paragraph placed at the beginning of the "Warnings/Precautions for Use" states that "addiction and physical and/or psychic dependence may develop even at therapeutic doses. The clinical need for analgesic treatment should be reassessed on a regular basis. For opioid-dependent patients and patients with a history of abuse or dependence, treatment should be of short duration and under strict medical supervision." It is then repeatedly stated that dependence as well as withdrawal syndromes can occur, even when the drug is taken for a short duration and at therapeutic doses.

In light of these findings, tramadol appears to be an atypical analgesic – both highly effective and distinct from other painkillers – that poorly suited to routine general practice, due to both its short-term risks (in terms of side effects especially) and its long-term risks of dependence, particularly when prescribed for chronic pain. In fact, to understand its success, it is necessary to look beyond the individual consultation and examine the way tramadol has been presented to practitioners.

An Industry-Led Success Story – Or How Pharmaceutical Companies Made Tramadol a Mainstream Painkiller

In the 2000s, the promotional campaign for tramadol was at its height: each new formulation of tramadol (pediatric formula, extended-release form, new combination with acetaminophen, etc.) was the subject of an article, and promotional advertisements grew steadily in number, as evidenced by the analysis of all issues of *Le Quotidien du médecin* published in January between 1975 and 2011 (Figure 1). Indeed, the number of advertisements for tramadol-based products increased markedly during the 2000s, from two in January 2000 to eleven in January 2008, while the overall number of advertisements for analgesics decreased significantly, as there were around twenty analgesic advertisements each January from 1975 to 2004, compared with an average of only eight each January between 2005 and 2011. Ultimately, between 2005 and 2009, almost all painkiller advertisements in *Le Quotidien du médecin* were devoted to the promotion of tramadol.

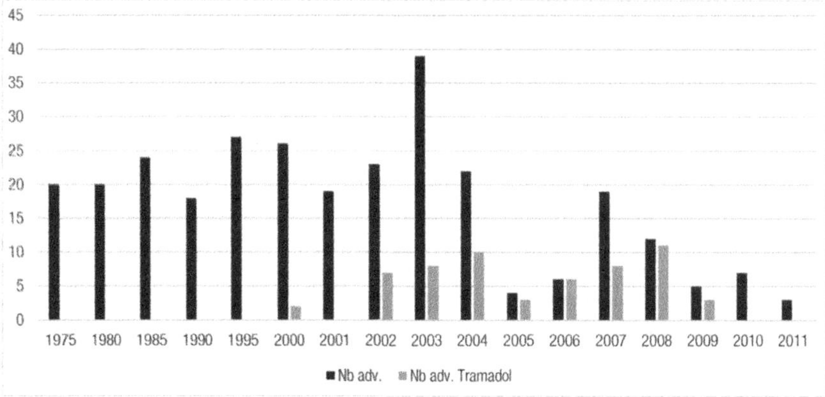

Figure 1. Number of advertisements for a painkiller (all painkillers combined, including tramadol-based) and for a tramadol-based painkiller in *Le Quotidien du médecin* from 1975 to 2011. Source: Issues of *Le Quotidien du médecin* available at the Bibliothèque Nationale de France for the months of January 1975 to January 2011.

Furthermore, the decrease in the total number of ads for painkillers hides the increase in their size: the count refers to the number of advertisements not to the number of pages on which they appeared. Over the period under study, the average size of advertisements increased: while at the beginning of the period there may have been four or five advertisements on one page (often the size of a postcard or smaller), toward the end there were only half-page or full-page advertisements. In short, by the late 2000s, tramadol had a virtual monopoly on painkiller advertising. The physicians surveyed also recalled the intensity of this promotional campaign:

> I remember one day saying to my boss, "Well, the patient is in pain," and he asked me to prescribe Ixprim for him [tramadol + acetaminophen], and I remember that because I wrote it with an X, an apostrophe and "prime" and I said to him, "What on earth is this stuff?" And he answered: "oh, it's a new thing that works great." [...] So that's it, it's because the medical visitors had come before. Clearly, they flooded the market at that point. *Interview with CB, 40/45-year-old woman, GP in a group practice in Burgundy.*

To understand why the pharmaceutical industry launched such a large-scale promotional campaign for tramadol in the 2000s, it is important to recall that in the early 2000s, Di-Antalvic was still the weak-opioid analgesic most prescribed by general practitioners (and even specialists), far ahead of tramadol, codeine and opium powder (see Figure 2). Indeed, if we examine the number of prescriptions for weak opioid analgesics as well

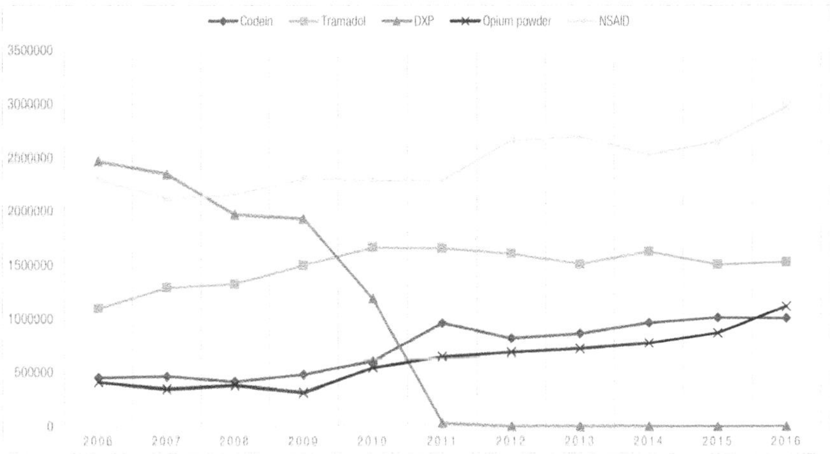

Figure 2. Number of prescriptions for weak opioid analgesics as well as non-steroidal anti-inflammatory drugs (NSAIDs) from spring 2006 to spring 2016 (where "spring" corresponds to the months of March, April, and May). Source: Panel EPPM – IMS Health.

as non-steroidal anti-inflammatory drugs (NSAIDs) from spring 2006 (i.e., March, April, and May) to spring 2016, the combination of dextropropoxyphene (DXP) and acetaminophen accounted for nearly 2.5 million prescriptions in spring 2006, slightly more than the number of prescriptions for NSAIDs (which are nevertheless available over the counter in France). Over the same period, tramadol reached around 1 million prescriptions, while codeine and opium powder accounted for approximately 500,000 prescriptions each. From spring 2006 to spring 2009 (a period during which DXP underwent several evaluations) the number of prescriptions for DXP-based drugs declined slightly, falling to around 2 million in spring 2009. In contrast, prescriptions for tramadol increased rapidly, reaching approximately 1.5 million, while those for codeine and opium powder remained stable. This highlights the extent to which, even at the height of the controversy, DXP continued to occupy a central position in France, to the point that it accounted for more prescriptions than all other weak analgesics (tramadol, opium powder, and codeine).

The DXP-based products were a cornerstone of analgesia in France: they were one of the ten most sold drugs in pharmacies,[16] until their withdrawal from the market in 2011 because DXP's efficacy was deemed insufficiently

16 Data from "Analyse des ventes de médicaments aux officines et aux hôpitaux en France," available for each year.

documented relative to the risks associated with its use.[17] The dominant position of DXP among analgesics highlights the difficulty for new products entering the market to displace Di-Antalvic and the success of pharmaceutical companies in getting tramadol onto physicians' prescriptions.

While the way pharmaceutical companies manage to shape prescribing patterns has already been widely documented by the social sciences,[18] this chapter analyzes both the role played by the context in which the drug was promoted and the strategies used by companies to place the drug at the heart of doctors' prescribing practices.

To do so, I have chosen to study the trajectory of two tramadol-based analgesics that occupy a prominent place on the market. The first is Ixprim, first marketed in 2003 by Sanofi, the company that held the patent for the famous Di-Antalvic; and the second is Zaldiar, marketed the same year by Grünenthal, the German company by which tramadol was first manufactured in the 1970s. Both Ixprim and Zaldiar are combination products – they are composed of tramadol and acetaminophen: this is the most widely prescribed and consumed form of tramadol in France, instead of tramadol alone (with immediate or extended release), which is widely used by German physicians.[19]

Analyzing the promotional strategies deployed by each of these companies allows us to examine different facets of the placement of tramadol in combination in different contexts: that of a pharmaceutical laboratory (Sanofi) that already marketed the dominant painkiller, and that of a company (Grünenthal) that (like all the others) had to place a drug with atypical pharmacological characteristics.

17 Even though most of the discussion in the media focused on the evaluation of DXP-related risks across different countries, it was in fact the lack of efficacy, or more precisely, the near absence of supporting data, that led the EMA to withdraw DXP from the market.

18 Jean-Paul Gaudillière and Ulrike Thoms, "Pharmaceutical firms and the construction of drug markets: From branding to scientific marketing," *History and Technology: An International Journal* 29, no. 2 (2013): 105–15; Jeremy A. Greene and Elizabeth Siegel Watkins, *Prescribed : Writing, Filling, Using and Abusing the Prescription in Modern America* (Johns Hopkins University Press, 2012); Jeremy A. Greene, *Prescribing by Numbers: Drugs and the Definition of Disease* (Johns Hopkins University Press, 2008); Sergio Sismondo and Jeremy A. Greene, eds., *The Pharmaceutical Studies Reader* (Wiley Blackwell, 2015).

19 K. Hedenmalm, J. Slattery, I. Skibicka-Stepien, X. Kurz, and D. Morales, "Prescribing Patterns of Tramadol in Adults in IMS® Primary Care Databases in France and Germany between 1 January 2006 and 30 June 2016," *European Journal of Clinical Pharmacology* 75, no. 5 (2019): 707–16.

Ixprim as the Successor to Di-Antalvic

During the intense promotional campaign for tramadol, the physicians interviewed recall that the pharmaceutical sales representatives themselves compared Di-Antalvic and tramadol and told them that Di-Antalvic would soon be discontinued. Some respondents explained how the pharmaceutical companies promoted Ixprim as the product that would replace DXP, a few months before Di-Antalvic was discontinued:

> **CB:** [...] this is what happened with Ixprim. [...] So, afterwards, did doctors start to be alerted [to the suppression of Di-Antalvic], and so they started to look for something else? When you know something is going to be gone soon then you try to find something else if you need it.
>
> Me: There was no switch to Lamaline [opium powder + acetaminophen + caffeine], [...] do you remember any visits from pharmaceutical sales representatives to promote it?
>
> **CB:** No, you're right, we didn't have many ads on Lamaline ...
>
> **Me:** What about codeine?
>
> **CB:** Whoa, codeine, there's very little advertising. A little bit, but not much.
>
> *Interview with CB, 40/45-year-old woman, GP in a group practice in Burgundy.*

This excerpt shows that Ixprim was seen as a response to the imminent withdrawal of Di-Antalvic, but also that other potential competitors were crowded out by the intense promotional campaign around tramadol.

Sanofi, which marketed the famous Di-Antalvic, organized a transfer of reputation from this product to Ixprim. Thanks to this promotional strategy, Sanofi did not have to market tramadol *ex nihilo* or, therefore, to highlight its intrinsic characteristics. Product placement was ensured at a lower cost since, by creating a continuity between the two products, the advantageous characteristics that physicians attributed to Di-Antalvic were supposedly transferred to Ixprim.

This continuity that Sanofi sought to create between Di-Antalvic and Ixprim is evident in the advertisements published in *Le Quotidien du médecin* in the 2000s. Indeed, advertisements promoting analgesics often rely on the same images or metaphors: they depict pain as a ferocious or indomitable beast which the patient, often tense or withdrawn, must struggle against. The advertisements promoting Di-Antalvic in *Le Quotidien du Médecin* during this period are, however, in stark contrast: far from violence or force, they depict soothing landscapes of a calm nature (a boat or a snowy landscape) printed on a double page of glossy paper. If we compare these advertisements with those for Ixprim, they are strikingly similar: we find the same landscape photographs showing a calm lake, a snow-covered mountain, or sunlit countryside.

It is undeniable that the advertisements for the two products are quite similar and thus create an impression of continuity which is found even in the slogan used: the tagline of Di-Antalvic featured on its advertisements, "It is so much more beautiful when it does not hurt," resonates with the slogan "Without pain, emotion is expressed," which appears on advertisements for Ixprim. Advertising can create or ensure a marketing continuity between two products, which practitioners are expected to see as equivalent. This strategy proved quite effective: one of the respondents, NV – a general practitioner in a group practice in Paris who defined himself as "not very advertising-minded" and even confessed to "hating it," despite "being immersed in it with medical magazines" – remembers very clearly "these ads [that] are very easy to spot": "They were great photos, really beautiful photos [...] they were really striking ads. [...] They were really atypical, very beautiful. I remember them well."

It is worth noting that although Sanofi did not initiate the withdrawal of Di-Antalvic – which was decided by the European Medicines Agency following a lengthy re-evaluation process – the company had, at best, anticipated it, since it never provided the missing efficacy data needed to justify the drug's therapeutic benefits and continued market authorization. At worst, Sanofi may have taken advantage of this opportunity, given that tramadol was sold at twice the price of dextropropoxyphene.

The Trivialization of Tramadol: The Example of Zaldiar

For Grünenthal, as for the other companies marketing tramadol in combination, the challenge was quite different, as they did not have a flagship product from which to organize a transfer of reputation. The promotion of tramadol was therefore based on a simple strategy: making it a normalized part of everyday prescribing practice.

Advertisements in medical journals are revelatory of this strategy. The advertisements depict scenes from day-to-day life (a woman playing sports, going to work, getting ready) in which tramadol becomes an everyday adjunct, as highlighted by the slogan "It takes too long to feel pain." Far from being a powerful analgesic reserved for severe pain, the drug is presented here as an asset for coping with a busy daily life, and therefore a substance intended to facilitate day-to-day life rather than to treat an actual condition.[20] Therefore, tramadol should become part of the ordinary pharmacopoeia, the self-medication that we carry with us for everyday ailments. In one example, the advertisement is divided into four quadrants, each prominently featuring a box of Zaldiar: it protrudes from the pocket of a pair of jeans in the first, from a lab coat in the second, from a man's suit in the third, and from a woman's purse alongside a pair of glasses, a wallet, and a pen in the fourth. In these ads, the patient in pain and their individual characteristics are absent, leaving only the drug and its daily use, as emphasized by the central slogan: "Relief – better have it in your pocket."

In this respect, the strategy for the placement of tramadol is based on references to three elements – firstly, the fact that the product has few undesirable effects; secondly, that it functions as a "facilitator" of daily life before being a drug; and thirdly, that women would be its primary beneficiaries – which are actually *topoi* that are regularly described in studies on the history of medicines analyzing the marketing strategies used to promote them. This is especially true for analgesics but also psychotropic drugs (amphetamines,[21] antidepressants,[22] or tranquilizers[23]), or medications that lie at the intersection of these two categories, as in the case of Librium studied by Andrea Tone,[24] which was promoted for a range of basic indications – from mild to moderate anxiety to tension headaches, and including gastrointestinal, cardiovascular, gynecologic, or dermatologic disorders for "everyday patients" (from mothers to children). For example, the promotion of Zaldiar echoes CIBA's launch of the sleeping pill Doriden in the mid-1950s in West Germany: CIBA had to place this new barbiturate-free hypnotic on a market dominated by thalidomide, which was regarded as harmless before its danger was discovered[25]. The advertisements for Doriden largely promoted the idea that it would not "free" the patient from his stressful life but would support

20 Elizabeth Siegel Watkins, "How the Pill Became a Lifestyle Drug: the Pharmaceutical Industry and Birth Control in the United States since 1960," *American Journal of Public Health* 102, no. 8 (2012): 1462–72.

21 Nicolas Rasmussen, *On Speed: The Many Lives of Amphetamine* (New York University Press, 2008).

22 Lucie Gerber and Jean-Paul Gaudillière, "Marketing Masked Depression: Physicians, Pharmaceutical Firms, and the Redefinition of Mood Disorders in the 1960s and 1970s," *Bulletin of the History of Medicine* 90, no. 3 (2016): 455–90.

23 David Herzberg, *Happy Pills in America: From Miltown to Prozac* (Johns Hopkins University Press, 2008).

24 Andrea Tone, *The Age of Anxiety: A History of America's Turbulent Affair with Tranquilizers* (Basic Books, 2008).

25 Nils Kessel, "Doriden von CIBA – Sleeping Pills, Pharmaceutical Marketing and Thalidomide," *History and Technology* 29, no. 2 (2013): 153–68.

him in his daily activities by adapting to his pace of life (because of its rapid and predictable action). But other similarities can be found with the promotion of Miltown in the 1960s, as described by David Herzberg.[26] The advertisement for Zaldiar echoes elements already present in the advertisements for Miltown: the minor tranquilizer which targets the troubles of the white middle class with intellectual and skilled jobs (with an additional difficulty for women who have to reconcile the imperatives of their careers with those of their families).

This strategy of trivializing tramadol has not gone unnoticed by practitioners: in the interviews, several respondents describe the triumph of tramadol in similar terms. This is what AF, a general practitioner near Paris, explains very well: "[Pharmaceutical companies] were pushing us to prescribe [...]. Ixprim and tramadol were trivialized at the beginning. But they are almost atomic bombs; I never prescribed them the way they advised us to."

This analysis echoes the work of Quentin Ravelli, who studied the promotion campaign for pristinamycin in France[27]. He examined the role played by advertising and argued that it widens the gap between the "latent use value" (what the drug can really be used for, which is found in the user instructions) and the "manifest use value" (what is suggested by the advertising). In the case of combination tramadol, the "manifest use value" suggests that tramadol is a mainstream drug that can be used daily for pain that is not unusual in its intensity or location, in the same way as Di-Antalvic. And yet, the "latent use value" of the drug is in fact much more limited, since the indications for both Zaldiar and Ixprim – which appear in small print on the advertisements and in the user instructions – state that the drug can be used for "moderate to severe pain requiring the use of tramadol." In addition to being tautological (how can a type of pain be defined by the molecule intended to treat it?), this indication contradicts the promotional messages used to advertise tramadol. Physicians' observations in clinical routine also point to the fact that tramadol is a powerful drug compared to equivalent analgesics: it causes more frequent and numerous side effects that seem more unpredictable, which makes it more difficult to manage. Such misleading advertising thus brings into the daily pharmacy a drug whose addictive potential and withdrawal difficulties are well documented.

26 Herzberg, *Happy Pills in America*.

27 Quentin Ravelli, *La Stratégie de la bactérie. Une enquête au coeur de l'industrie pharmaceutique* (Le Seuil, 2015).

Tramadol: A Drug that is "One Step Away" from Codeine?

The strategy of making tramadol a standard treatment has been successful because tramadol has found its place in a relatively small market in France: that of weak opioids or step II analgesics – to use the WHO terminology that all respondents refer to. Popularized in 1987 for the management of cancer pain and subsequently extended to the management of non-cancer pain, this typology is based on three levels of pain – "mild," "mild to moderate," "moderate to severe" – to which the three steps of painkillers are attached.

However, if we look at the main pharmacology textbooks commonly used by medical students in France,[28] we find that the three-step pain ladder is either absent or mentioned very briefly, as in the textbook by Moulin and Coquerel,[29] which only mentions it once. These textbooks all use the opioid/non-opioid typology, although in reality they all classify analgesics in their own way, often using a variation of the WHO classification.

In addition, the WHO classification has been the subject of much criticism.[30] Useful at the time of its publication to generalize the use of analgesics for patients suffering from insufficiently relieved pain, the simplicity of its three-step classification was essential to ensure its dissemination. But today the three-step ladder is criticized for being too restrictive because it does not take into account the different clinical expressions of pain and therefore it prevents physicians from using all the available pharmacopoeia in the best way. In short, the three-step WHO classification overlooks products that relieve certain types of pain (antispasmodics, antidepressants, antiepileptics, etc.) and reduces the landscape of painkillers to those whose analgesic value is based on the presence (or notable absence) of an opioid substance. Conversely, in the alternative classifications, tramadol occupies a marginal position due to its "mixed" molecular structure.[31]

However, the three-step ladder is widely used by respondents, who refer to it repeatedly to describe both the products and the way they prescribe them for pain. In all the records I was able to consult, it is in advertising that

28 Yves Landry and Jean-Paul Gies, *Pharmacologie : Des cibles vers l'indication thérapeutique* (Nouvelle. Dunod, 2003); Michael W. Neal, *Pharmacologie médicale*, 2nd ed. (De Boeck, 2003); Heinz Lullmann and Klaus Mohr, *Atlas de poche de Pharmacologie*, 5th ed. (Lavoisier, 2016); Maurice Moulin and Antoine Coquerel, *Pharmacologie*, 2nd ed. (Masson, 2002).

29 Moulin and Coquerel, *Pharmacologie*.

30 Arthur D. Lipman, Pierre Beaulieu, David Lussier, Frank Porreca, and Anthony H. Dickinson, *Pharmacology of Pain* (IASP Press, 2010).

31 Lipman et al., *Pharmacology of Pain*.

it is most widely used, and it seems, moreover, that its continued use serves the interests of pharmaceutical companies.

The strategy of promoting tramadol in combination also relied on the WHO classification. For example, in some advertisements for Ixprim, one can read "to be used immediately in case of moderate pain," a formula that uses the exact terms of the WHO classification and its logic. Similarly, in the advertisement for Zaldiar the drug is indicated "in the treatment of moderate to severe pain,"[32] which also recalls the original WHO typology. Moreover, the slogan indicates that Zaldiar is "a first-line step 2 analgesic." These references to the three-step WHO ladder serve both as a reminder of tramadol's position in the small weak opioid market and as a first-line pain medication (playing on the fact that the physician's attention will be captured by this "first-line" classification rather than by the idea that it applies only to the step II category).

Therefore, the classification of tramadol as a step II painkiller has helped position it as comparable to other opioid analgesics already on the market and commonly used by prescribers as all-purpose painkillers. In addition, it has obscured its unique molecular structure by reducing it to its opioid nature. This may help explain why, in interviews with practitioners, tramadol's side effects are often described as unusual and unpredictable, partly because it is perceived only as an opioid analgesic and not also as having properties similar to those of an antidepressant. This dual perception helps account for both its characteristic side effects and its place in an alternative classification of analgesics.

Consequences of the Normalization of an Atypical Painkiller

The trivialization of tramadol has direct consequences on the management of the risks inherent to its prescription. On the one hand, while most of the physicians interviewed currently avoid prescribing tramadol and favor other painkillers, some continue to prescribe it, by choice or by necessity, and incorporate the risks associated with its use into their prescribing strategy through a gradual increase in dosage and detailed instructions to patients:

> You start with very small doses, at night, and if you're puking after forty minutes, well, at least you're going to bed, so that's it. But be careful if you take it every day. [...] You have to start with small doses, I say half or one in the evening ... Especially not at bedtime because [otherwise] we won't know if it works or not. [...] So an hour before going to bed, so he has

32 The term "modérées" (mild) is written in bold, and in a different color from that used for the rest of the text, emphasizing the first term and thus participating in the trivialization of the drug.

> time to see if there is a side effect or not, and if it works on the pain or not. And then after that, he can take one, one and a half or two. But he's got to increase the dose gradually. *Interview with AF, a 60/65-year-old man, GP in a single practice in the Paris region.*

> I told the patient "you take one pill at a time [...] and then you see what happens; if it's really not effective, you take two at a time but when you take two at a time, you stay home, you don't step away from your house, you don't drive, nothing at all and you see what happens. *Interview with EV, a 55/60-year-old man, GP in a single practice in Burgundy.*

We can be surprised at how constraining the advice and precautions for managing the risks associated with tramadol use can be (limiting driving, taking it an hour before going to bed, not being home alone when taking it), especially for such a commonly prescribed drug that is supposed to make life easier for the patient. This advice is presented as obvious, as if prescribing this drug went hand in hand with specific precautions, which is far from being usual. When asked about it, general practitioners appear to be so used to dealing with the unwanted effects of tramadol that they automatically give this advice when prescribing it and seem surprised at the idea of reporting them to pharmacovigilance authorities. This leads to an unexpected consequence: the poor handling of tramadol is sometimes attributed to the patients – as if the problem was not with the drug itself but with the many users who do not tolerate it and who must be identified so that they are not prescribed it again;[33] or to the prescribers themselves, since some fear that their warnings act as a form of nocebo effect, as this practitioner indicates:

> I've seen so many patients who are intolerant to tramadol that we're going to be very careful and prescribe it with the usual precautions, but then we don't know if the patient can't tolerate it because you've warned them [laughs], you've really warned them, or are they not tolerating it because they don't have the enzymes to tolerate it. *Interview with AL, a 35/40-year-old man, GP in a group practice in Burgundy.*

In this case, the situation is completely reversed: the practitioner acknowledges that he has seen many patients who are intolerant to tramadol, but for him, the question is whether this is due to the many patients who do not tolerate it or due to his warnings. He does not even consider that the cause may lay in the very prescription of a molecule that is far from harmless even though it is presented as such.

33 Anne-Chantal Hardy, "Oser l'incertain. L'imputation des effets indésirables médicamenteux," *Anthropologie et Santé* 19 (2019).

How can we explain the apparent gap between physicians' awareness of tramadol's risks and their tendency to distance themselves from it in interviews on the one hand, and the still high national prescription rates for this drug on the other hand? First, the general practitioners interviewed represent a particular subset: they are those who agreed to participate in a social science study about their analgesic prescribing practices. These are often practitioners who see fewer patients per day and are more willing to reflect critically on their clinical practices, thus, they tend to be more attentive to the risks associated with the medications they prescribe, especially for a drug as common as tramadol. Even within this sample, however, those who remain favorable to tramadol are often practicing in contexts that shape their risk perception differently. For example, physicians working regularly in emergency departments are more likely to prescribe tramadol, partly because patients rarely return for follow-ups, which alters their perception of risks and benefits as they need a strong analgesic but are less attentive to the risks it may pose, since the patients who will experience those risks will already have been discharged from the ER. Other physicians in highly disadvantaged areas consider tramadol to be more controlled and manageable than over-the-counter codeine (especially in cough syrups) which was widely misused by young people until codeine-based products became prescription drugs in 2017.

Second, national data show that tramadol prescriptions have been declining over the past decade, while prescriptions for other options – like opium powder, codeine, or NSAIDs – have increased. This trend can be attributed to a combination of factors: growing public health warnings; tighter regulatory restrictions on tramadol's prescription and packaging; the publication of clinical guidelines in widely read medical journals; and, finally, the slow but steady diffusion of experiential knowledge among practitioners, which, over time, tends to consolidate around commonly used molecules.

Tramadol Addiction: An Overlooked Risk in General Practice Medicine?

In the long term, trivializing tramadol and presenting it as a weak opioid painkiller similar to codeine or opium powder has led both physicians and patients to downplay the risks of dependence that it generates. On the one hand, physicians are particularly wary of prescribing strong opioids, as they often associate morphine with end-of-life care or dependence – a fear they attribute to their patients but which they also admit to sharing. This apprehension can be explained by the very strict legislation that governed the prescription of strong opioids until recently, since the youngest physicians, even when they have been trained in the use of analgesics during a palliative care course, admit to being reluctant to prescribe them. Indeed, until 1999 in France, doctors had to use a counterfoil book to prescribe strong opioids, i.e., booklets dedicated to the prescription of narcotics that the physician had to order in advance. To write a prescription, it was therefore necessary to fill out several sheets (one kept by the pharmacist, the second by the patient, and the third by the doctor).

At the same time, general practitioners display very little awareness of the issue of dependence induced by weak opioids, which is often discovered in a fortuitous manner, by a call from a pharmacist worried about a patient with several prescriptions from different doctors, by a memo left by a substitute colleague, or even by a question during an interview with a sociologist.[34]

Yet, like any opioid substance, tramadol can lead to addiction. For example, according to data from the medicines agency's addiction monitoring system,[35] tramadol is the opioid analgesic most commonly subject to falsified prescriptions: between 2010 and 2017, 616 suspicious prescriptions containing tramadol were reported, compared to 504 for codeine. It is also the leading substance in all deaths attributable to analgesics as in 2016, for example, 37 deaths were attributable to tramadol compared to 22 for morphine, 16 for codeine and 8 for oxycodone[36]. For the practitioners surveyed, tramadol addiction is particularly difficult to manage, as summarized by this practitioner.

> **EV:** Yes, with tramadol, I had a grandma who was addicted. I took her off the tramadol and she went into withdrawal syndrome! The pain came back, and then on top of all this, she became depressed. [...] So I put her back on it. Because we have nothing against these addictions! Nothing to replace them with. [With other analgesics,] by gradually decreasing the dosage, we have no problem with withdrawal, we manage perfectly well. [...] I have noticed that I worry much more about tramadol, especially in its chronic use, than about morphine. Tramadol poses problems and, in addition, it induces a kind of state of well-being, which is a bit devious. Some people who have used tramadol for a long time find it very difficult to stop taking it. And then there's the idea of the drug! Because patients don't expect to be addicted to tramadol. [...] I have two patients on tramadol who have

34 Joséphine Eberhart, "De la peur de la morphine à la dépendance au tramadol: les médecins généralistes face au mésusage des antalgiques," *Douleurs* 23, no. 3 (2022): 117–25.

35 E. Monzon and N. Richard, *État des lieux de la consommation des antalgiques opioïdes et leurs usages problématiques* (ANSM, 2019).

36 Based on data from "enquête Décès Toxiques par Antalgique" (Toxic Analgesic Deaths survey). See also David Herzberg, *White Market Drugs. Big Pharma and the Hidden History of Addiction in America* (Chicago University Press, 2020).

become addicted and I haven't found a substitute. So we're stuck, whereas an anxiolytic, when you're persuasive with the patient and you take good care of him, it's long, it's not easy, but you manage to wean him off. But with tramadol, I have two cases that cannot be weaned off the drug.

Q34: And what do you do then?

EV: Well, I prescribe them minimal effective doses, that is to say, I prescribe doses that remain low, with the constraint of renewing their prescription regularly and not having the pharmacy issue any additional supply. So we try to control the dosage as best we can. Because stopping was catastrophic, well, the attempt to stop ... Two people ... [...] Insomnia, a state of general malaise that was really striking! Whereas by taking another tramadol tablet... poof!

Interview with EV, a 55/60-year-old man, GP in a single practice in Burgundy.

This excerpt highlights two elements that are related to the mixed nature of the molecule and that greatly complicate the management of tramadol dependence. Due to its antidepressant nature, tramadol produces positive psychoactive effects in some patients, which makes it all the more attractive. In the interview extract, the comparison with withdrawal from anxiolytics is not insignificant. This also contributes to the invisibility of the dependence phenomenon, since for some practitioners, this psychoactive effect is no longer perceived as a risk, but rather as a side effect of the drug – literally, which is ultimately valuable, since it sometimes allows patients to "cope" in a stressful or harmful professional environment, or when faced with a complicated family situation. Tramadol was not introduced for its psychotropic effects, but they appear as an emerging effect as patients request prescription refills and the psychological component of their pain (most often chronic) seems to take precedence over the physical component that the practitioner intended to target at the outset. This is part of the reason why physicians have such difficulty in identifying patients who are "addicted" to tramadol: they do not fit the practitioner's image of the psychoactive substance user (such as the "grandma" in the interview who is very isolated and suffers from loneliness).

But because of its antidepressant nature, the practitioner interviewed also points out a second element regarding the risks induced by tramadol: the fact that complete withdrawal is particularly delicate to achieve. For this respondent, as for others interviewed during the study, the last tramadol tablet seems to be impossible to remove. While this is already a factor in the drug agency's warnings, all of the practitioners interviewed seem to have become aware of this issue through their practice.

The fact that tramadol appears to be a weak opioid analgesic like any other has changed the way practitioners consider the risks inherent in its prescription: in the short term, its iatrogenic effects have been integrated into the advice given by prescribers, while in the long term, the invisibility of its psychotropic effects has led to cases of dependence that are particularly insidious and are not thought of as such by practitioners.

Conclusion

Tramadol has become the leading "weak" opioid prescribed by French general practitioners, surpassing codeine and opium-based preparations, both of which have long been known and available on the market. Its mixed molecular structure (part opioid, part antidepressant) gives rise to a risk/benefit profile that is both unusual and difficult to predict: vomiting, delirium, hallucinations, or euphoria, etc. seem to be more frequent and unpredictable than with other painkillers, while the drug's addictive potential led regulators to tighten its surveillance only a few years after its launch. European pharmacovigilance data confirm these concerns, and reports from North Africa and the Middle East even describe tramadol as a "legal drug" widely consumed for its psychoactive effects. Why, then, has a product carrying such short- and long-term risks become so successful in everyday primary care?

To answer this question, we examined the way in which the pharmaceutical industry has reframed tramadol's risks and benefits, making it a mainstream painkiller through two examples. First, Sanofi's Ixprim inherited the reputation of the wildly popular Di-Antalvic, encouraging prescribers to transfer their confidence from the withdrawn product to its tramadol-acetaminophen successor. Second, Zaldiar cast tramadol as the analgesic of choice for young, active people, as a common product that everyone should have in their pocket, purse, or briefcase.

This strategy of normalization has relied on the use of the three-step pain ladder which positions tramadol in the (very small) weak opioid market. This WHO classification structures the way practitioners think about analgesics and how they compare to one another. The centrality of this classification, which is largely maintained by the pharmaceutical industry, contributes to the invisibility of the original molecular structure of tramadol by reducing it to its opioid character. By foregrounding tramadol's Step II status, promotion recast an ambivalent drug, with pronounced psychoactive properties, into a reassuring medicine whose benefits ostensibly outweighed its harms.

These examples demonstrate that the promotional strategies deployed by pharmaceutical companies are embedded in a specific socio-regulatory configuration that is structured around legal (strict legalization of strong opioids), economic (a market for analgesics with few products, one of which stands out), and scientific factors (general practitioners' insufficient medical training in pain management, which allows for the triumph of a product classification that leads to a biased view of the reality of the available pharmacopoeia).

Within this configuration, industry messaging effectively neutralized risk, allowing tramadol to be widely prescribed while its hazards were either actively managed or rendered invisible. Some physicians responded by abandoning tramadol; others have integrated advice and monitoring protocols into their routine practice. Yet dependence remains largely overlooked because it is assumed to be a problem caused by strong opioids only, a blind spot that is particularly dangerous for a molecule whose psychoactive effects can foster insidious, long-term use.

The trajectory of tramadol in France thus seems to have all the characteristics of what David Herzberg calls "white market drugs,"[37] i.e., drugs that benefit from a marketing authorization and whose use is largely "medically" and thus socially validated by doctors' prescriptions because with such drugs they can resolve various problems that patients present with – but which also have psychoactive effects and different risks, including addiction that is particularly difficult to identify both by the physician and the patient. Tramadol's trajectory reminds us that, when assessing therapeutics, we must look beyond pharmacology alone and pay attention to the social work that stabilizes – or destabilizes – the balance between benefit and risk.

Appendix

Codoliprane – 400 mg acetaminophen / 20 mg codeine

Codeine-related:
At therapeutic doses, the adverse effects of codeine are comparable to those of other opioids but are rarer and more moderate.
Possibility of:
- sedation, euphoria, dysphoria;
- miosis, urinary retention;
- hypersensitivity reaction (pruritus, urticaria and rash);
- constipation, nausea, vomiting;
- somnolence, dizziness
- bronchospasm, respiratory depression (see Contraindications);
- acute abdominal pain syndrome of the biliary or pancreatic type, suggestive of a spasm of the sphincter of Oddi, occurring particularly in cholecystectomized patients;
- pancreatitis: very rare cases of pancreatitis have been reported. There is a risk of withdrawal syndrome in case of abrupt discontinuation, which can be observed in the user and the newborn of a mother intoxicated with codeine (see Fertility/Pregnancy/Nursing).

37 Herzberg, D. 2020. *White Market Drugs: Big Pharma and the Hidden History of Addiction in America*. Chicago University Press.

Ixprim – 325 mg acetaminophen/ 37 mg tramadol

The most frequently reported adverse reactions in clinical trials with tramadol-paracetamol combination are nausea, dizziness, and somnolence, which are observed in more than 10% of patients.

Within each frequency grouping, adverse events are presented in descending order of severity.

Psychiatric Disorders:

- Common (1 to 10% of patients): confusion, mood changes, anxiety, nervousness, euphoria, sleep disturbances.
- Uncommon (0.1 to 1% of patients): depression, hallucinations, nightmares, amnesia.
- Rare (0.01% to 0.1% of patients): drug dependence.

Post-Marketing Surveillance:

- Very rare (less than 0.01%): abuse.

Central and peripheral nervous system disorders:

- Very common (more than 10% of patients): drowsiness, dizziness.
- Common (1–10% of patients): headache, tremor.
- Uncommon (0.1 to 1% of patients): involuntary muscle contractures, paresthesias.
- Rare (0.01% to 0.1% of patients): ataxia, convulsions, syncope.

Visual disturbances:

- Rare (0.01% to 0.1% of patients): blurred vision. Hearing and inner ear disorders:
- Uncommon (0.1% to 1% of patients): tinnitus.

Cardiac System Disorder:

- Infrequent (0.1 to 1% of patients): arrhythmia, tachycardia, palpitations.

Vascular System Disorder:

- Infrequent (0.1 to 1% of patients): hypertension, flushing.

Respiratory, thoracic, and mediastinal disorders:

- Uncommon (0.1 to 1% of patients): dyspnea.

Gastrointestinal disorders:

- Very common (more than 10% of patients): nausea.
- Common (1 to 10% of patients): vomiting, constipation, dry mouth, diarrhea, abdominal pain, dyspepsia, flatulence.
- Infrequent (0.1 to 1% of patients): dysphagia, melaena.

Skin and subcutaneous tissue disorders:

- Common (1 to 10% of patients): sweating, pruritus.
- Uncommon (0.1 to 1% of patients): skin reactions (e.g., rash, urticaria)

Renal and urinary system disorders:

- Infrequent (0.1 to 1% of patients): urinary disorders (dysuria and urinary retention), albuminuria.

General Disorders and Administration Site Conditions:

- Infrequent (0.1 to 1% of patients): chills, chest pain.

Investigations:
- Infrequent (0.1 to 1% of patients): increased transaminases.
Although not observed in clinical studies, the occurrence of adverse reactions known to be related to the administration of tramadol or paracetamol cannot be excluded:
Tramadol:
- Orthostatic hypotension, bradycardia, collapse.
Post-marketing data for tramadol have identified rare changes in the effect of warfarin, in particular an increase in prothrombin time.
- Rarely (0.01% to 0.1% of patients): allergic reactions with respiratory symptoms (e.g., dyspnea, bronchospasm, wheezing, angioedema) and anaphylaxis.
- Rarely (0.01% to 0.1% of patients): change in appetite, muscle weakness, and respiratory depression.
- Worsening of asthma has been reported, although a causal relationship has not been established.
- Withdrawal symptoms have been reported rarely, but including panic attacks, severe anxiety, hallucinations, paresthesias, tinnitus, and other CNS symptoms.

Chapter Nine

Change for Continuity: Temporalities of Risk and Benefit in the French Appetite Suppressant Scandal of Mediator (1976–2009)[1]

Solène Lellinger

Using the case study of the French pharmaceutical agent, Mediator (benfluorex), which led to a major health scandal and a significant reform of drug regulation in France, this chapter demonstrates the manner in which a pharmaceutical agent that was regarded as therapeutically ineffective and labeled "does not harm"[2] by prescribers, and yet remained on the market for decades before being withdrawn, causing harm to thousands of individuals.

Benfluorex was synthesized in the 1960s by the French pharmaceutical company Les Laboratoires Servier (hereafter referred to as *Servier*), as part of its research into the therapeutic potential of amphetamine derivatives for

1 Over the past fifteen years, I have benefited greatly from my exchanges with Nils Kessel, and I would like to express my sincere gratitude to him. His insights have continually informed and enriched my thinking. I am also grateful for his careful reading, which allowed me to strengthen the work presented here. Finally, I would like to thank Nils, David Herzberg, and Joseph M. Gabriel for inviting me to contribute to this book and for their dedicated efforts in preparing and editing it.

2 Anne Crignon, "MEDIATOR. Qui savait quoi?," *Le Nouvel Obs*, November 4, 2011.

the treatment of metabolic disorders. In 1954, trained pharmacist Jacques Servier rebranded his family business in Orléans as Les Laboratoires Servier. The company initially focused its research on cardiovascular therapies, later expanding into the field of metabolic disorders – a category encompassing hormonal dysregulation such as diabetes and lipid metabolism abnormalities.

Benfluorex became a commercial success for *Servier* under its brand name Mediator. Between its market introduction in 1976 and its forced withdrawal in 2009, approximately 145 million packages were sold. In 2009, however, the drug was withdrawn from the French market due to serious cardiopulmonary complications, including drug-induced valvular heart disease (DIVHD) and primary pulmonary hypertension (PPH), both of which caused severe harm – and in many cases, death – among patients.

This paper shows how pharmacology and clinical medicine were used to "reinvent" the drug at three different moments in time by providing new explanations that protected the drug from its withdrawal. *Servier* introduced Mediator in 1976 without acknowledging its potential classification as an amphetamine derivative, for two main reasons. First, the company was already marketing another amphetamine-based appetite suppressant, Ponderal (fenfluramine). Second, it is reasonable to assume that *Servier* executives were aware of the scandals involving amphetamines in West Germany in the late 1960s, as well as in the early stages of a broader reassessment of amphetamine-based appetite suppressants during the 1970s.[3]The company subsequently managed to prevent the drug from being withdrawn from the market in France by strategically dissociating it from the amphetamine category. This was achieved during the fen-phen diet drug controversy in the United States in the late 1990s, despite growing scientific criticism and an official inquiry by the French drug safety agency into the drug's properties. Subsequently, at a third moment in the early 2000s, Mediator became primarily prescribed for weight loss, an off-label use since it had become obsolete in the treatment of "metabolic disorders,"[4] its initial therapeutic indication given for market authorization.

This case prompts numerous inquiries into the regulatory and therapeutic status of a substance over time. Mediator was presented as a revolutionary drug – by hiding its chemical group. The drug's case demonstrates how pharmacological knowledge, such as the classification of substances into specific classes and subclasses, was employed by the manufacturing firm and its

3 Nils Kessel, "Arzneimittelschäden zwischen Regulierung und Skandal. Das Beispiel des Appetithemmers Phentermin 1971," in *Arzneistoffe im 20. Jahrhundert*, ed. Nicholas Eschenbruch, Viola Balz, Ulrike Klöppel, and Marion Hulverscheidt (Transcript, 2009), 283–308.

4 We will return to this classification, which includes diabetes, hypercholesterolemia, hypertriglyceridemia, hyperlipidemia, and hyperuricemia.

affiliated scientists to maintain the drug's market presence. *Servier*'s marketing strategy, which involved altering the classification of the medication in question, proved effective in persuading the French drug regulatory authorities and medical prescribers to perceive the medication as a single entity, despite the presence of contradictory scientific evidence. In the French context, this therapeutic ineffectiveness, coupled with the perception that the drug "can't do any harm," became a way for regulators and prescribing physicians to manage risks.

This chapter thus establishes a nexus between the concepts of risk and benefit associated with pharmaceuticals and the temporal frameworks that govern regulatory mechanisms and market dynamics. The paper, which is supported by archival evidence, published materials concerning this France's major drug scandal,[5] and the results of a survey administered to French cardiologists,[6] suggests that understanding benefits and risks as performative practices is an evolving process that occurs over time. In this process, regulatory agencies, as well as prescribers and manufacturers, play a key role.

From S992 to Mediator: From the Laboratory Bench to Pharmacy Counter

To comprehend the recalibrations in Mediator's benefit-risk balance, it is imperative to delve into its historical origins and the scientific and social milieu that surrounded the discovery of benfluorex. Indeed, the context in which the molecule was developed is a critical factor in comprehending the relationship between its pharmacological profile (its physiological effects on the consumer's body) and its market positioning (which may not correspond to its pharmacological profile). This market positioning gives rise to two profiles: an administrative profile, which is determined by the marketing authorization granted by the regulatory agency, and a commercial

5 In addition to compiling scientific publications on Mediator and anorectic amphetamine derivatives, a key resource for this study is the report by the French General Inspectorate of Social Affairs (IGAS) – which includes a 3000-page tome of appendices containing Mediator's administrative archives, seized by the courts as part of the criminal proceedings. Anne-Carole Bensadon, Etienne Marie, and Aquilino Morelle, "Enquête Sur Le Mediator®: Rapport Définitif" (IGAS, 2011); Anne-Carole Bensadon, Etienne Marie, and Aquilino Morelle, "Enquête sur le Mediator®: Tome annexe" (IGAS, 2011).

6 Solène Lellinger, "Innovation Thérapeutique et Accident Médicamenteux. Socio-Genèse Du Scandale Du Benfluorex (Mediator) et Conditions de Reconnaissance d'une Pathologie Émergente : Les Valvulopathies Médicamenteuses" (PhD dissertation, University of Strasbourg, 2018).

profile, which is determined by the laboratory's advertising. These profiles may overlap to a certain extent.

Research on metabolic diseases, particularly diabetes, has been a long-standing and strategic focus at *Servier*. In 1956, *Servier* introduced Glucidoral, the first hypoglycemic sulfonamide available in France. The company's success compelled it to prioritize diabetes research,[7] culminating in the establishment of a dedicated "diabetes and obesity" department in 1963. The emphasis on metabolic diseases and obesity is firmly rooted in the broader international scientific context. The concept of risk factors first emerged in the 1950s,[8] after the initial results of the Framingham Heart Study.[9] The primary results of the study indicated a correlation between hypertension, obesity, hypercholesterolemia, and an elevated risk of coronary heart disease,[10] thereby signifying a paradigm shift in the realm of cardiovascular health.

7 Sophie Chauveau, *L'invention pharmaceutique: la pharmacie française entre l'État et la société au XXe siècle* (Institut Synthélabo, 1999).

8 Robert A. Aronowitz, *Making Sense of Illness: Science, Society, and Disease* (Cambridge University Press, 1999).

9 "History | Framingham Heart Study," accessed October 16, 2023, https://www.framinghamheartstudy.org/fhs-about/history/. This prospective Study was organized between 1947 and 1949, as part of a public health program concerning cardiovascular disease, a major cause of mortality. The initial cohort of 5209 Framingham residents, aged between twenty-eight and sixty-two, was recruited between 1948 and 1952. The value of such a cohort lies in the fact that it provides a varied, unselected population, intended to be as representative as possible of the American population. For the team of researchers conducting the study, this was fundamental, enabling the inclusion of both healthy and sick people. Since 1948, study subjects have been examined every two years. In 1971, the second generation was included, i.e., the children and spouses of the original participants, while the third generation joined the study in 2002. See Luc Berlivet, "'Association or Causation?' The Debate on the Scientific Status of Risk Factor Epidemiology, 1947–c.1965," in *Making Health Policy: Networks in Research and Policy after 1945*, ed. Virginia Berridge (Rodopi, 2005), 39–74; Gerald M Oppenheimer, "Profiling Risk: The Emergence of Coronary Heart Disease Epidemiology in the United States (1947–70)," *International Journal of Epidemiology* 35, no. 3 (2006): 720–30; Jeremy A. Greene, *Prescribing by Numbers: Drugs and the Definition of Disease* (Johns Hopkins University Press, 2007); Carsten Timmermann, "Appropriating Risk Factors: The Reception of an American Approach to Chronic Disease in the Two German States, c. 1950–1990," *Social History of Medicine* 25, no. 1 (2012): 157–74; Élodie Giroux. "The Framingham Study and the Constitution of a Restrictive Concept of Risk Factor," *Social History of Medicine* 26, no. 1 (2013): 94.

10 Thomas R. Dawber, Felix E. Moore, and George V. Mann, "II. Coronary Heart Disease in the Framingham Study," *American Journal of Public Health*

The advent of the concept of risk factors has transformed the perception of obesity, shifting it from a purely aesthetic issue to a medical concern. The issue of obesity and its metabolic consequences has become a significant challenge for pharmaceutical companies such as *Servier*. The link between obesity and the new nosological category of "metabolic disorders" (which is a general term that encompasses diabetes, hypercholesterolemia, hypertriglyceridemia, hyperlipidemia, and hyperuricemia) is diversifying the pharmacological families of interest beyond sulfonamides. Amphetamines are one such family.

The development of amphetamines in the 1920s, and their subsequent widespread use during the Second World War,[11] led to the exploration of their potential in the treatment of obesity. Researchers in the pharmaceutical industry sought to isolate desirable effects, such as appetite suppression, while minimizing adverse effects, including dependency. *Servier*'s research concentrated on compounds with anorexigenic properties: fenfluramines. This opened a vast area of research: "the unusual pharmacological properties and clinical usefulness of fenfluramine ... have stimulated further study of a large number of related compounds."[12] *Servier* commercialized fenfluramine in France as Ponderal in 1968. The Food & Drug Administration (FDA) approved it as Pondimin and Ponderol in the United States in 1973.[13]

In 1966, by "continuing the screening of fenfluramine congeners,"[14] this group of *Servier* researchers were interested in a derivative referred to as S992.[15] The substance was first presented in 1969, at the International Symposium on Amphetamines and Related Compounds, alongside numerous other experimental molecules and was regarded as a highly promising prospect[16]: this compound "shows properties similar to those of fenflura-

and the Nation's Health 47, no. 4.2 (1957): 4–24. The medical term for this is *arteriosclerosis*. For more details, see Harry M. Marks. *The Progress of Experiment: Science and Therapeutic Reform in the United States, 1900–1990* (Cambridge University Press, 1997).

11 Nicolas Rasmussen, *On Speed: The Many Lives of Amphetamine* (NYU Press, 2008).

12 L. Beregi et al., "Structure-Activity Relationships in CF3-Substituted Phenethylamines," in *International Symposium on Amphetamines and Related Compounds*, ed. Erminio Costa and Silvio Garattini (Raven Press, 1970), 22.

13 Alicia Mundy, *Dispensing with the Truth: The Victims, the Drug Companies, and the Dramatic Story Behind the Battle Over Fen-Phen* (St. Martin's Press, 2001), 39.

14 J. Duhault and C. Malen, "Effect of a fenfluramine derivative (S 992) on lipid and glucose metabolism," in *International Symposium*, ed. Costa and Garattini, 619.

15 Laszlo Beregi, Pierre Hugon, and Jean-Claude Le Douarec, "Brevet spécial de médicament. PV n°112.833 N°6.564 'Médicaments à base de nouveaux dérivés du phényl-amino propane,'" issued December 23, 1968.

16 See Beregi et al. "Structure-Activity Relationships in CF3-Substituted Phenethylamines," 39–45. "We chose compound 70 (S992), which appeared

mine, but 10 times less toxic,"[17] due to apparently low absorption rates (identified based on remaining urinary concentrations). Although the notion of "toxicity" was not clearly explained during the symposium, it appears to be due to the product's rapid metabolism and because of a "lack of untoward effects."[18] This study showed that this molecule reduced food intake in rats and influenced blood glucose and triglyceride levels. This makes the molecule a potential treatment for several metabolic disorders.

In 1971, the WHO assigned the International Nonproprietary Name S992 to "benfluorex". Two years later, in November 1973, *Servier* submitted a marketing authorization application for Mediator to the Service central de la pharmacie et des medicaments (Central Department of Pharmacy and Medicines), under the authority of the Minister of Public Health and Social Security.[19] This regulatory step turns the molecule, a scientific entity, into a commercial one, the authorized product. While the literature has extensively shown how drugs are "looking for diseases" and their markets, it can be argued that drugs are also looking for their "public" profile.[20] When submitting a market approval application, the laboratory indicates the intended uses of the drug. This may result in a discrepancy between the pharmacological and administrative profiles of the drug. The molecule is designed to address a specific clinical situation and therefore falls into a particular nosological category.

Professor Guignard was commissioned on December 20, 1973, to report back within fifteen days. In accordance with several 1972 decrees, in a post-thalidomide context,[21] the evaluation constraints are manifold, and these "specify the protocols to be applied to the analytical, toxicological, pharmacological, and clinical appraisals of drugs."[22] The report should summarize the information in the file, especially the toxico-pharmacological and clinical assessments. The report concluded in the case of Mediator that "the present

---

to be the most effective orally, both in rats and in dogs, in order to compare its intensity and duration of action with fenfluramine. … Whether S992 is active *per se*, or its activity is a result of metabolic conversion by undergoing a rapid *in vivo* hydrolysis of the re-arrangement of this drug could be accepted, the active entity is clearly a potent anorexic."

17 Duhault and Malen, "Effect of a fenfluramine derivative (S 992)," 619.

18 Beregi et al., "Structure-Activity Relationships," 39 and 45.

19 Bensadon, Marie, and Morelle, "Enquête sur le Mediator®," 646–50, ANNEXE 2-3: "Dossier de présentation Mediator."

20 Rein Vos, *Drugs Looking for Diseases: Innovative Drug Research and the Development of the Beta Blockers and the Calcium Antagonists. Developments in Cardiovascular Medicine* (Kluwer Academic Publishers, 1991).

21 See Nils Kessel's chapter in this book.

22 Chauveau, *L'invention pharmaceutique*, 477.

application for a new drug in the fenfluramine family with anti-atheromatous metabolic properties ... appears acceptable from a toxico-pharmaco-clinical point of view."[23] The rapporteur emphasizes, with his conclusion, that benfluorex belongs to the pharmacological family of fenfluramines, which are anorexigenic derivatives of amphetamines. On April 1, 1974, the compagnie was asked to provide additional information, "according to the dossier, a metabolic study should be carried out in view of the chemical links between the molecule and fenfluramine." *Servier*'s response distances benfluorex from fenfluramines. This leads the rapporteur to conclude that "the metabolism of Mediator does not pass through the fenfluramine stage." Guignard also notes that "further investigation of the clinical and biological tolerability of this product, which is intended for long-term use, is necessary."[24] Treatments for metabolic disorders require long-term use. French regulations were influenced by new European standards from 1965 and 1970, but these standards were not the main factor. Rather, it was quite clear from the beginning that tolerance in long-term treatment was an issue.

So, the relationship between fenfluramine and benfluorex was not an argument for marketing authorization, nor was it emphasized by *Servier*. *Servier* subsequently set aside this link in scientific and commercial communications to position the drug in a therapeutic area other than weight loss. Thus, while the chemical relationship with anorectic amphetamine derivatives has been established, it does not condition the molecule's marketing authorization, or the benefits promoted by the company. Although its pharmacological profile establishes it as an anorexigenic agent, its administrative profile – at the manufacturer's request – is for "metabolic disorders, atherogenic carbohydrate-lipid metabolic disorders," "lipid metabolism disorders," and "carbohydrate metabolic disorders." This avoids self-competition. As noted above, for example, *Servier* had already marketed Ponderal as an obesity treatment at that time. This self-competition is less clear-cut when it comes to Glucidoral, an anti-diabetic drug already on the market. Mediator is presented as acting on the entire metabolism, not just the carbohydrate metabolism. This approach may seem surprising given that, during that time, clinicians treated its various risk factors separately and manufacturers sought to offer different treatments for each metabolic entity. Jeremy A. Greene, for example, has described these kinds of strategies.[25] Finally, the multiple positioning of *Servier*'s drug means that its molecules are complementary.

23 Bensadon, Marie, and Morelle, "Enquête sur le Mediator®," 649, ANNEXE 2–3: "Dossier de présentation Mediator."

24 Bensadon, Marie, and Morelle, "Enquête sur le Mediator®," 651, ANNEXE 2–4: "Courrier du 1er avril 1974 Laboratoires Servier au ministère de la Santé."

25 See Greene, *Prescribing by Numbers.*

Evaluators clearly saw what *Servier* tried to prevent the authorities and prescribers from seeing during the following decades. As its name suggests, benfluorex is a derivative of amphetamines and, as such, is potentially dangerous for long-term use. The discrepancy between the pharmacological and administrative profiles can result in overlooking the risks associated with this type of molecule. These risks have been identified, as we will now see.

Amphetamine- and Drug-Induced Valvular Heart Disease: A Long Story

The cardiotoxicity of amphetamines became apparent in the 1960s. In 1965, aminorex was introduced in Switzerland, Germany, and Austria under the brand name Menocil.[26] This molecule, whose structure is similar to adrenaline, was used to treat overweight individuals.[27]

Following this, "a surprising number of young people – mainly in their twenties and thirties, and 80 percent of them women – began coming to cardiology clinics gasping for breath."[28] They were suffering from primary pulmonary hypertension (PPH), a rare lung disease characterized by abnormally high blood pressure in the pulmonary artery, which carries blood from the heart to the lungs. The main symptom is shortness of breath. A study showed that 80% of the 500 to 850 cases occurred in patients who had taken Aminorex. This correlation was discussed at a hearing in the Mediator criminal trial on October 1, 2019.

Another example is phentermine, which was approved in the United States in 1959. During the same period, this molecule was also commercialized as an anorectic drug in Germany. In 1971, two women who had taken drugs containing phentermine died from PPH.[29] Some researchers blamed phentermine for having the same effects as aminorex and called for the withdrawal of all amphetamines in anorectic drugs by establishing a reasoning of

26 Nils Kessel, "Umstrittene Expertise. Der Beirat 'Arzneimittelsicherheit' in der bundesdeutschen Arzneimittelregulierung 1968–1976," *Medizinhistorisches Journal* 44, no. 1 (2009): 61–93.

27 Edward Byrne-Quinn and Robert F. Grover, "Aminorex (Menocil) and Amphetamine: Acute and Chronic Effects on Pulmonary and Systemic Haemodynamics in the Calf," *Thorax* 27, no. 1 (1972): 127–31.

28 Rasmussen, *On Speed*, 240.

29 Nils Kessel, "Arzneimittelschäden Zwischen Regulierung und Skandal. Das Beispiel des Appetithemmers Phentermin (1971)," in *Arzneistoffe im 20. Jahrhundert. Historische Skizzen von Lebertran bis Contergan*, ed. Nicholas Eschenbruch et al. (Transcript, 2009), 283–308.

chemical analogy. However, there were far too few case reports to establish scientific evidence. Nevertheless, in response to government pressure, pharmaceutical companies replaced phentermine with other therapeutic agents in their anorectic drugs.

Servier has not been untouched by the identification of amphetamine toxicity in the cardiovascular system. In 1985, the same manufacturer introduced a new version of fenfluramine with only one isomer – the active one – called dexfenfluramine.[30] It was marketed as Isomeride in France. The FDA authorized this molecule in the US in 1996 under the name Redux.[31] Both fenfluramine and dexfenfluramine were met with great success due to their significant weight loss effects when combined with phentermine. In fact, this diet drug combination was known as the "Fen-phen Cocktail," wherein "the anorexigenic effects of fenfluramine could be duplicated and its side effects minimized by the use of smaller doses of the drug in combination with phentermine." From 1992 to 1996, the annual number of prescriptions increased from 2,000,000 to 11,000,000 for phentermine and from 69,000 to 7,000,000 for fenfluramines.[32]

The first observation of a link between fenfluramine and PPH was published in 1981,[33] before dexfenfluramine had been commercialized. Ten years later, French doctors conducted a five-year retrospective study of seventy-three patients with PPH and observed that 20% had taken fenfluramine. In 67% of these cases, they found a correlation between consumption of the drug and the disease.[34] Following these findings, *Servier* launched the International Primary Pulmonary Hypertension Study (IPPHS).[35]

30 It is a purified form of fenfluramine thought to have fewer side effects and lower toxicity than fenfluramine.

31 Camille Tragos, "Fen-Phen Litigation Against American Home Products Corporation: The Widespread Use of Fenfluramine (Pondimin) and Dexfenfluramine (Redux) for Weight Loss, The Health Problems Associated with Those Drugs, the Resulting Litigation Against American Home Prod" (Masters Paper, Harvard Law School, 2000), 32, http://dash.harvard.edu/bitstream/handle/1/8965626/Tragos%2c_Camille.html?sequence=2.

32 Leslie Iversen, *Speed, Ecstasy, Ritalin: The Science of Amphetamines* (Oxford University Press, 2008), 42.

33 J. G. Douglas et al., "Pulmonary Hypertension and Fenfluramine," *British Medical Journal (Clinical Research Edition)* 283, no. 6296 (1981): 881–83.

34 F. Brenot et al., "Primary Pulmonary Hypertension and Fenfluramine Use," *British Heart Journal* 70, no. 6 (1993): 537–41.

35 L. Abenhaim et al., "Appetite-Suppressant Drugs and the Risk of Primary Pulmonary Hypertension. International Primary Pulmonary Hypertension Study Group," *The New England Journal of Medicine* 335, no. 9 (1996): 609–16.

The IPPHS showed that anorexigenic drug use, particularly fenfluramine use, increased the risk of developing PPH. As a result, the French regulatory system restricted the use of amphetamines and fenfluramines in 1995. Meanwhile, dexfenfluramine (Redux) was introduced to the US market. In 1997,[36] the first publication discussing a link between fenfluramine and valvular heart disease was published, describing observations made at the Mayo Clinic. The physicians had observed a group of twenty-four patients with valvular heart disease who had also taken fen-phen. The physicians observed damaged valves thickened by fibrous material that did not function normally. This type of damage resembled that caused by carcinoid cancer or migraine medications (ergotamine or methylergometrine).

The drugs were withdrawn by the FDA, drawing much media attention. Class action lawsuits have been filed against the manufacturer in the US and Canada. However, the drug was withdrawn from the market in France without any compensation for victims. The difference in reaction between France and the US regarding fenfluramines can be explained by their different judicial structures and cultures of judicialization of medicine. In France, all amphetamine derivatives have been withdrawn from the market, except for Mediator. However, the effects of the administrative dissociation between benfluorex and fenfluramine can also explain why Mediator remained on the market.

Apart from the Agency's dysfunctional approach, an aggravating factor is the positioning of Mediator as something other than an amphetamine, which is a direct consequence of the commercial profile forged by the laboratory. Additionally, a lack of pharmacological knowledge amongst some doctors meant that they could not "read" the international non-proprietary name of Mediator, benfluorex, and misinterpreted the suffix -orex.

Finally, benfluorex was marketed in more than fifty countries (in southern Europe, and countries in Latin America, South Asia, and Africa) from 1976 as a treatment for a metabolic disorder.[37] This prevented the emergence of

36 Heidi M. Connolly et al., "Valvular Heart Disease Associated with Fenfluramine–Phentermine," *New England Journal of Medicine* 337, no. 9 (1997): 581–88; L. B. Cannistra, S. M. Davis, and A. G. Bauman, "Valvular Heart Disease Associated with Dexfenfluramine," *New England Journal of Medicine* 337, no. 9 (1997): 636.

37 Refusal report published on June 16, 2006, by the FDA. After contacting the Division of Drug Information of the Food and Drug Administration in February 2015 regarding this matter, it appears that they were unable to provide me with any information on this finding because access to marketing authorization files for rejected drugs is not available: "Because Benfluorex is not an FDA-approved drug, any information on Benfluorex that has been submitted to the FDA is considered confidential and cannot be released to the public."

a potential signal regarding benfluorex that was unrelated to the attention given to this family of molecules in the United States. The risk associated with a molecule from another continent was completely overlooked. The initial administrative dissociation only grew stronger throughout Mediator's time on the market. This moves it further and further away from its initial pharmacological profile. A decade-long story then began about changing Mediator indications that also responded to the need to dissociate Mediator from amphetamines.

Chameleon Marketing: How to Adapt Pharmacological Information to Commercial Interest

In its request, *Servier* planned to start marketing the product in October 1974, but Mediator was not marketed until 1976. I hypothesize that some of this time was devoted to preparing the promotional campaign for Mediator, thereby creating its commercial profile. During this initial period, Mediator was promoted by *Servier* as a treatment for metabolic disorders. This campaign presents Mediator as a "discovery" that is the "logical treatment for atherogenic lipids and carbohydrate overload" and which "directs lipids towards the Krebs cycle."[38] The benefit-risk balance, that is, is tilted in favor of the prevention of cardiovascular disease, where this treatment is presented and defended as acting on the whole metabolism.

In addition to this positioning choice, we could study the company's "scientific marketing." Gaudillière and Thoms describe scientific marketing as comprising promotional techniques that go beyond brand promotion as practiced in other sectors. These techniques mobilize "science" in two ways: first, the science of marketing is used to design campaigns; second, scientific arguments are used within the campaigns themselves, such as research data and graphical representations, to present drugs as innovative[39] – or, in the case of Mediator, as "revolutionary." This study of the promotional campaign reveals that the chemical relationship of the product with fenfluramines has been erased, thereby removing it from the amphetamine family. This opens the door to a risk-based interpretation of the product.

Marketing authorization for Mediator was granted on July 16, 1974. This evolved during the years the drug was on the market (Table 1). Approved in

38 See Lellinger, "Innovation Thérapeutique et Accident Médicamenteux," 98–105.

39 Jean-Paul Gaudillière and Ulrike Thoms, *The Development of Scientific Marketing in the Twentieth Century: Research for Sales in the Pharmaceutical Industry* (Routledge, 2013).

1974 for the treatment of "metabolic disorders, atherogenic glucido-lipidic metabolic disorders," "lipid metabolic disorders," and "carbohydrate metabolic disorders," the molecule was only given the indication "adjuvant of adapted diet in overweight diabetics" when it was withdrawn in 2009.

Table 1. Changes in Mediator marketing authorization in France over the years.

Years	Prescription indications
1974	"metabolic disorders, atherogenic carbohydrate-lipid metabolic disorders" "lipid metabolism disorders" "carbohydrate metabolic disorders"
1979	"endogenous hypercholesterolemia and hypertriglyceridemia in adults, isolated or associated, when an adapted and assiduous diet has proved insufficient or when cholesterol levels after dieting remain high and/or there are associated risk factors; continued dieting is always essential" "adjuvant of diet in asymptomatic overweight diabetes"
1987	"adjuvant of adapted diet in hypertriglyceridemia" *loss of indication for diabetes that was not applied*
1995	**Prohibition is only on compounded preparations**
1997	"adjuvant of adapted diet in hypertriglyceridemia" *withdrawal of indication for diabetes (not applied)*
2001	"adjuvant of adapted diet in hypertriglyceridemia" "adjuvant of adapted diet in overweight diabetics"
2007	"adjuvant of adapted diet in overweight diabetics"
2009	**Withdrawal**

This review of the indications suggests that there is another factor besides the distancing from fenfluramines and therefore amphetamines in the identification of the risks of benfluorex. We see that in 1979 overweight diabetics were mentioned. At that time, the focus was not on treating overweight individuals but on addressing the associated risk factors. In other words, this does not bring us closer to understanding its anorexigenic nature.

Mediator was evaluated by several committees of the agency responsible for regulating medicines. In fact, the committee responsible for the marketing authorization and re-evaluation of this authorization was divided by therapeutic class. As part of an update to drug dossiers in 1987, following the implementation of a European directive, a second modification took place. Mediator was initially reevaluated alongside drugs in the "drugs used in cardiovascular medicine" class. It was then approved as an "adjuvant to an appropriate diet for hypertriglyceridemia." Mediator lost one of its indications (the one relating to diabetes) and was only classified as an "adjuvant."

This classification implies that Mediator is not a treatment in its own right, but rather a supplement for patients already undergoing treatment. Two years later, Mediator was reevaluated and placed in the class of "antidiabetics and hyperglycemic agents." However, this evaluation did not reach the same conclusion, and the change did not take effect. Two committees issued different recommendations about the same molecule in a completely disconnected manner. The second committee does not mention the first committee's conclusions at all. The same problem occurred between 1997 and 2001 when the diabetes indication was not lost.

In 1995, Mediator was banned from compounded preparations, which are medicines prepared directly by pharmacists in pharmacies as opposed to ready-to use treatments. This was a direct consequence of the identified adverse effects and the withdrawal of fenfluramines, as mentioned above. Post-withdrawal administrative investigations identified this as a major dysfunction because the ready-to-use version was not affected. At that time, the dissociation of the pharmacological profile from the administrative and commercial profile of Mediator had direct consequences.

The history of Mediator illustrates the tensions that can exist between pharmacological profile of a molecule, administrative profile, and commercial profile. The pharmaceutical company submits a marketing authorization application for certain indications, which the administrative authority validates based on a dossier combining scientific, technical, and pharmacological aspects. Therefore, it is up to the laboratory to decide which indication to apply for, and consequently, which benefit to pursue. These indications are not acquired forever, but are subject to regular re-evaluations that impact the pharmaceutical company's strategy. Additionally, these indications are based on studies designed with a specific goal in mind by *Servier* researchers (Figure 1), which will also guide the promotion process, in a scientific marketing approach.

The key issue is not so much the quantitative analysis of the data (which reveals that the number of publications remains limited), but the study of the periods of more intense publication. This inventory retraces all publications over the period 1969–2013. Most of these studies were funded and published by *Servier* researchers from the "diabetes and obesity" department.[40] Let's examine two significant time periods. Most publications date back to the mid-1970s. These publications were intended to accompany the marketing of Mediator, which may explain the two-year gap between the granting of marketing authorization and the launch of the product. Marketing efforts included a large-scale advertising campaign with brochures distributed to doctors that highlighted the promising results of these studies and extolled

40 Lellinger, "Innovation Thérapeutique et Accident Médicamenteux," 136–37.

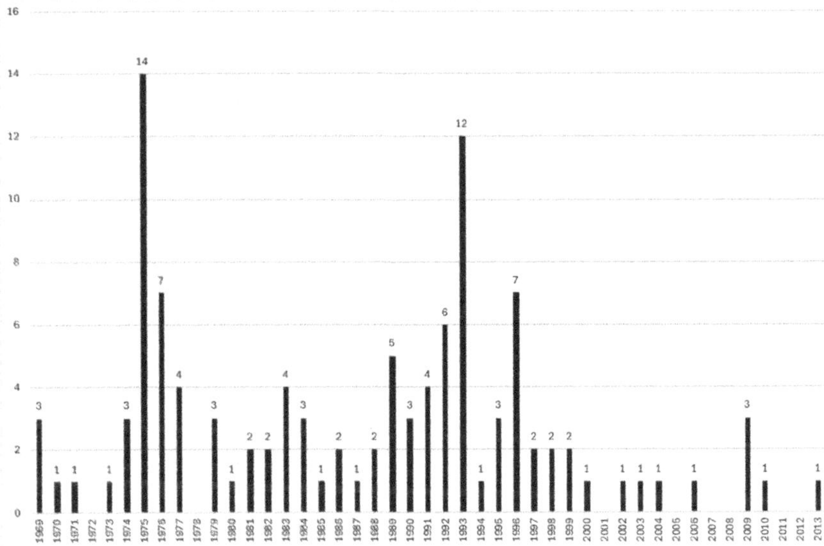

Figure 1. Number of publications per year on benfluorex/S992/780SE from 1969 to 2013. This overview of publications was initially compiled using PubMed to find publications, and then the bibliographies of those publications were used to create a database.

the benefits of Mediator in response to cardiovascular risks faced by people with metabolic disorders. There was also a press conference, traces of which can be found in the medical press in the form of a special issue.[41]

A second turning point occurred after the re-evaluation of Mediator in the 1990s. After the risk of losing the diabetes indication at the end of the 1980s, there was an increase in publications highlighting the beneficial effects of Mediator for this indication. This strategy is more quantitative than qualitative when considering the recognition indices of the medical journals in question. Re-evaluations of drugs are carried out on the basis of 1) new pharmacovigilance data (new risk assessment), 2) a request from the company to include new indications based on post-marketing clinical trials, or 3) drug regulation (every five years) and their evolution (particularly the link with the emergence of European drug regulations[42]) (administrative assessment).

In this case, these are not pharmacovigilance signals, but rather a downward reassessment of the drug's clinical efficacy. This has prompted the

41 *La Médecine Praticienne* no. 643, special issue on Mediator (November 1976): 2.

42 Boris Hauray, *L'Europe du médicament: politique, expertise, intérêts privés* (Presses de la Fondation nationale des sciences politiques, 2006).

laboratory to attempt to regain lost indications. This has changed the focus of scientific studies. In the early 1990s, *Servier* responded to the loss of diabetes indications with publications from *Servier* researchers linking to the benefits of Mediator for this condition. It also led to an "adaptation" of the pharmaceutical company's marketing strategies to promote the drug.

The last period, from 2009 onward, with one exception in 2003, which we will examine in more detail later, focuses primarily on the risks of Mediator. There was a change in tone, as well as a change in participants, involving researchers other than those from *Servier*.

From Off-Label Use of a "Useless" Drug to Drug Scandal.

Following the withdrawal of amphetamine derivatives from the French market, several factors contributed to keeping Mediator on the market in a context where the risk of cardiopulmonary pathologies (PPH and DIVHD) had been identified.

First, as mentioned above, the market positioning of Mediator as a treatment for metabolic disorders distanced it from its kinship with fenfluramines, which slowed the recognition of side effects. Second, the Mediator case exemplified the problem of conflicts of interest between manufacturers and the agency responsible for drug regulation, as demonstrated in previous work.[43]. The Mediator case reveals a dichotomy between doctors' perceptions and judicial investigations, highlighting the normalization of conflicts of interest. Doctors view conflicts of interest as someone else's problem, not their own. The judicial system individualizes responsibility, distancing doctors from systemic problems, viewing transparency measures and legal proceedings as superficial responses rather than real solutions to conflicts of interest.

Another factor that is somewhat related is the perception of Mediator among healthcare professionals and their ability to identify its toxic effects. As we have seen, Mediator was initially approved for the treatment of metabolic disorders. General practitioners and endocrinologists mainly prescribed

43 Solène Lellinger and Christian Bonah, "'This Corporation Has "Anesthetized" the Actors in the Drug Chain'. Influence Peddling and the Normality of Conflicts of Interest in the Mediator® Scandal," in *Conflict of Interest and Medicine: Knowledge, Practices, and Mobilizations*, ed. Boris Hauray, Henri Boullier, Jean-Paul Gaudillière, and Hélène Michel (Routledge, 2021), 181–200.

this treatment.[44] Cardiologists, on the other hand, monitor cardiac pathology caused by Mediator. Cardiologists are not necessarily aware of all the treatments patients are taking for various reasons. For example, patients may not mention treatments prescribed by another specialist or may not consider them relevant to this consultation. In the case of Mediator, however, it is considered "shameful" to use the drug off-label for weight loss (prioritizing its pharmacological profile over its administrative and commercial profile).

From 2012 to 2015, a survey was conducted among French cardiologists to identify how they relate to and diagnose DIVHD.[45] The survey aimed to understand the under-recognition of DIVHD caused by benfluorex during its thirty years on the market. It tested the hypothesis of etiological crossover, which leads to confusion between DIVHD and another declining type of pathology: rheumatic heart disease. Among other things, this survey questioned cardiologists' relationship with Mediator. Although they rarely prescribe this drug,[46] they are nevertheless specialists in the organ affected by its consequences for several patients.[47] This raises the question of "fragmentation" in patient care provided by different specialists.

The cardiologists were asked about their perception of the drug before it was withdrawn. The results, based on a multiple-choice question, show that the perception of the drug varies according to cardiologists' graduation period (Figure 2).[48]

44 According to the user survey (see Lellinger, "Innovation Thérapeutique et Accident Médicamenteux"), confirmed in a telephone conversation with the French health insurance company.

45 Solène Lellinger, "Naissance et Reconnaissance d'une Pathologie Nouvelle : Le Cas Des Valvulopathies Médicamenteuses Sous Benfluorex (Mediator®). Enquête Sur Les Pratiques Des Cardiologues Français" (Masters dissertation, Université de Strasbourg, 2012); Lellinger, "Innovation Thérapeutique et Accident Médicamenteux." The survey was completed by 173 people.

46 Lellinger, "Innovation Thérapeutique et Accident Médicamenteux," 324. Over 94% of cardiologists surveyed said they had not prescribed Mediator (around 2% were unsure), over 86% had not prescribed it again (7.5% were unsure), and over 58% had not extended a prescription (around 17% were unsure).

47 Published data estimate that one in every 1,000 patients exposed to Mediator develops drug-induced valvulopathy. See Alain Weill et al., "Benfluorex and Valvular Heart Disease: A Cohort Study of a Million People with Diabetes Mellitus," *Pharmacoepidemiology and Drug Safety* 19, no. 12 (2010): 1256–62.

48 Number of cardiologists trained between 1970 and 1979 = 14; between 1980 and 1989 = 69; between 1990 and 1999 = 51; between 2000 and 2009 = 34; after 2010 = 5. The indicator is the date of graduation.

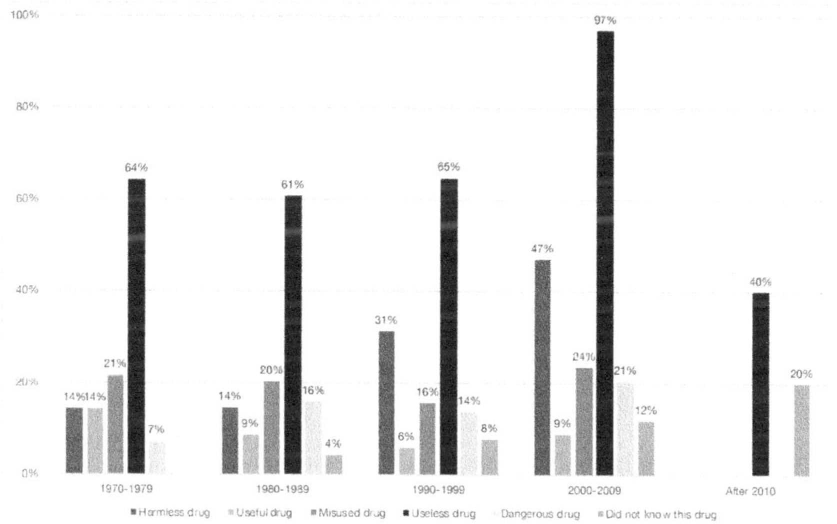

Figure 2. Surveyed cardiologists' opinions of the usefulness of Mediator according to the period in which they obtained their graduation.

Among the cardiologists surveyed who graduated in the 2000s, Mediator was widely perceived as a useless drug, though almost half of the cardiologists questioned deemed it harmless. A similar phenomenon, though to a lesser extent, was observed among cardiologists who had graduated in the previous decade. The highest proportion of cardiologists who considered the drug useful occurred in the period from 1970 to 1979, as did the lowest proportion who considered it dangerous. This period was closest to when the molecule was first marketed.

The proportion of surveyed cardiologists who felt the drug had been misused remained relatively constant across all time periods except among those who graduated in the 1990s, when it was slightly lower. However, it is difficult to draw conclusions from the small sample size of cardiologists who graduated after 2010. Overall, the drug was perceived as useless and relatively harmless. In this case, the theoretical benefit that would justify a drug's presence on the market is unclear. As long as there are no identified risks, benefit is not a prerequisite for market presence. One may question the need to prescribe a drug with no apparent benefit. Here, we are assuming that the benefit is more social than physiological. First, the drug provides a therapeutic response (albeit minimal) to metabolic diseases, a public health problem. Second, it addresses patients' demands from their doctor. Even if the drug has little or no effect, it provides patients with a sense of care. For many patients, it is easier to take a pill than to change their eating habits. Third, prescribing is influenced by doctors' perceptions of a molecule and their relationships with its manufacturer. In the case of Mediator, we know that the pharmaceutical company's influence on prescribers, as well as marketing and medical visits to promote the drug to healthcare professionals, played a significant role amongst prescribers, who are not trained – or are only minimally trained – to critically evaluate information about drugs provided by the pharmaceutical industry. The fact that a molecule has been approved is sufficient proof of its benefit.

Additionally, knowledge of Mediator indications varies among different groups of cardiologists, reflecting changes in the drug's marketing authorization. Nevertheless, between 25% and 30% of surveyed cardiologists, regardless of their graduation period, indicated that Mediator was prescribed for overweight patients without associated diabetes. This indication is based on off-label use.

After other amphetamine derivatives were withdrawn from the market in the late 1990s, Mediator was prescribed and used for purposes other than those for which it was intended. Consequently, the drug's benefits have reverted to its original purpose as an appetite suppressant. This phenomenon has been observed in certain regions, as evidenced by data from the French health insurance system and by cardiologists such as Dr. G., who has stopped prescribing Mediator: "I had to convince certain patients that taking off-label drugs was unreasonable, and the use of Mediator to lose weight was endemic in Provence [South of France]."[49] This reading incorporates the idea of user responsibility in prescribing the molecule while setting aside the issue of risk. Long perceived as a "useless but harmless" drug, the benefit/risk balance of this drug was reassessed during the last period of its commercial life and found to tilt more and more towards risk.

The withdrawal of Mediator exemplifies a clash of cultures between doctors' reporting of clinical situations and the management of marketing authorization by agencies and manufacturers.[50] In 1999, Dr. Georges Chiche, a French cardiologist, submitted the first pharmacovigilance report concerning valvulopathy caused by Mediator. However, the agency disregarded his report while informing *Servier*.[51] In turn, they pressured the declarant via his former department head to revise his declaration.

49 Lellinger, "Innovation Thérapeutique et Accident Médicamenteux," 329.

50 Solène Lellinger, "Des Petits Nombres à l'Amorce d'un Scandale Sanitaire," *Revue d'Anthropologie des Connaissances* 18, no.4 (2024): https://journals.openedition.org/rac/35983.

51 Bensadon, Marie, and Morelle, "Enquête Sur Le Mediator®: Rapport Définitif," 71.

Following that, one case was reported in a Spanish medical review in 2003, and another one later in Italy. The Spanish review states:

> We report the first case of valvular heart disease due to benfluorex. A 50-year-old woman who had been taking the anorectic agent benfluorex intermittently for one year developed severe fibrosis and regurgitation of the mitral, aortic and tricuspid valves. Clinical, echocardiographic and histopathological findings were analogous to those reported with fenfluramine and dexfenfluramine. The similarity between the histopathological lesion documented in patients treated with the appetite suppressants fenfluramine, dexfenfluramine and benfluorex and the valvular lesions reported in valve disease associated with ergot alkaloid use and carcinoid heart disease suggest a common pathophysiological mechanism and a central role for serotonin in the development of the disease.[52]

In 2005, *Servier* decided to remove this medication from Spain and Italy. Since 2007, a few cases have been identified and published in France, going beyond a pharmacovigilance report.

This case raises questions about weak signals and how to detect them, especially when these signals are "diluted" (in this case, presented to several risk management bodies). Cases are often compared with drug sales data, which essentially compares a few risk signals with millions of boxes sold. One of the lessons learned from the Mediator case is that there is a dissonance between, on the one hand, the regulatory framework and pharmacovigilance procedures, and on the other, the reality of practice, which leads to the reversal of the burden of proof on the safety of a drug. The shortcomings in the effectiveness of pharmacovigilance are not unique to Mediator or to France. Daniel Carpenter has illustrated the challenges of monitoring within the FDA by using oral contraceptives as an example.[53]

The withdrawal of Mediator is the result of an alert launched by a team at Brest University Hospital (in north-west France), and, in particular, by pneumologist Irène Frachon. After a thorough clinical investigation, the team reports any side effects to the relevant pharmacovigilance center, as required by French law since the 1980s. Initially, there were reports through the official pharmacovigilance channel suggesting a causal link between taking Mediator and a certain type of serious cardiopulmonary pathology. Starting in February 2007, Dr. Frachon observed several patients taking

52 Josefa Rafel Ribera et al., "Valvular heart disease associated with benfluorex," *Revista Espanola De Cardiologia* 56, no. 2 (2003): 215–16.

53 Daniel P. Carpenter, *Reputation and Power: Organizational Image and Pharmaceutical Regulation at the FDA* (Princeton University Press, 2010), 585–634.

Mediator who suffered from PPH. She joined forces with colleagues and, together, they studied five cases of PPH and one case of heart valve damage under benfluorex treatment. These cases were reported to the regional pharmacovigilance center. However, the regulatory procedure is inoperative for constituting an alert; action goes beyond this notification. The first step is to remove the report from the administrative arena and publish it in a pulmonary medical journal, which is a common practice in the field of medicine. Another step is taken when this team is called upon to report its observations to the regulator outside its practice. Two years after the initial notification, the observations were presented at a meeting of the drug agency's "risk management" group in June 2009 and to the national pharmacovigilance committee the following month.

Based on these Brest publications and others emerging at the time, the French regulatory agency, AFSSAPS (Agence Française de Sécurité Sanitaire des Produits de Santé), decided to remove the drug from the market in November 2009.[54] These studies demonstrate the link between fenfluramine and benfluorex; both drugs are metabolized into norfenfluramine,[55] which causes DIVHD. She goes beyond the standard reporting procedure by presenting and publishing the cases to the agency. This procedure is intended to allow the benefit-risk ratio to be questioned, but it is dysfunctional, as evidenced by Dr. Chiche's report.

The withdrawal of the drug is not very different from the standard process of removing a drug from the market. It involves the agency providing information to health professionals and a brief mention in the press. It doesn't automatically turn into a health scandal. Particularly in France, where trials against drug companies or the regulatory authorities were rather rare, due to different legal systems compared to the United States, for example. In principle, the information stops there. The marketing authorization is suspended, and the drug is withdrawn from pharmacies. Health professionals, informed by the AFSSAPS, are responsible for following up with patients who have taken benfluorex. This information occasionally appears in the press, but it doesn't immediately lead to a scandal or widespread mobilization.

54 K. Boutet et al., "Fenfluramine-like Cardiovascular Side-Effects of Benfluorex," *European Respiratory Journal* 33, no. 3 (2009): 684–88; Irène Frachon et al., "Benfluorex and Unexplained Valvular Heart Disease: A Case-Control Study," *PLOS ONE* 5, no. 4 (2010): e10128; Christophe Tribouilloy et al., "Restrictive Organic Mitral Regurgitation Associated with Benfluorex Therapy," *European Journal of Echocardiography: The Journal of the Working Group on Echocardiography of the European Society of Cardiology* 11, no. 7 (2010): 614–21; Weill et al., "Benfluorex and Valvular Heart Disease."

55 Boutet et al., "Fenfluramine-like Cardiovascular Side-Effects of Benfluorex," 686.

But, in June 2010, Irène Frachon published *Mediator 150mg. Combien de morts?* (How Many Deaths?),[56] recounting her scientific investigation and the battle she and her team waged over pharmacovigilance reporting. Frachon stepped outside her professional sphere, deliberately appealed to public opinion, and assumed the role of "whistleblower,"[57] even though she was not familiar with the term coined by sociology. Through her actions, Irène Frachon transformed from a "doctor fulfilling her role in pharmacovigilance" into a "whistleblower."

The third stage in the Mediator affair was the estimation of the number of potential victims. This began with the results of a pharmacy thesis that estimated Mediator had caused between 500 and 1,000 deaths since its approval.[58] This estimate was published in June 2010 and taken up by Socialist Member of Parliament Gérard Bapt in an August 2010 article for *LeMonde.fr*. He concludes his article by stating that: "For the sake of public health, a project must be launched to address the shortcomings of pharmacovigilance, the lack of transparency, the handling of conflicts of interest, and the inadequacy of monitoring and alert responsiveness."[59]

In this way, we shift our focus from information about withdrawal to the lessons it teaches us about how the drug system works. This shift in focus toward understanding the dysfunctions of the drug agency gives rise to a new interpretive framework that focuses on the influence strategies deployed by drug manufacturers, particularly conflicts of interest. It is as if that were the only factor that enables the benefits of a treatment to be overestimated and the molecule to remain on the market.

At the same time, the French national health insurance fund requested an official report to estimate the potential number of drug-related victims.[60] After receiving this report, the newly appointed Minister of Health, Xavier Bertrand, referred the matter to the Inspectorate General of Social Affairs (IGAS). On November 29, 2010, the IGAS was commissioned by the French Ministry of Labor, Employment, and Health to conduct "a

56 Irène Frachon, *Mediator 150 Mg. Combien de Morts?* (Éditions dialogues.fr, 2010).

57 Francis Chateauraynaud and Didier Torny, *Les sombres précurseurs: une sociologie pragmatique de l'alerte et du risque* (Presses de l'EHESS, 2010).

58 Flore Michelet, "Utilisation de nouveaux outils en pharmacovigilance : à propos du retrait du Médiator® (benfluorex)" (PhD dissertation, University of Rennes, 2010).

59 Gérard Bapt, "Mediator : Combien de morts?," *Le Monde.fr*, August 24, 2010, http://www.lemonde.fr/idees/article/2010/08/24/mediator-combien-de-morts_1402014_3232.html.

60 Alain Weill et al., "Benfluorex, Valvulopathies Cardiaques et Décès," CNAMTS, September 28, 2010.

fact-finding and assessment mission concerning Mediator and the reform of pharmacovigilance in France."[61] The submission of the IGAS report, on January 15, 2011, marked the fourth stage in the build-up to the scandal, and was widely covered in the media. The conclusions are clear:

> To use an expression that came up several times in the testimonies gathered by the committee of inquiry, this corporation "anesthetized" the actors in the drug chain and even, according to two former marketing authorization application committee chairs, "completely pulled the wool over their eyes."[62]

Parliamentary inquiries were then conducted,[63] and consultations were held between various stakeholders in the drug supply chain.[64] The goal was to reform the drug regulation and monitoring system in France. These efforts culminated in a reform in December 2011.

In this health scandal, the usefulness of the molecule itself is not really being questioned. Rather, it is the laboratory's strategies that are being questioned, particularly its attempts to pressure the regulatory agency. Fundamentally, the issue is not the molecule's practical uselessness or the presence of molecules with no therapeutic benefit on the market.

Conclusion

As I have emphasized in this chapter, pharmacological profile, administrative profile, and commercial profile are theoretically linked and flow from one another, governing the benefit-risk balance. In practice, dissociation between this different kind of profile can occur.

First, belonging to a chemical family allows us to anticipate certain known risks based on the drug's pharmacological profile. In addition to the theoretical chemical properties of a family of chemicals, the scientific dossier is

61 Bensadon, Marie, and Morelle, "Enquête Sur Le Mediator®: Rapport Définitif," 125.

62 Bensadon, Marie, and Morelle, "Enquête Sur Le Mediator®: Rapport Définitif," I.

63 Jean-Pierre Door, "Rapport d'information déposé en application de l'article 145 du Règlement par la Commission des affaires sociales en conclusion des travaux de la mission sur le Médiator et la pharmacovigilance" (Assemblée nationale, 2011); Marie-Thérèse Hermange and François Autain, "Rapport d'information fait au nom de la mission commune d'information sur 'Mediator: évaluation et contrôle des medicaments'" (Sénat, 2011).

64 Edouard Couty and Thomas Lesueur, "Rapport de synthèse des assises du medicament" (Les assises du medicament, 2011).

based on the effects observed in *Servier*'s studies. At this stage, the "scientific facts" observed and interpreted by *Servier*'s researchers determine how the drug will be classified and presented. This is where the administrative profile begins to emerge. The administrative profile is defined as the way in which the molecule is described in official documents, such as pharmacological and toxicological data and scientific publications, in order to obtain marketing authorization. Translating scientific facts into a regulatory dossier marks an initial distancing from the initial data. This dissociation becomes more pronounced in the final stage: the marketing campaign. The goal of this phase is to develop the drug's commercial profile, i.e., the image formed among healthcare professionals (and the public through) promotional arguments. The commercial profile, which is distinct from the administrative profile, highlights certain advantages of the drug. Thus, a transformation takes place, allowing the transition from S992, which was synthesized in the context of research on anorectic amphetamine derivatives, to treatment, Mediator, a "discovery" that "revolutionizes" the treatment of metabolic disorders. This process illustrates how each stage, pharmacological, administrative, and then commercial, reinforces the dissociation between scientific facts and the public image of the drug.

Thus, *Servier*'s strategy of refuting benfluorex's classification as an amphetamine was successful. This dissociation is reinforced by pharmaceutical company marketing strategies in a specific socio-medical context. This molecule was brought to market in response to an identified need relating to the prevention of cardiovascular risk factors, in a specific scientific context. Rather than focusing on the multifactorial causes of obesity and its health consequences, the emphasis was placed on managing the consequences while disregarding the socioeconomic factors impacting the disease (e.g., food access, precariousness). In this context, the drug fits into a specific nosological framework and provides a therapeutic response. This strategic choice not to position Mediator for what it is – an anorectic – is reinforced by the fact that this manufacturer already has a molecule on the market for weight loss, Pondéral (fenfluramine).

Nevertheless, prescribing and usage practices can help to reconfigure the way in which the benefits of a drug are interpreted. While benefits may be redefined during the marketing period, as a result of re-evaluations by the Agency and requests from the pharmaceutical industry to broaden the range of indications, the definition of risks is attenuated, contributing to the maintenance of ignorance or even agnotology in Proctor's sense.[65] This example

65 Robert Proctor and Londa L. Schiebinger, eds., *Agnotology: The Making and Unmaking of Ignorance* (Stanford University Press, 2008).

illustrates that a drug does not need to have benefits to remain on the market, beyond failing to identify a risk.

There had been about 300,000 boxes of Mediator sold per year in France at the time of its withdrawal (and 145,000,000 boxes sold throughout the marketing period).[66] Based on extrapolated sales and reimbursement data, it is estimated that around 5 million people have used this molecule. Measures have been put in place to identify victims of this drug, as well as compensation schemes (out-of-court settlement or legal proceedings). The withdrawal of the drug has also led to an overhaul of drug regulation, with particular emphasis on conflicts of interest management and pharmacovigilance. It has paved the way for new ways of managing drug risk through new tracking systems, on the one hand, involving users in the reporting of adverse events and, on the other, making more systematic use of health insurance databases for pharmaco-epidemiological studies.

66 Catherine Hill, "Mortalité Attribuable Au Benfluorex (Mediator®)," *La Presse Médicale* 40, no. 5 (2011): 462–69.

Part Four

Resisting Systems of Risk and Benefit

Chapter Ten

Lying about Opioids? Rescuing Risk and Benefit from the Addiction Paradigm[1]

David Herzberg

Introduction

Cultural and regulatory authorities approach "addiction" differently than other drug risks such as weight gain or high blood pressure. This is because addiction has long served as a boundary concept, useful for a wide range of political actors and agendas only tenuously linked to documentable drug effects. As numerous historians have shown, addiction was articulated in its modern form in the early twentieth century by an alliance of anti-"vice" crusaders and therapeutic reformers responding to a sharp increase in sales and use of opioids and cocaine. Having to navigate increasingly criminalized markets led many drug consumers to engage in a range of predictable behaviors that came to be associated with the state of "addiction."[2] Addiction came to be an amalgam of measurable biological phenomena such as tolerance

1 I am fortunate to be a unionized faculty member at a public university, which affords me the time and resources to do projects like this one. Special thanks to my co-editors Nils and Joe for their hard work and good spirits, and also to our wonderful contributors for their patience with this long-brewing volume.

2 See, e.g., David Courtwright, *Dark Paradise: A History of Opiate Addiction in America* (1982; repr., Harvard University Press, 2001); Joseph Spillane, *Cocaine: From Medical Marvel to Modern Menace in the United States, 1884–1920* (Johns Hopkins University Press, 1999); Caroline Jean Acker, *Creating the American Junkie: Addiction Research in the Classic Era of Narcotic Control* (Johns Hopkins University Press, 2002).

and withdrawal; subjectively expressed phenomena such as desire and craving; and socially produced phenomena such as shame, lying, criminality, and downward social mobility.[3]

This addiction paradigm was no less real for having been socially constructed. The structure and policing of drug markets made it likely that people who experienced tolerance, withdrawal, and desire were also people who lied about their drug use, broke the law, and were downwardly mobile. The forces linking these phenomena were so robust that it was nearly impossible to disaggregate biological, psychological, and social elements. For opioids, narratives of benefit and risk inevitably included psychological and social elements. Tolerance and dependence were practically interchangeable with lying and criminality.

Addiction was thus no mere side effect. It was absolute abjection – the negation of all possible good. There was no equation where benefits could be made to balance out this asymptotic risk. Therapeutic authorities warned physicians that addiction was so horrifying that opiates should be generally withheld even from patients suffering a mortal illness until their life "can be measured in weeks."[4] And because addiction hinged on consumers' active desire, avoiding it required stronger stuff than professional regulation. Criminal prohibitions were needed to ensure that everyone, not just physicians, made the right choices. Criminalization completed the self-reinforcing circuitry connecting the biological, the psychological, and the social. The moral arc attributed to opioid use from relief and pleasure, to desire, to ruin, became a "natural history" so sturdy that it could be applied to a host of substances other than opioids to which it fit only awkwardly at best. If the pharmacological elements did not match, the social elements could easily be supplied – as, for example, in the case of cannabis, which for much of the twentieth century was legally and culturally categorized as an addictive narcotic.

This chapter examines a moment of partial disruption at the heart of this addiction paradigm and its associated framework of risk and benefit: the introduction of Demerol, the first fully synthetic opioid, in 1944. As I have argued elsewhere, authorities were initially uncertain about how the potentially revolutionary new drug fit into the addiction paradigm. Perhaps the scientific wizardry that had freed opioids from the poppy plant had also

3 For a theoretical overview and exploration of this "constructionist" approach to addiction, see, e.g., Suzanne Fraser and David Moore, eds., *The Drug Effect: Health, Crime and Society* (Cambridge University Press, 2011).

4 M. J. Schiffrin, *The Management of Pain in Cancer* (L Year Book, 1956), 7–8, 13–33, cited in Marcia Meldrum, "A Capsule History of Pain Management," *JAMA* 290, no. 18 (2003): 2470–75.

vanquished opioids' addictiveness.[5] Circumstances favored this optimism. As a synthetic drug with no existing non-medical supply chains, Demerol was initially available only to the most privileged type of US drug consumer: white middle-class "patients." Even as criminalization hardened in the early twentieth century, so-called "medical addicts" typically received more empathy and care than their racialized urban peers.[6] For both these reasons, Demerol's early consumers were partially sheltered from the harsh teleology of the addiction paradigm.

Drawing from a collection of Federal Bureau of Narcotics (FBN) reports, I argue that these consumers had at least some room to make sense of experiences like tolerance, withdrawal, and desire on their own terms. In doing so they articulated alternatives to the addiction paradigm, often disassembling it by severing opioids' pharmacological effects from their social and psychological effects. Risks such as tolerance and withdrawal could be understood and navigated differently if they were not inevitably accompanied by desire, moral decline, and social ruin.

Using the same FBN reports, however, I also argue that even this limited freedom to reimagine opioid use was not to last. The FBN's push to expand the Harrison Anti-Narcotic Act to cover synthetic opioids left little room for early Demerol consumers' alternative ways of experiencing and making sense of the drug's effects. Indeed, the FBN deliberately shut down consumers' imaginings, insisting that they were the typical lying of "addicts." In 1948, after a determined lobbying campaign supported by a popular media blitz about the addictive threat posed by Demerol, the FBN won its battle: the Harrison Act was expanded and challenges to the addiction paradigm were largely silenced.

To properly understand the short lifespan of Demerol dreams, we must reckon with the reasons the FBN shut them down. The FBN, of course, is best known for its sensationalized crusades against racialized "junkies" and foreign traffickers. But the FBN was also a pioneering regulatory agency that had won unusually robust power to govern the pharmaceutical industry – much stronger than its better-known cousin the Food and Drug Administration (FDA).[7] The FBN's two missions were connected: only by harnessing the political power of the anti-narcotic crusade had the agency been able to win regulatory power over a major industry in the business-friendly US. For decades, FBN chief Harry J. Anslinger had used that regulatory power to prevent pharmaceutical companies from launching a parade

5 David Herzberg, *White Market Drugs: Big Pharma and the Hidden History of Addiction in America* (University of Chicago Press, 2020), 102–15.

6 Herzberg, *White Market Drugs*, 46–83.

7 This paragraph drawn from Herzberg, *White Market Drugs*, 84–134.

of new would-be miracle opioids that they claimed were less addictive or even nonaddictive. Anslinger saw Demerol as just the latest of these. The manufacturer, Winthrop Chemical Company, promoted the drug as the long-sought nonaddictive painkiller through aggressive medical advertising, lobbying regulators, and lining up favorable media coverage from influential physicians and friendly journalists. Indeed, this marketing campaign was surely at least partially responsible for clearing a space for consumers to imagine themselves free of some aspects of the addiction paradigm.

Demerol consumers and Winthrop Chemical were engaged in very different projects, but it is easy to understand why they looked like two sides of the same coin to an FBN long jaded by previous "miracle opioid" hypes. Both created wiggle room in the addiction paradigm, weakening the basis of the Bureau's power over opioid manufacturers and its power to protect a potentially misinformed public from dangerous drugs. The FBN's robust regulatory power over a major industry was a rare and tenuous achievement in the business-friendly US, and it was not paranoid to be zealous in protecting it. Subsequent events, moreover, have shown the devastating consequences when large-scale corporate purveyors of what historian David Courtwright calls "limbic capitalism" are permitted to operate freely.[8]

The point of this chapter is not to idolize Demerol consumers and demonize the FBN. Rather, it is to see what can be learned by taking both seriously. This can be difficult for twenty-first-century readers. Trained by the addiction paradigm to expect self-serving lies from "addicts," we could easily share the FBN's scorn for Demerol consumers' claims about their drug use. But we do not have to see this as a binary choice. Drug policy does not have to be – should not be – a zero-sum game, with the only options being the twin catastrophes of false marketing hype or prohibitionist sensationalism. History can help us find alternatives, giving us an opportunity to learn from the ways that people who use drugs understood and managed their experiences. Exploring such alternatives is not itself without risk, of course, as the twenty-first-century opioid crisis makes clear; one must always be wary of the miles that industry marketers can take when they are given an inch. This is a reason for caution, however, not for the absolutist zeal of the FBN, which led to its own destructive consequences. In a history with few appealing precedents, glimpses of the potential to operate between the extremes are particularly worth exploring.

8 David Courtwright, *The Age of Addiction: How Bad Habits Became Big Business* (Belknap, 2021).

Demerol Dreams

When Demerol first came on the market, Winthrop Chemical was not alone in believing that it was truly different from "narcotics" like morphine. Many consumers, too, hoped that it could provide the benefits of opioids with fewer or even none of opioids' risks – that it truly was nonaddictive, causing none of the biological, psychological, or social elements of the addiction paradigm. The rosiest of these hopes turned out to be false; Demerol is no more or less likely to produce addiction than any other opioid. This does not mean, however, that consumers' Demerol dreams were simply ignorant, self-deceiving, or the stereotypical dishonesty of "addicts." They can also be understood as efforts to re-narrate the experience of using an opioid, reinterpreting basic experiences such as tolerance and desire in ways that are potentially problematic but arguably less so than the addiction paradigm. This section explores these most hopeful narratives – narratives that, even when acknowledging Demerol's effects, made sense of them without reference to addiction.

The hopes that consumers could invest in Demerol was poignantly expressed by Mrs. C. in a letter to Anslinger in 1944. She explained that she "became a morphine addict" nearly a decade ago after a serious bout of illness. "For three long years," she wrote, "I tried to improve my general health and my nerves in order to have the strength to overcome this vicious habit. Finally after a two months withdrawl [*sic*] treatment I was able to do so, but only after such horrible suffering as only God and I know about." Nine years later she claimed to be "entirely free of addiction" despite some use of opioids for "very serious illnesses." But now she was facing surgery that called for extended pre- and post-operative opioids, and she feared becoming re-addicted. She had heard of Winthrop's Demerol being used "as a substitute for morphine addiction" and pleaded with the FBN to send her "very reputable and very conscientious doctor" a substantial enough supply to "carry me through the treatment and hospitalization. It means so much to me, my whole future, my husband's and my adopted son's. Its [*sic*] more than life to me, because living under the shadow of addiction is not living, its [*sic*] merely a horrible existence."[9]

Putting on our FBN hat, we might read this letter through the lens of the addiction paradigm. Mrs. C., an "addict," rationalized continued opioid

9 Mrs. A. D. Clement to Mr. H. J. Anslinger, February 21, 1944 (Subject Files of the Bureau of Narcotics and Dangerous Drugs, 1916–1970, Record Group 170, National Archives II, College Park, MD [*hereinafter "FBN Papers"*], File 0480-190, Folder 2 "Drugs: Demerol (Dolantin): Isonipecaine: January 1944–March 1944").

use by claiming "very serious illnesses," and asked authorities for a legal supply of the drug she craved. One could also see the entitlement of a white market consumer, rather than brave honesty, in sending such a request to the nation's premiere anti-narcotics cop. But there is no evidence for this reading. Indeed, given how new and unavailable Demerol was, Mrs. C. was unlikely to have known that it had the same qualities as other opioids. From this perspective, her letter reads differently. She recognized the need for opioids' benefits (i.e., pain control), but hoped for a way to disconnect those benefits from the misery of a "vicious habit." We know, of course, that Demerol was not the miracle opioid she hoped it could be, but her goal of using opioids without addiction was perfectly reasonable and, in fact, is the most likely outcome even for long-term pain patients.

We will never know whether Mrs. C. used Demerol, and if so, whether it rekindled her unwanted desire. But the FBN's records do provide evidence that similar hopes could survive the experience of using Demerol. For example, Mrs. McC., a "chronic invalid from asthma" who had been using Demerol for several months, described the drug as "reliev[ing] these awful spasms which occur with almost clock like accuracy every 3 to 4 hours ... it has afforded me more relief in shorter time than any drug yet used." Mrs. McC. did not understand herself as experiencing withdrawal, but rather "awful spasms" when the medicine wore off – to her, an indication that Demerol was working, not that it was problematic. As such, her main challenge was simply purchasing Demerol. In a letter to Eleanor Roosevelt, she asked "if there is any way in which you could issue me a permit to get my requirements I would certainly appreciate it as would my husband and my little daughter."[10] To the FBN this might have sounded like the maneuvering of an "addict," but a stable, predictable supply does reduce the psychological and social risks associated with long term opioid use. We do not know what Mrs. McC was thinking, but she was at least not wrong to guess that her future would be better with that stable supply of a non-stigmatized drug. In other words, while it is easy to sneer at her seemingly naïve misreading of abstinence syndrome, it is also easy to see that, under some circumstances, that misreading might have led to a better outcome for her than the alternative (i.e., the addiction paradigm, which might have increased her risk of experiencing the worst outcomes of opioid use).

An FBN District Supervisor encountered a similar situation with a neighbor of his who had been given Demerol to ease abdominal pain after "several surgical operations." The neighbor's physician "assured her Demerol

10 Mrs. James H. McClury to Mrs. Roosevelt, July 30, 1944 (FBN Papers, File 0480-190, Folder 2 "Drugs: Demerol (Dolantin): Isonipecaine: April 1944–").

was harmless," and she swore that "she has never had a craving for it." Nonetheless, "her physician now prescribes the tablets in quantities of one hundred and she has noted the original dosage does not now afford as much relief of pain as when she started using the drug."[11] Here the neighbor rejected the derogatory term "craving" and instead emphasized how Demerol eased her abdominal pains. This reframing of her relationship to the drug was not pollyanna; she recognized, for example, what appears to have been a developing tolerance. Again, there is nothing pharmacologically distinctive about Demerol. The drug's social status, not its chemical qualities, made it possible for the FBN agent's neighbor to tell a different and more pragmatic story about its risks and benefits.

The prospect of a non-addictive opioid proved especially appealing for people hoping to free themselves of a currently existing addiction. Arkansas physician Dr. G., for example, had been using morphine for medical reasons until one day he became "very anxious to reach a state where he would not be dependent on any drug." He checked himself into a hospital where he received Demerol to help him through morphine withdrawal. He continued to use a reduced dose of Demerol for a while and "achieved a reasonable degree of comfort." For Dr. G., however, this comfort was not enough. He did not explain why, but he decided to check himself into a sanatorium in another effort to completely free himself of drugs.[12] Another addicted doctor, Dr. P. of Massachusetts, had worse luck; he "tried to use a preparation called DEMEROL" to wean himself off another pharmaceutical opioid, Roche's Pantopon, "but it had little or no effect on his desire for Pantopon."[13] If nothing else, these cases show that people apparently experiencing opioid addiction were not mindless zombies but could make rational efforts to balance their risks and benefits.

Interestingly, one did not have to believe that Demerol was nonaddictive to find it valuable for managing an addiction. One could simply find it to be less risky than the alternatives. A number of consumers and prescribing physicians seem to have done this, using Demerol to reduce tolerance, to manage withdrawal, or to simply substitute a less stigmatized drug. Helen C. of Bangor, Maine, for example, explained that she only used her illegally procured Demerol (obtained by requesting it from Winthrop on stationary

11 A. B. Grisler, District Supervisor, to Mr. H. J. Anslinger, June 14, 1946 (FBN Papers, File 0480-190, Folder 2 "Drugs: Demerol: Paul de Kruif").

12 Report by Narcotic Inspector Harley E. Anderson, February 28, 1946 (FBN Papers, File 0480-190, Folder 2 "Drugs: Demerol (Dolantin): Isonipecaine: March–Dec 1946").

13 Report by Narcotic Agents Meade and Murphy, June 13, 1944 (FBN Papers, File 0480-190, Folder 2 "Drugs: Demerol (Dolantin): Isonipecaine: April 1944–").

from a local hospital) to tide her over when she was without the morphine that was her primary drug of addiction. The rest went to her father who suffered from a heart ailment and was allergic to morphine.[14] In Konawa, Oklahoma, Dr. W. told an undercover FBN informant that he would sell him opioids if he agreed to take "a new drug known as DEMEROL along with the morphine." He would provide 100 tablets of each, and, Dr. W. explained, "the new drug would take the place of morphine and after he had taken it for some time, he could leave off the morphine." (The informant's cover was blown before the sale could take place.)[15] Further north in Grand Forks, Minnesota, a physician decided to stop treating a "medical addict," Raymond B., upon realizing that Raymond could not be convinced to stop using opioids. Another physician took a different tack, prescribing Demerol "in an effort to overcome the effect of the withdrawal of morphine." Raymond successfully switched from morphine to Demerol, but he was not entirely pleased with the change; "it seemed to him," an FBN agent reported, "that Demerol only lessened the withdrawal effects of morphine but did not give the effect of morphine."[16] Mrs. Lloyd K., from a "very prominent family" and married to a "prominent attorney" in Morton, Texas, had been receiving clandestine morphine maintenance for years before a young physician successfully weaned her off. When her husband suffered a stroke and she pleaded with the physician for more morphine, he decided to provide Demerol instead, which "he did not consider ... as harmful as morphine."[17] A physician in Laconia, New Hampshire, wrote Anslinger to

14 Report by Agent Kelly, February 17, 1944 (FBN Papers, File 0480-190, Folder 2 "Drugs: Demerol (Dolantin): Isonipecaine: April 1944–").

15 Case Report, March 30, 1944 (FBN Papers, File 0480-190, Folder 2 "Drugs: Demerol (Dolantin): Isonipecaine: April 1944–").

16 Reports by Agent Dietz, June 10 and 29, 1944 (FBN Papers, File 0480-190, Folder 2 "Drugs: Demerol (Dolantin): Isonipecaine: April 1944–").For authorities, this dissatisfaction suggested a different opportunity: Demerol tablets, an FBN agent reported, "are not very popular with the addicts," at least not compared to the "liquid taken hypodermically" which "seems to provide a greater kick." "If the Winthrop Chemical Company would confine the manufacture of the product to the table form its value as a substitute for morphine would be materially lessened." H. T. Nugent, Confidential Memorandum for Mr. Anslinger, May 2, 1944 (FBN Papers, File 0480-190, Folder 2 "Drugs: Demerol (Dolantin): Isonipecaine: April 1944–").

17 "DEMEROL" (FBN Papers, File 0480-190, Folder 2 "Drugs: Demerol (Dolantin): Isonipecaine: March–Dec 1946").

report that he was treating his son-in-law, "a hopeless alcoholic," by "administering Demerol," but did not provide any further information.[18]

We know little about these Demerol consumers beyond the brief reports from skeptical and relatively unsympathetic FBN agents. But the common patterns identified here are telling. The reports show people who, in one way or another, tried to escape or at least disassemble the addiction paradigm – to disconnect the relief of suffering from the inevitability of psychological and social ruin. We do not have to believe that these consumers were sincere, or that they were right about Demerol's uniqueness (they were not), to recognize that their approaches were not obviously less realistic or less effective than the draconian "common sense" of the addiction paradigm. Pharmacologically, Demerol was no miracle opioid, but it still created an opportunity for some of its consumers or would-be consumers to imagine new ways to access opioid benefits while pragmatically managing their risks.

Demerol Purgatory

In July 1944, the *Bulletin of the Menninger Clinic* announced "the only case of spontaneous addiction to Demerol so far reported in this country": a thirty-eight-year-old, affluent, married school teacher and church volunteer with multiple degrees and no children who was "an attractive, friendly, capable person with a good sense of humor" with "many acquaintances and friends." After five major operations and multiple hospitalizations over thirteen years, however, she had been introduced to Demerol by a physician (and later a pharmacist) who assured her it was "not habit-forming." Over time she increased the dose tenfold. The authors concluded that "addiction to Demerol does occur," and warned that "as soon as the supply increases, case reports of ... addiction to Demerol ... will appear more often."[19]

The *Bulletin*'s presentation of the case was unusual in that it recognized the phenomena of tolerance and, implicitly, desire, and labeled them "addiction," but did not link them to the socially stigmatized elements of the phenomenon. This was, in part, an artifact of Demerol's own unusual status as an entirely white market medicine that had not (yet) been linked to racialized stereotypes of "addiction." The FBN, however, was not happy about that unusual status and was already hard at work categorizing Demerol as an addictive opioid just like the others. Ultimately, after Demerol had been

18 Untitled Memo, October 2, 1946 (FBN Papers, File 0480-190, Folder 2 "Drugs: Demerol (Dolantin): Isonipecaine: March–Dec 1946").

19 Jerome M. Schneck, "A Case of Addiction to Demerol," *Bulletin of the Menninger Clinic* 8, no. 4 (1944): 122.

added to anti-narcotic statutes in 1948, this meant cracking down on consumers' access to Demerol, especially long-term use. Consumers increasingly faced a choice: stop using Demerol, or take illegal actions to secure a supply. In other words, FBN policies began to make the world more like the FBN already believed it to be. Demerol consumers who experienced tolerance and dependence became increasingly likely to experience the rest of the addiction paradigm – desire, shame, lying, criminality, and downward social mobility.

This section explores Demerol consumers' experiences as the FBN began its crackdown. While some consumers were convinced or pressured to stop using the drug, I argue, others found that space remained to accept and manage the realities of tolerance, dependence, and desire without accepting stigmatization and criminalization. Despite the FBN's regulatory strength as compared to the FDA, governance of pharmaceutical white markets at the retail level remained relatively weak, especially before 1948. Moreover, because most Demerol consumers could claim an identity as "patients," their illegal activities did not always resemble those common in prohibition markets. They did not typically "deal" drugs, engage in property crime, become sex workers, or interact socially with racially stigmatized or poor communities. Instead, they did things like forge prescriptions or siphon off legally prescribed drugs from a relative, or they were physicians who prescribed for themselves. These transgressions did not fit the addiction paradigm perfectly and thus left open a space – albeit tenuous and rapidly narrowing – to resist the psychic and social consequences imposed on consumers by the FBN and other narcotic authorities.

Many consumers, even long-term ones, stopped using Demerol as it became more firmly linked to addiction. Dr. McN. of New York, for example, was one of those with a previous addiction to another opioid (morphine), who hoped Demerol would allow him to avoid other opioids. After being treated for his morphine addiction he began to "occasionally take Nembutal [a barbiturate] for sleeping and, recently, had resorted to the irregular use of Demerol" (several tablets per week). Informed that Demerol was in fact a narcotic according to New York law and that many physicians considered it habit-forming, Dr. McN. agreed to try to stop using it even though, he said, his own physician "used demerol extensively in his surgery and doesn't share the fear as to its habit forming properties."[20]

Dr. McN. remained unconvinced of Demerol's risks, but as time went on, others who stopped using Demerol for similar reasons represented themselves as having escaped an addiction. Take the case of twenty-nine-year-old Bethel, North Carolina, father of two J. W., a so-called "medical

20 Letter-Report of Agent Cross, December 28, 1942; and Letter Report of Agent Costarella, March 25, 1944 (FBN Papers, File 0480-190, Folder 2 "Drugs: Demerol (Dolantin): Isonipecaine: April 1944–").

addict" whose physician had been prescribing him morphine since 1942 for chronic asthma. J. W. was introduced to Demerol during addiction treatment at a sanitarium and continued to buy it afterwards, sometimes without a prescription. He described its effects as different from morphine: "it relaxes me, makes my head feel light and relieves all pain in about 5 minutes," he said. But there was a cost: an "extreme craving for another shot of Demerol which takes place in about an hour or less." These were, he emphasized, extremely powerful cravings. "I have been addicted to the use of morphine," he said, and "I have also used some hypnotics, however none have ever produced the cravings, in so short a period of time, as Demerol." J. W. explicitly framed his desire in the language of addiction ("craving") and understood his Demerol use as fundamentally similar to his earlier morphine use. Realizing that "I couldn't possibly get loose from Demerol," he returned to the sanitarium, where they weaned him off Demerol and returned him to morphine – a less intense addiction, he felt. "I do not ever expect to take another dose of it [Demerol]."[21]

Another consumer who initially embraced Demerol but ultimately identified it as addictive and chose to stop taking it was B. P., who was being treated for pneumonia in Berkeley, California, when he was discovered to be "addicted to the use of Demerol" after "demand[ing] that he be given large doses" of the drug. B. P. admitted to having taken Demerol for at least a year, some secured from his wife, who was dying of cancer, and some from various physicians' prescriptions. A psychiatrist evaluated him and found "no evidence of psychosis," just an effort to manage the stress and insomnia that accompanied caring for his dying spouse. At first, B. P. defended his Demerol use, citing a *Reader's Digest* article claiming that Demerol was "not habit-forming" and reasoning that it was "silly for him to be nervous when he can derive such a peaceful feeling from Demerol." Later, however, when he tried to stop, B. P. suffered "somewhat severe" withdrawal symptoms and "certainly would have re-established the habit" had not "alert physicians" been "instant in their denial." Now having "finally lost any desire for the drug," B. P. told the FBN they were welcome to use his story "in any way you wish" to combat false assurances about Demerol. "Having gone through the experience of Demerol addiction," he explained, "I am most anxious and willing to do all possible to assist in the dissemination of information for complete control and proper use of the drug."[22]

21 Jasper Wynne Jr. statement to Narcotic Agent Wm. T. Atkinson, May 27, 1944, 3492; H. J. Anslinger to Dr. Lawrence Kolb, May 30, 1944 (FBN Papers, File 0480-190, Folder 2 "Drugs: Demerol (Dolantin): Isonipecaine: April 1944–").

22 Memorandum for file, October 15, 1946, 3803; 4431–35; 4426–28 (FBN Papers, File 0480-190, Folder 2 "Drugs: Demerol: Paul de Kruif").

Not everyone wanted to, or was able to, stop using Demerol even after it had been identified as an addictive opioid. For them, the FBN's tightening net meant turning to illegal activity to secure a supply. Leland H. of Denver, Colorado, for example, was caught scheming to pass forged prescriptions. H. had suffered from tuberculosis since childhood and was introduced to morphine through medical treatment. He used morphine "until he felt it was getting the best of him" and requested hospital treatment for addiction. His physician was skeptical that he could "get along without the drug" and advised that "as soon as Demerol could be obtained it would help him in place of morphine." He had been taking Demerol ever since. At one point, he took more than he was supposed to and his physician cut his supply "almost in half." That was "when it began to bother him" and he turned to the false prescriptions.[23] Boston physician Dr. George K. had a similar experience. He had begun taking Demerol after a severe injury and infection to his right arm and was soon "definitely addicted." He "cursed the drug vehemently" and described it as "even more habit forming than morphine" to the FBN agent interviewing him after he was caught prescribing himself Demerol in the name of patients. Indeed, he said, "it is one of the most habit forming drugs I know of."[24]

As suggested by the appearance of these men's stories FBN records, federal authorities were well aware of this type of behavior. Indeed, fraudulent prescriptions were usually the reason authorities discovered cases of illegal Demerol use. But it was not entirely clear what could or should be done about these crimes. Because Demerol was a white market medicine, most consumers caught transgressing the law could claim a status as a "patient" with a past or present medical condition; many were physicians.[25] Both could

23 Report of District Supervisor A. M. Bangs, October 28, 1944 (FBN Papers, File 0480-190, Folder 2 "Drugs: Demerol (Dolantin): Isonipecaine: April 1944–"). Even some consumers who denied that Demerol was addictive, such as Dr. Robert F. of Deer Park, Washington, ended up forging prescriptions; see Report by Narcotic Agent John H. Young, March 29, 1945 (FBN Papers, File 0480-190, Folder 2 "Drugs: Demerol (Dolantin): Isonipecaine: April 1944–").

24 Report by Narcotic Agents John Sheehan and M. I. Goodman, December 13 and 17, 1947 (FBN Papers, File 0480-190, Folder 2 "Drugs: Demerol (Dolantin): Isonipecaine: March–December 1946").

25 For cases of forged prescriptions with a claim of medical justification, see, e.g., the case of Herbert M., who supplemented his physician's legal prescriptions because he deemed them "insufficient to sustain [his] need" (Report by Narcotic Agents Morgan, Newey and Nickell, July 21, 1944 [FBN Papers, File 0480-190, Folder 2 "Drugs: Demerol (Dolantin): Isonipecaine: April 1944 –"]); Mrs. Ruby A. of Phoenix, Arizona, who "developed a craving" for

be seen as what had formerly been called "medical addicts," that is, people who had contracted addiction through no moral fault of their own but solely through their dutiful obedience to medical advice. True, there was no legal distinction made between prescription forgers and other types of "dope fiends," but in practice authorities often responded to these cases more leniently – with treatment rather than punishment (although, of course, the line between the two could be difficult to discern when it came to addiction). This was especially so early on, when Demerol's political categorization as an addictive opioid was less certain. It was, ironically, another way that the otherwise unremarkable opioid truly could offer reduced risks for consumers.

Dr. M., for example, who used "about 60%" of the Demerol he prescribed for his invalid wife, was allowed to take a "cure" but appears to have faced no other discipline or consequences.[26] Dr. Ernest M. from Hot Springs, Arkansas, who began using Demerol before it was placed under Harrison controls, similarly appears to have evaded punishment for passing fraudulent prescriptions despite being "generally known" as addicted in the town.[27] A nurse, Mrs. Helen J. of Binghamton, New York, "acquired a desire for Demerol" after using the drug for weeks before and after surgery for an injured arm. When she was caught stealing prescription blanks from her employer she received treatment for addiction rather than being

Demerol and forged prescriptions despite her physician's assurances that it was not habit-forming in providing it to her after four major surgeries (Report by Narcotic Agent Early A. Smith, May 27, 1946 [FBN Papers, File 0480-190, Folder 2 "Drugs: Demerol (Dolantin): Isonipecaine: March–December 1946"]); William G. of Norfolk, VA was caught soliciting Demerol prescriptions from multiple physicians; he had used various opioids briefly after each of a series of operations for appendicitis, but was unable to stop Demerol after surgery to remove his gall bladder (John Balas to Mr. B. M. Marting District Supervisor, July 12, 1946 [FBN Papers, File 0480-190, Folder 2 "Drugs: Demerol (Dolantin): Isonipecaine: March–December 1946"]); Mary W., a St. Louis nurse, had developed a reliance on Demerol due to migraine headaches and was caught forging prescriptions at her hospital; she promised to stop but said she would seek a legal supply of the drug "if it became evident that she could not carry on without it" (E.B. Quarles, MD to Mr. H.J. Anslinger, October 30, 1946 FBN Papers, File 0480-190, Folder 2 "Drugs: Demerol (Dolantin): Isonipecaine: March–December 1946"]).

26 Report by Narcotic Agent L. A. Morgan, January 10 and 26, 1945 (FBN Papers, File 0480-190, Folder 2 "Drugs: Demerol (Dolantin): Isonipecaine: April 1944–").

27 Report by Narcotic Inspector Harley Anderson, March 28, 1946 (FBN Papers, File 0480-190, Folder 2 "Drugs: Demerol (Dolantin): Isonipecaine: March–December 1946").

arrested or punished.[28] Another nurse, New Yorker Mrs. H. E. J., received similarly lenient – even sympathetic – treatment. She used Pantopon for two weeks after a severe heart attack, and "acquired a desire for Demerol" soon thereafter when she used it for several weeks to ease the pain of an accidental arm injury at work. She was caught stealing prescription blanks but faced no punishment; instead, another physician offered to medically supervise her cure.[29] A Denver, Colorado, nurse claimed to have developed a "habit" and "craving" for Demerol in less than a week's use following a surgery. It gave her "unending endurance" to "handle twice as many patients as before," but she also eventually began to steal from the hospital pharmacy to maintain her supply. She went not to prison but to a sanitarium, after which she swore off the drug entirely: "the fear of Demerol addiction is far greater than any desire for it could ever be."[30]

Not all Demerol consumers got such lenient treatment, but even those subjected to harsher penalties still tended to fare better than many during an era of intensely punitive drug policing. Mrs. Thelma N. from Brooklyn, for example, was arrested after forging a prescription for Demerol. She had suffered a severe spinal injury in 1939 and after numerous surgeries Demerol was "the only thing that relieves her suffering." When her physician "refused to issue [Demerol] prescriptions as a regular routine matter," she stole his prescription pad. According to the FBN agent, however, "this woman is not a criminal type and undoubtedly would not have committed this offense were it not for the severe pain she suffers." The FBN allowed her to continue to receive prescriptions for Demerol until yet another scheduled surgery, after which she would go for addiction treatment at the federal prison/hospital in Lexington, Kentucky.[31] A similar case involved Jerome T. from

28 Report by Narcotic Agent A.D.Crimmins and State Investigator Sidney Joffe, June 21, 1946 (FBN Papers, File 0480-190, Folder 2 "Drugs: Demerol (Dolantin): Isonipecaine: March–December 1946").

29 June 17, 1946, Frank J. Smith, Supervisor to Commissioner H.J. Anslinger (FBN Papers, File 0480-190, Folder 2 "Drugs: Demerol: Paul de Kruif").

30 December 29, 1946, Narcotic Agents Jack Merrill and Leroy Sutherland to Mr. A. B. Crisler District Supervisor (FBN Papers, File 0480-190, Folder 2 "Drugs: Demerol (Dolantin): Isonipecaine: March–December 1946"). A similar discovery was made by a New York City man who had helped a friend get treatment for morphine addiction. The friend had emerged from the sanitarium "with a strong determination that he would not take any more narcotics," but soon began to take Demerol. See J. Newcomb Blackman to Anslinger, July 25, 1946 (FBN Papers, File 0480-190, Folder 2 "Drugs: Demerol (Dolantin): Isonipecaine: March–December 1946").

31 Report by Narcotic Agent Bernard Sporn, May 10, 1946 and Letter report of Chief Probation Officer Printzlein, July 18, 1946 (FBN Papers, File 0480-190, Folder 2 "Drugs: Demerol (Dolantin): Isonipecaine: March–December 1946").

Mayview, Pennsylvania, who had started using opioids in 1937 for sinusitis. After arrest and conviction for narcotics violations he received a suspended sentence, probation for five years, and a term at the Lexington narcotics farm. In protecting him from the worst legal consequences of his actions, the FBN agent noted that he had "no previous record; has a wife and two children to support; suffers from continued headaches, and bears a good reputation in the local medical world."[32]

In these cases, consumers themselves identified their long-term Demerol use as addiction, but authorities remained willing to entertain the possibility that not all elements of the paradigm applied. Options for Demerol consumers were narrowing; authorities increasingly insisted that all long-term use come to an end. Yet those who did not or could not follow this dictate were, for the most part, treated as if they were suffering from a harmful medicine's side effect rather than being seen as threatening criminals. Of course, it helped that so many were either physicians or could claim a status as "patient" – both presumptively white categories at that time and neither seen as particularly threatening. Within these constraints, at least some Demerol consumers had space to implement their vision of addiction as a drug risk like others, to be managed, rather than an abject cultural nightmare that dwarfed all possible benefits.

Demerol Nightmares

Even this limited room to think differently about addiction was tenuous and ultimately did not last. One crucial element of most cases of Demerol addiction was the consumers' claim of ignorance about the drug's qualities, at least when use began. But part of the FBN's crackdown was a public awareness campaign that made good faith claims of ignorance increasingly difficult. The campaign intensified in 1946 after popular health writer Dr. Walter Alvarez, supplied with information by Winthrop, wrote a puff piece in *Reader's Digest* claiming that Demerol was a "magic" drug that could "comfort millions of pain-racked human beings" without producing any addiction. The FBN flooded popular media with aggressive debunking of what Anslinger called "dangerous propaganda to push sales of this drug,"

32 October 25, 1939, provided by Narcotic Inspector D. W. Roush, Dec 14, 1946 (FBN Papers, File 0480-190, Folder 2 "Drugs: Demerol (Dolantin): Isonipecaine: March–December 1946"). Dr. Harry K. followed a similar if slightly harsher trajectory: arrested and sentenced to 15 months at the Lexington, KY narcotics farm, followed by two years probation ("Demerol Addicts," n.d. [FBN Papers, File 0480-190, Folder 2 "Drugs: Demerol (Dolantin): Isonipecaine: March–December 1946"]).

and, behind the scenes, bullied the offending reporter and magazine to ward off any recurrence.[33] These actions heralded a tougher attitude towards Demerol transgressions at the retail and consumer level, with punishments more common than sympathy and treatment. This section explores the closing of the imaginative space for Demerol consumers as the FBN increasingly derided as a set of self-serving fantasies or outright lies.

In some cases, this was as simple as insisting on enforcing the law despite circumstances that might previously have been seen as mitigating. Take, for example, Irene K. in McAlester, Oklahoma, arrested for providing codeine to a friend in recovery from addiction. She had befriended a local physician who prescribed her Demerol in another woman's name; the physician knew Irene had just been released from addiction treatment, but claimed not to know that she was "addicted to demerol" nor "how serious the condition might be." This was a fairly typical story. But the outcome was surprising: "Prosecution recommended as to each defendant."[34] In another case, William B. was given a one to fourteen-year sentence in a federal penitentiary for stealing a prescription pad and using it to buy Demerol.[35] Barbara C. in Detroit was arrested and pled guilty to a narcotics violation when she was caught passing false prescriptions, even though she had a quasi-plausible story: her husband was a druggist and she had simply "found" the blank prescriptions; she only took drugs for pain and nausea and chose Demerol because it was more helpful than the barbiturates she had been prescribed; and she claimed that "she was not addicted to Demerol" because "when she did not take it she did not miss it."[36] W. A. J., who had checked himself into a hospital in Detroit for a severe leg infection due to needle injections, was similarly arrested despite having

33 Herzberg, *White Market Drugs*, 112–14. I have not seen evidence determining the extent to which Alvarez was working collaboratively with or for the manufacturer.

34 Report by Narcotic Agent H. B. Westover, April 10, 1945 (FBN Papers, File 0480-190, Folder 2 "Drugs: Demerol (Dolantin): Isonipecaine: April 1944–"). See also Report by Narcotic Agent H. B. Westover, May 31, 1945 (FBN Papers, File 0480-190, Folder 2 "Drugs: Demerol (Dolantin): Isonipecaine: April 1944–"), for evidence of other ways that Irene K. procured Demerol.

35 Demerol "doesn't seem to be so habit forming as the other narcotics," B. mused, "but you do crave the drug. All you want to do is keep shooting it all day. It gives you such an abnormally relaxed feeling"; R. W. Artis District Supervisor to Anslinger, September 13, 1946 (FBN Papers, File 0480-190, Folder 2 "Drugs: Demerol (Dolantin): Isonipecaine: March–December 1946").

36 Report by Narcotic Agents Newey, Nickell and Rudd, and State Drug Inspector Herbert Reid, July 17, 1946 (FBN Papers, File 0480-190, Folder 2 "Drugs: Demerol (Dolantin): Isonipecaine: March–December 1946").

begun using Demerol for a gall bladder condition and claiming to have been misled about the drug by the *Reader's Digest* article.[37]

The records do not indicate how these cases turned out, but criminal prosecution was in itself a significant escalation. The FBN was transitioning from collecting stories about Demerol addiction – useful in bullying Winthrop into behaving – to real narcotics policing with the goal of identifying and punishing transgressors. This included adopting tactics such as "sting" operations in which undercover agents attempted to make suspicious purchases from physicians. For example, FBN agents visited Dr. Kramer G. in Chandler, Arizona, and requested Demerol for a fictitious ill wife. Dr. G. expressed concern that the agent's fictitious wife might be addicted; the informant promised to wean her off opioids once she was back on her feet and Dr. G. gave in.[38]

Stricter foot-leather policing also came with stricter discursive policing to shut down alternative narratives of Demerol's effects – narratives that, under the circumstances, increasingly appeared to be marketing schemes by Winthrop or duplicitous defenses by "dope fiends." As the stories told by Demerol users came to seem as false as their prescriptions, the FBN more openly derided them and categorized transgressors as typically dishonest "addicts" rather than relatively sympathetic "medical addicts." "I have found," wrote an FBN district supervisor to Anslinger,

> that many of these drug addicts have learned, through publicity which has been given to Demerol in various ways, that they have hit upon something which will satisfy their addiction if they minimize the results of the use of Demerol. For that reason there is no assurance that they will give authentic information. This is an old trick of addicts.[39]

The supervisor then proceeded to revisit several cases, re-narrating them as classic cases of addiction and mocking consumers' efforts to portray them as anything else. Dr. L., for example, who had used Demerol for a year, claimed it was non-addictive. "If this drug did not cause addiction," the supervisor noted, "it would not be necessary for him to submit to

37 August 2, 1948, "Excerpt from case report Mich-3333-Walter Augustine Jonas" (FBN Papers, File 0480-190, Folder 2 "Drugs: Demerol: Paul de Kruif").

38 August 5, 1946, Report by Narcotic Agents A. M. Monroy and Early A. Smith (FBN Papers, File 0480-190, Folder 2 "Drugs: Demerol (Dolantin): Isonipecaine: March–December 1946"). For another case of a "sting" purchase by an agent, see Report by Narcotic Agents Monroy, Kelly and Crook, August 6, 1946 (FBN Papers, File 0480-190, Folder 2 "Drugs: Demerol (Dolantin): Isonipecaine: March–December 1946").

39 July 10, 1946, R. W. Artis to Anslinger (FBN Papers, File 0480-190, Folder 2 "Drugs: Demerol: Paul de Kruif").

treatment." In Paul G., a person with heroin addiction who "carried himself over periods with Demerol," the supervisor did not see a person rationally managing tolerance and dependence, but rather "conclusive proof that demerol will maintain a drug addict at what he calls his normal level." Of Robert W., sentenced to the federal penitentiary for forging a Demerol prescription, the supervisor argued that he was "certainly an addict," and "if the Demerol would not take care of his addiction, wouldn't it have been just as easy for him to forge a prescription for morphine?" In each case, the supervisor collapsed the wide range of ways that Demerol's consumers might have understood their own use into a one-dimensional, stereotypical story of addiction, with any discrepancies attributed to the irrationality and dishonesty to be expected of "addicts."[40]

We can read the FBN's actions through the lens of "drug war" historiography as yet another example of the moralistic and inflexible approach to drug use that proved so useful for culture warriors and white supremacists across the twentieth century. Or, through the lens of pharmaceutical historiography, we might see this as another example of the Bureau's uniquely robust power to counter the multiple levels of drug company marketing hype. Both of these are useful interpretations. But from the cross-cutting perspective of risk and benefit we can see a third story: of how policy choices affect the balance of a drug's risks and benefits and even, in this case, introducing entirely new dangers only tenuously connected to drug effects.

Conclusion

One way that historical narratives reinforce a divide between "medicines" and "drugs" is through the narrative device of constructing two different archetypal drug trajectories. One, applied to pharmaceuticals generally, is a predictable cycle wherein new medicines go through successive phases of therapeutic excitement and overuse, backlash and restriction, and finally, more or less rational use that balances benefits and risks.[41] The other, applied only to psychoactive substances such as LSD, cannabis, heroin, and cocaine, is the criminalization arc, wherein the risks are too dire, and too inextricably connected to the benefits, to be balanced out, and so the second stage – backlash and restriction – leads to prohibition rather than rational use.

40 July 10, 1946, R. W. Artis to Anslinger (FBN Papers, File 0480-190, Folder 2 "Drugs: Demerol: Paul de Kruif").

41 See, e.g., Stephen Snelders, Charles Kaplan, and Toine Peters, "On Cannabis, Chloral Hydrate, and Career Cycles of Psychotropic Drugs in Medicine," *Bulletin of the History of Medicine* 80, no. 1 (2006): 95–114.

At this point the stories diverge significantly, with radically different implicit or explicit interpretations of almost all the key actors (manufacturers, sellers, regulators, and consumers). These differences hinge on acceptance that there is an actual radical divergence in the balance of benefits and risks between the two types of drugs.

Yet these narratives are not as separate as they at first appear – and neither are the risk/benefit stories they rely on. Most psychoactive drugs, like Demerol, have remained available to at least some degree in medical white markets. Some, like LSD and cannabis, were restricted solely to research. Others, like heroin, were fully criminalized, but nearly identical drugs remained widely available in white markets. And, of course, the story does not end with criminalization; many formerly criminalized drugs are now making white market comebacks.[42] In short, these narratives are both historically and historiographically constructed – they are the product of work both in history and by historians.

Consumer experiences with the first synthetic opioid Demerol can help us understand this work and imagine alternatives to the binary scheme of dividing drug benefits and risks. This is because Demerol, like most other opioids, fits neither narrative perfectly. Its overall trajectory fits the "pharmaceutical" narrative better, since it was never fully criminalized and remained an important medicine. Yet few pharmaceuticals leave a trail of arrests and incarcerations in their wake. Demerol's distinctive path highlights the way these trajectories are not natural but were built through authorities' active decisions to shape drug benefits and risks.

What it meant to use Demerol for an extended period of time, for example, was powerfully influenced by regulatory decisions. In clamping down on Demerol, the FBN eliminated alternate ways of understanding toleration, dependence, and desire – an effective strategy to reinforce the moral simplicity that undergirded the agency's power to regulate a powerful industry. The risk of addiction was not found but was built, in response to the long-running cat and mouse game between pharmaceutical companies and government regulators in the context of a racist drug war.

As this chapter has shown, Demerol consumers did not always understand their experiences with the drug as "addiction." Some recognized the phenomena of tolerance, dependence, and desire, but they used different frames for understanding them. Others accepted that they were or had been addicted, but sought more pragmatic and less moralistic ways of managing what they portrayed as a troublesome side effect rather than a totalizing condition.

42 See, e.g., Lucas Richert, *Strange Trips: Science, Culture and the Regulation of Drugs* (McGill-Queens University Press, 2018).

Because of the way US authorities linked addiction so deeply to race and class hierarchies, the fact that Demerol consumers were primarily white, middle-class men and women, with health professionals over-represented, allowed room for their alternative frames, at least briefly. Authorities sometimes implicitly accepted that Demerol consumers were either literally experiencing something different from other "addicts." Or they allowed the possibility that consumers were genuinely confused and did not recognize their own addiction.

But especially as Winthrop's marketing campaign ramped up, the FBN began to crack down on such ambiguities as threats to the moral simplicity the agency relied on in its quest for power to police racial boundaries and to regulate a powerful industry. This crackdown ensured that long-term Demerol use became increasingly likely to produce all the elements of the addiction paradigm, including not just tolerance, dependence, and desire, but lying, shame, criminality, and downward social mobility. This style of drug policing literally made drugs more dangerous.

This story has echoes in the early twenty-first century, when some reformers pushed to recognize a distinction between opioid "dependence" and opioid "addiction." They did so for the laudable purpose of protecting pain patients and people in opioid substitutive treatment such as methadone or buprenorphine (i.e., long term white market opioid consumers) from the stigma of addiction. But why single out these opioid consumers for special protection from the many risks created by stigmatization and criminalization? Why not protect all people who use opioids from these risks? Doing so does not mean embracing the utopian hype of pharmaceutical marketers. Instead, following many of the consumers documented here (and the lived expertise of the generations of opioid consumers who followed them), it can mean approaching opioid effects pragmatically, recognizing and managing the very real risks of tolerance, withdrawal, and desire without forcing all who experience them to face the destructive consequences of stigma and criminalization. This approach is only possible if we, like opioid consumers, reconnect stories of risk and benefit separated by the medicine/drug divide.

Chapter Eleven

"Why Must We Again be the Guinea Pigs in this Genocidal Mentality?": Toward a Historical Understanding of Black Popular Resistance to Harm Reduction

Samuel Kelton Roberts Jr.

In the late 1990s, Black harm reductionist Imani Woods described her frustration at the challenges of turning harm reduction into a viable social and political movement within African American politics. Woods had been doing the work for over a decade, having begun at the Narcotic and Drug Research Institute (NDRI) in 1986, moving on a year later to a pathbreaking harm reduction organization named the Association for Drug Abuse Prevention and Treatment (ADAPT). Both organizations operated in New York, where Woods quickly gained recognition as a brilliant social worker, organizer, and leading harm reduction activist. Indeed, Woods was one of the original cadre of harm reduction activists in New York, part of a small but growing circle led in part by Edith Springer, under whom Woods trained and worked for several years. Eventually, Woods moved to Seattle, Washington, to become the Executive Director of the Street Outreach Services (S.O.S.) program. In Seattle, she worked among Black, Latinx, and White people who used drugs, helping them to find not only clean needles but also connections to social services such as medical attention, pre- and post-natal care, vocational opportunities, and addiction recovery services.

Reflecting on her years of experience and the current moment, Woods categorized the challenges of Black harm reduction work roughly into two categories. First was a taboo subject which has plagued multi-ethnic social justice movements since the anti-slavery campaigns of the mid-nineteenth century: the marginalization and alienation of people of color as leaders and even as rank and file. The "efforts by well-meaning harm reductionists of European descent," she wrote, "to design programs for and introduce them into African American communities will be regarded with suspicion and distrust by the members of those communities. Moreover, I have found that despite (or in some cases as a result of) their good intentions, white harm reductionists tend to reenact patterns of white-dominance-black-submission in their attempts to work with their black counterparts. U.S. society as a whole is being forced to reevaluate us black folks, and the harm reduction movement is no exception." White people in the movement therefore needed to understand the differing subject positions maintained by Black people. Evoking DuBois's theorization of double consciousness, Woods noted that Black harm reductionists

> experience our "two-ness" as our white counterparts' expectations become overbearing. My experience has been that those of us black folks who are involved in the harm reduction movement are constantly taken to task, as white folks grow impatient with our prudence and caution. Our racial authenticity is challenged as we seek the normality that transcends cultural commitment and allows for independent thinking. Our actions in proceeding prudently and thoughtfully serve not only ourselves, but the members of our community, who catch hell every day ... Meanwhile, our white counterparts require and demand the full benefit of our symbolic participation ... We are constantly aware that we are not just harm reduction advocates; we are black harm reduction advocates – a rare but powerful commodity![1]

This first problem exacerbated the second, which was the daunting challenge of overcoming Black popular resistance to harm reduction and of introducing into the Black public sphere a discussion of the nature and potential benefits of harm reduction practiced for and by Black people. Many bristled even at the idea that the War on Drugs and the relentless persecution of people who use drugs was ill-conceived and misdirected. Incredulous, they immediately pointed to drug-related property crimes. "Who's going to pay

1 Imani P. Woods, "Bringing Harm Reduction to the Black Community: There's a Fire in My House and You're Telling Me to Rearrange My Furniture?," in *Harm Reduction: Pragmatic Strategies for Managing High-Risk Behaviors*, ed. G. Alan Marlatt (Guilford Press, 1998), 319.

for my stolen TV?" they demanded, rhetorically. "We're being robbed and knocked down in the street for drugs," was an accusation aimed directly at Woods, "and you want to talk about giving out needles and keeping people alive?!" Others pointed to the human toll of drug use, and could not imagine a movement which was critical of the criminalization of drug use. Middle-aged adults complained: "I've been taking care of my little grandbaby for 8 years ... Don't you know my son and his woman [are] in jail because of [their drug use]?" Such logic often conflated the direct effects of drug use with those of the War on Drugs, although Woods's interrogators were not unaware of the patent unfairness of the drug war and its particular focus on communities of color. Convinced that drug use was probably as high or higher in other communities, yet also opposed to harm reduction in Black communities, many angrily expressed their belief that "White folks' kids get jobs even after they do all that!"[2]

And then there were the allegations of genocide. As Woods put it:

> People look at me like I'm crazy when I go to the black community to explain harm reduction. I am accused of supporting a policy that makes peace with genocide. How can one talk about "reducing harm" to a people under siege? The scourge must be lifted; the villain must be vanquished. Harm reduction is seen as settling, giving up, accepting failure, and bargaining with the devil.[3]

Indeed, many Black New Yorkers placed harm reduction on the same historical continuum with the Tuskegee Syphilis Study, during which for forty years the US government actively prevented 200 Black men and their sexual partners from receiving treatment simply in order to discover the long-term effects of syphilis infection. For Black America, the 1972 revelation of the Tuskegee abuses was not just symbolic but emblematic of generations of official neglect and structural violence. Black New Yorkers a generation later asked Woods how providing syringes to people using heroin was much different. "Who are those white folks trying to come in our neighborhood with needles?" some asked, leaving Woods to wonder whether the question were rhetorical or actual. "They just trying to kill us. And you're missin' it!"[4]

As we know now, and as Woods knew then, syringe exchange and harm reduction have little in common with the Tuskegee Study, and even less with genocide. However, as Woods herself learned, popular Black protest against harm reduction practices and policies invites us to consider seriously the subjective and objective bases – the lived experience and structural realities – for

2 Woods, "Bringing Harm Reduction to the Black Community."

3 Woods, "Bringing Harm Reduction to the Black Community," 301.

4 Woods, "Bringing Harm Reduction to the Black Community."

widespread suspicion within the Black public sphere. Why, Woods's interlocutors asked, after spending years and millions of dollars in chasing "junkies" and dealers should the state, organized public health, and, perhaps more generically, White people now be taken on their word that syringe provision represented an adequate or trustworthy response? If government had not cared enough to secure for Black citizens fundamental rights to health or opportunities for work, education, and housing, how could any Black person believe that the same government now had undertaken the responsibility of preserving Black lives? After all, in New York and many of the other cities which adopted syringe exchange, the officially recognized and aboveground programs began as geographically and numerically limited studies conducted under the auspices or oversight of health departments. So, too, had Tuskegee, a friend challenged Woods:

> "You say harm reduction is a public health model! This public health system here in the U.S.! Those are the same people that used us for 40 years!
>
> "Imani, think about it, they used us to find out how to keep themselves *alive*! They didn't want us to have penicillin, so why *now* do they want to give us clean needles?"

Woods herself was forced into nearly dumfounded self-reflection. "My passionate pleas fall on the ears of skeptics. And why should they believe me?" she wrote, comparing herself to the Black woman who had assisted the physicians at Tuskegee, "I could be the Nurse Rivers of harm reduction."[5]

This essay is not about Imani Woods. She instead introduces us to a rather thorny and commonly unaddressed problem: the meanings of genocide in Black political critiques of harm reduction. I argue that allegations of "genocide" were a discursive register within Black politics, signaling concerned recognition of the historical and present risks posed by medical abuse and neglect and by structural violence. Since the nineteenth century, African Americans have participated in discussions of race and risk. Beginning in the late 1800s, debates regarding so-called racial differentials in disease morbidity and mortality, for example, directly impacted the insurability of Black lives. A similar management of risk is the example of redlining practices, initiated by mortgage lenders and real estate interests (and adopted by the federal government during the New Deal) to safeguard the value of real property through the exclusion of Black, Latinx, Asian, and Jewish Americans from "greenlined" areas.

In Black political culture of late-industrial America, one easily may have found critique of what we may think of as *racialized risk inequity*. In contrast

5 Woods, "Bringing Harm Reduction to the Black Community."

to the assertion of early risk society theorists that risk of harm caused by the industrial products of reflexive modernity (as Anthony Giddens termed the era), an acknowledgement of racialized risk inequity means consideration of the historically patterned, institutionally produced, and legally normalized unequal distribution of socially manufactured hazards and protections across racialized populations. Racialized risk inequity arises where modern risk governance allocates exposure, transfers burdens, and withholds protections so that harms and uncertainty concentrate among stigmatized groups while benefits, security, and insulation accrue to dominant ones. A staple of environmental justice thought since the 1960s, therefore, has been the recognition of benefits provided by the chemical and nuclear power industries with the risk taken up by communities of color.[6] And most Black and many White Americans in the 1960s and 1970s held views of the geography of Black working-class and poor communities ("the ghetto") as being one of especially *intense* risk for all manner of bodily and social harms (even if theories of how risk presented itself could vary widely). Indeed, by the early 1980s (the advent of Ulrich Beck's theorization of "risk society"), the floating signifier of "at-risk youth" in both policy and colloquial discussions was synonymous with urban Black children.[7]

6 Bernard E. Harcourt, *Against Prediction: Profiling, Policing, and Punishing in an Actuarial Age* (University of Chicago Press, 2007); Benjamin Wiggins, *Calculating Race: Racial Discrimination in Risk Assessment* (Oxford University Press, 2020); Samuel Roberts, *Infectious Fear: Politics, Disease, and the Health Effects of Segregation* (University of North Carolina Press, 2009); Douglas S. Massey and Nancy A. Denton, *American Apartheid: Segregation and the Making of the Underclass* (Harvard University Press, 1993); Richard Rothstein, *The Color of Law: A Forgotten History of How Our Government Segregated America* (Liveright, 2017); Robert D. Bullard, ed., *Unequal Protection: Environmental Justice and Communities of Color* (Sierra Club Books, 1994); Robert D. Bullard, *Dumping in Dixie: Race, Class, and Environmental Quality* (Westview Press, 1994); Dorceta E. Taylor, "The Rise of the Environmental Justice Paradigm: Injustice Framing and the Social Construction of Environmental Discourses," *The American Behavioral Scientist* 43, no. 4 (2000): 508–80; Dorceta E. Taylor, *The Environment and the People in American Cities, 1600s–1900s: Disorder, Inequality, and Social Change* (Duke University Press, 2009); Josiah Rector, *Toxic Debt: An Environmental Justice History of Detroit* (University of North Carolina Press, 2022).

7 Patricia Albjerg Graham, *Schooling America: How the Public Schools Meet the Nation's Changing Needs* (Oxford University Press, 2005); Maris Vinovskis, *From a Nation at Risk to No Child Left Behind: National Education Goals and the Creation of Federal Education Policy* (Teachers College Press, Columbia University, 2009); David P. Gardner and United States National Commission on Excellence in Education, *A Nation at Risk: The Imperative for Educational*

After a series of perceived defaults, the arrival of harm reduction, even though not propelled or even promoted by the government, therefore seemed like just another. Instead of addressing what critics believed were the root causes of the drug problem – the need for deep reforms in housing, education, and the economy – White America could offer only the band-aid solution of harm reduction, which hardly matched up to the unaddressed risk environments (to use a term coined decades later) in which Black Americans in cities struggled.[8] Opposition often invoked civil and economic rights, racial justice, and protection of the Black community. To be sure, Black political and civic leadership, whom I discuss later in this essay, often had cynical reasons for harm reduction – using a leadership position to move public opinion was politically risky and could endanger one's aspirations for re-election or reappointment. For many in the Black political laity, however, antipathy toward harm reduction was more genuine. Some of it is explained by the deeper historical legacies of what Evelyn Brooks Higginbotham calls a "politics of respectability," in which Black Americans since the nineteenth century have based citizenship claims on rejections of stigmas and stereotypes of Black social disorganization, sexual licentiousness, skewed gender norms, criminality, and use of intoxicants, in favor of the earnest adoption of (hyper-)normative values of upright comportment, morality/religiosity, temperance, and the deferral of gratification.[9] A historical phenomenon, respectability politics has served as a defensive measure against the weight of popular stigma and exclusion. However, as political scientist Cathy Cohen has noted of Black politics in the early years of HIV/AIDS, socially conservative Black leadership suffered from not just a lack of sympathy and vision, but also a dearth of options.[10] Elected officials in particular watched as shrinking tax bases left them increasingly in need of a similarly shrinking federal appropriation budget. Bucking the "Bennett Plan" (the zero-tolerance and militarized approach named after William Bennett, the director of President George H. W. Bush's Office of National Drug Control Policy) by

---

Reform: A Report to the Nation and the Secretary of Education, United States Department of Education (US Department of Education and the US Government Printing Office, 1983).

8 Tim Rhodes, "Risk Environments and Drug Harms: A Social Science for Harm Reduction Approach," *International Journal of Drug Policy* 20, no. 3 (2009): 193–201.

9 Evelyn Brooks Higginbotham, *Righteous Discontent: The Women's Movement in the Black Baptist Church, 1880–1920* (Harvard University Press, 1993); Kevin K. Gaines, *Uplifting the Race: Black Leadership, Politics, and Culture in the Twentieth Century* (University of North Carolina Press, 1996).

10 Cathy J. Cohen, *The Boundaries of Blackness: AIDS and the Breakdown of Black Politics* (Chicago, IL: University of Chicago Press, 1999).

supporting anything smacking of decriminalization was no way to maintain the possibility of federal funding for much needed services, especially the comprehensive addiction treatment programs Black leadership preferred to have over simple needle exchange. As such, African American opposition to harm reduction should be viewed as having a basis in both enduring social conservatism but also in the broader and dominant political logics of federal retrenchment, post-Fordist political economy, incipient hyperpolicing and mass incarceration, and the War on Drugs.

Thus the vociferous cries of protest and accusations of genocide in the 1980s and 1990s. When New York Health Commissioner Stephen Joseph announced the beginning of a limited study of syringe exchange in October 1988, to be initiated with the opening of four sites, the protest was significant. Police Commissioner Benjamin Ward sourly informed a television audience that "As a Black person we have a particular sensitivity to doctors conducting experiments, and they too frequently seem to be conducted against Blacks."[11] Bronx City Councilman Wendell Foster labeled the project a "planned assassination in the minority community ... a damnable, intolerable, unforgivable project."[12] Harlem's City Councilman, Hilton Clark, flatly declared, "This is a racist program. ... If the I.V. drug population was anywhere close to being [ethnically] integrated, you can be sure we would not have this program; we'd find money for drug treatment." Clark also announced his intention, should even a single overdose death emerge from the study, "to ask that the health commissioner be arrested for murder."[13] Clark likened the program to genocide, as did the Reverend Reginald Williams, director of Harlem's Addicts Rehabilitation Center, one of the nation's oldest addiction services ("Why must we again be the guinea pigs in this genocidal mentality?").[14] Revealing how law enforcement had become the dominant political paradigm in drug policy, in an open letter to Koch the City Council's Black and Hispanic Caucus wrote: "It is beyond all human reason and common sense for the city to hand out needles to drug addicts at a time when our police officers and citizens have become casualties in the drug war."[15] The *Amsterdam News*, New York's Black daily paper, called for Koch to resign, noting that Koch earlier had called for the death

11 Michel Marriott, "Needle Exchange Angers Many Minorities," *New York Times*, November 7, 1988.

12 Larry Bivins, "Koch, Joseph Lashed on Needle Swap," *Newsday* (Long Island, NY), October 28, 1988.

13 Sandra G. Boodman, "N.Y. 'Needle Exchange': Curbing AIDS or Condoning Drug Use?," *The Washington Post* (Washington, DC), March 6, 1989.

14 Marriott, "Needle Exchange Angers Many Minorities."

15 Marriott, "Needle Exchange Angers Many Minorities."

penalty for anyone guilty of killing a police officer while under the influence of drugs.[16] In late December 1988, the Harlem Drug Task Force (a coalition, formed by Councilman Clark, of former drug users, treatment professionals, law enforcement, and victims of drug-related crime) protested at the Health Department headquarters.[17]

Some critiques were simply social (dislike of people who use drugs), but even structural and political commentary (highlighting the hypocrisy of uneven social services while funding the needle exchange program, for example) did not regard those most at risk – Black gay men and people using drugs intravenously – as political agents and potential allies. On one hand, this should not be surprising, given the oppressing weight of criminalization and stigmatization borne by both groups – the late-twentieth-century expansion of rights for gays and lesbians is a direct result of the HIV/AIDS activism of the period, and people using narcotics illicitly are still criminalized (and often politically disenfranchised) in most states. On the other, that there were Black harm reductions there and then to point out this failure of political vision shows our own similar assessment to be not entirely ahistorical.

But that is not the point, which instead is that such thought, without regard as to whether it takes the historian in a direction of which we approve, demands to be considered thoroughly on its own terms. Indeed, even as historians and social scientists have described opposition to harm reduction, their failure to deal analytically with genocide-discourse-as-critique makes the need for such a historical examination particularly clear. As a member of a very small cohort of African American harm reductionists, Woods belonged to two communities which generally were quite distant from one another. Her subject position in this regard is not merely historically unique but also methodologically instructive. Woods's article, an early and powerful written example of Black harm reduction thought titled, "Bringing Harm Reduction to the Black Community," reveals her as a ranging and eclectic Black woman intellectual of sophisticated praxis – her analysis of race, drug politics, and harm reduction drew from her equal and synthetic investments in community work, social investigation and analysis, justice, public health, and a Black critical intellectual and political tradition (as evidenced by her allusions not just to DuBois, but also to Malcolm X, Derrick Bell, Lani Guinier, Bruce Wright, Farai Chideya, Naim Akbar, and Earl Ofari Hutchinson). Her dual challenge to White harm reductionists and the Black public just as well could

16 Wilbert A. Tatum, "Editorial: While Corruption Investigation Continues, Koch Must Resign – Koch's Needle Exchange Program," *New York Amsterdam News*, November 5, 1988.

17 "Task Force to Protest Needle Giveaway Proposals," *New York Amsterdam News*, December 3, 1988.

be one to public health scholars (including historians) who too quickly dismiss the political and social histories of the populations they study.

* * *

Syringe exchange was not the first historical drugs-related political context in which allegations of genocide had emerged. As Woods undoubtedly was aware, she had inherited a challenge faced by Black advocates for methadone maintenance treatment (MMT) since the late 1960s. MMT, originating in New York City in the mid 1960s and widely available there and in other metropolitan areas after 1970, also had fallen under similar suspicion in Black and Latinx communities. This was largely because its promoters never offered an analysis of the political economy of race and drug use, but instead preferred to simply medicalize addiction as a "metabolic disorder." MMT, as I've argued elsewhere, arrived after fifteen years of Black and Latinx grassroots activism to establish locally based treatment programs which framed addiction as something which an individual with community support (medical and psychiatric care coupled with after-care programs, vocational and educational services, social work, etc.) could confront but which nonetheless had to be understood more broadly in terms of the structural inequalities and racism which they believed constituted "root causes" of drug use.[18]

At bottom, whether one supported MMT or the social-psychological-cum-social-work perspective depended largely on how one viewed addiction itself. One medicalized "disease model" of heroin addiction in the 1960s and 1970s argued that it could be treated with a replacement drug administered by a qualified physician working in a hospital or at least a clinic. To critics, this was no less than a negation of the demands for community-based treatment which were part and parcel of a larger suite of demands for educational equity, affordable housing, an end to job discrimination, and an address of police corruption and brutality, all of which, critics insisted, were root causes of the addiction problem. In New York, the political pharmacology of methadone was one in which City Hall and Governor Nelson Rockefeller (and, later, President Richard Nixon) appeared more willing to support methadone maintenance as a cheap, large-scale, and technocratic "false cure" whose appeal derived more from its touted anti-crime properties (addicts using methadone will not need to steal to buy heroin) than its usefulness within an agenda stressing community participation and control not just in addiction treatment or even health care, but also in a wide range of facets of American life. In short, rather than pursuing reform to address

18 Samuel Kelton Roberts Jr., "'Rehabilitation' as Boundary Object: Medicalization, Local Activism, and Narcotics Addiction Policy in New York City, 1951–1962," *Social History of Alcohol and Drugs* 26, no. 2 (2012): 147–69.

the period's legal, social, and economic conditions, methadone advocates seemed to their critics more willing to displace the risks these contradictions produced onto those most vulnerable in the first place.

Articulations of the critique were as various as they were widespread. As clinics opened their doors across the country in the early 1970s, sociologists Dorothy Nelkin and Amitai Etizioni (both White), were among several who critically labeled methadone a "technological fix" for deeper social problems.[19] Implicitly commenting on a particular form of addiction medicalization represented in MMT, African American *Washington Post* columnist William Raspberry in 1971 expressed his deep skepticism at politicians' zeal for "the miracle drug that will cure the curse of heroin addiction," and worried that "methadone is not so much a means for treating addicts as a way of fighting crime. ... [M]ethadone not only blocks the effects of heroin in the addict; it blocks the effects of drug addiction on society, rendering addiction a merely personal problem."[20] Removing addiction from social context to the individual ("personal") might possibly have undesirable effects, principally a further disruption of the increasingly embattled postwar liberal consensus emphasizing investment in communities as the best pathway to individual betterment and social equality: "if methadone maintenance by itself shows promising signs of reducing crime, [providers] will be increasingly hard put to justify expenditures for [the supportive services of] psychiatrists, social workers, placement specialists and the rest. ... Some of our officials would just as soon narcotize the whole ghetto population on a cheap synthetic if that would stop crime."[21] In October 1972, US House of Representatives Delegate Walter E. Fauntroy (District of Columbia) held two days of hearings on MMT, airing his skepticism of the benefits for Black communities and Black patients alike. In his testimony, Ron Clark, the director of Washington, DC's, RAP, Inc., argued that MMT was "politically expedient," whereas real recovery was "supposed to 'rehabilitate' [the addict] back into the mainstream of the larger society which produced him in the first place. Presumably, he is better able to cope with the same contradictions in his community: the availability of drugs, inadequate employment conditions, inadequate education or none at all."[22]

19 Dorothy Nelkin, *Methadone Maintenance: A Technological Fix* (G. Braziller, 1973); Amitai Etzioni and Richard Remp, *Technological Shortcuts to Social Change* (Russell Sage Foundation, 1973).

20 William Raspberry, "Methadone Use: Another Blunder," *The Washington Post*, May 11, 1971.

21 William Raspberry, "Holdups or Hangups?," *The Washington Post*, June 25, 1971.

22 Peter Osnos, "Is It a Solution?: Controversy on Methadone as Heroin Solution Mounting," *The Washington Post*, December 26, 1972.

Historians of methadone maintenance have correctly pointed out that methadone's invention as an analgesic came some thirty years before its use as an officially sanctioned maintenance modality, and that MMT's arrival had less to do with scientific discovery than the propitious historical moment when a small but vocal and growing minority of physicians was willing to challenge not just the criminalization of addiction but also the premise of abstinence as the fullest measure of rehabilitation. In their analyses of MMT history, however, none of them has done so in the context of the important movements for medical and Civil Rights, or of the quickening leftist Black and Brown Power movements emphasizing community self-determination in the "domestic colony" of the American ghetto. The embrace of tricontinental (Third Worldist) and anticolonial politics was a staple feature in the dozens of groups in New York, San Francisco, Los Angeles, Washington, DC, Chicago, and elsewhere who comprised what I call the *radical recovery* movement. The members of Lincoln Detox, a community-based program with strong ties to Marxist-nationalist groups, included in its rehabilitation program tellingly-named "political education" classes in which members discussed, among other things, the connections between US militarism in Southeast Asia to the importation and domestic distribution of heroin via illicit smuggling channels facilitated by official corruption and structural inequality in the ghetto. The curriculum included Yale University historian Alfred McCoy's 1972 *The Politics of Heroin in Southeast Asia*, along with other books and pamphlets which circulated through radical political circles. *The Opium Trail: Heroin and Imperialism*, a slim volume published in 1972 by the Committee of Concerned Asian Scholars, plainly stated, in its authors' view, the historical connections and similarities between nineteenth-century British insistence on maintaining its opium trade in China (even to the point of waging two wars between 1839 and 1860 with China in order to protect its market) and twentieth-century official complicity in importation of heroin from Southeast Asia. The Committee also pointed out that American law enforcement proponents who emphasized supply-side actions, meaning the pursuit and prosecution of street-level drug peddlers, rarely seemed to view a re-evaluation of foreign policy as an appropriate step in drug control.[23]

Even more popular and assertive was Michael Cetawayo Tabor's *Capitalism Plus Dope Equals Genocide*, an eleven-page pamphlet published independently by the New York Black Panther Party in 1970. Tabor was one of the "New York 21," who were eventually acquitted of murder and bombing conspiracy charges in 1971 (by which time Tabor had fled to Algeria).

23 Committee of Concerned Asian Scholars, *The Opium Trail: Heroin and Imperialism*, 2nd ed. (New England Free Press, 1972).

Like the Committee of Concerned Asian Scholars, Tabor was critical of US foreign policy. He also addressed something that was widely known in many Black communities but unaddressed by White power structures: the problem of official corruption and police complicity in the drug trade. *Capitalism Plus Dope Equals Genocide* linked these and neglect to both demand and supply: drug use was the expected though dysfunctional individual response to the physical and structural violence experienced on the individual and community levels, while the supply was aided by police themselves.

As had the widely read *Black Power* (written in 1967 by activist Stokely Carmichael and Columbia University political scientist Charles V. Hamilton), Tabor's treatise read the American ghetto as an "internal colony," a theory reflecting the influence of Third World Marxism and the arguments of World Systems theorists (principally Oliver Cox and Immanuel Wallerstein). Combined with a critique of colonial occupation and violence (e.g. in the work of Frantz Fanon), the idea moved easily within Left political circles.[24] Most critically – and here is a point which emerges in contemporary critical harm reduction movements, though less so in mainstream liberal ones – Tabor described anti-drug policy and politics as modalities of racialized class conflict. He further argued that prevalent views of drug use or assumed definitions of addiction reflected the larger power structures in which they were formed but not the lived reality of people using drugs or the communities in which they existed. The incipient War on Drugs (officially declared in 1971) itself was therefore a brutal resolution of contradictions in what political theorist and historian Cedric Robinson a decade later labeled *racial capitalism*, and one which, as in most colonial regimes, needed the ardent complicity of appointed indigenous leaders: "Given the fact that Black people have abandoned the non-functional and ineffective tactics of the 'Civil Rights' era and have now resolved to attain their long overdue liberation by any means

24 Stokely Carmichael and Charles V. Hamilton, *Black Power: The Politics of Liberation in America* (Random House, 1967); Harold Cruse, "Revolutionary Nationalism and the Afro-American," in *Rebellion or Revolution?* (Morrow, 1968), 74–96; William K. Tabb, *The Political Economy of the Black Ghetto* (W. W. Norton & Co., 1970); William K. Tabb and Larry Sawers, *Marxism and the Metropolis: New Perspectives in Urban Political Economy* (Oxford University Press, 1978). See also Laura Pulido, *Black, Brown, Yellow, and Left: Radical Activism in Los Angeles* (University of California Press, 2006); Manning Marable, *How Capitalism Underdeveloped Black America: Problems in Race, Political Economy and Society*, 1st ed. (South End Press, 1983); Manning Marable, *Race, Reform and Rebellion: The Second Reconstruction in Black America, 1945–1982* (University Press of Mississippi, 1984); Cedric Johnson, *Revolutionaries to Race Leaders: Black Power and the Making of African American Politics* (University of Minnesota Press, 2007), 23.

necessary," Tabor declared, "it has become necessary for the oppressor to deploy more occupation forces into the Black colony." The unfortunate irony was what Tabor viewed as the complicity of "responsible negro community leaders" whose understandable desire for crime reduction and ardor for law enforcement made them fail to "remember who put the [heroin] plague in Harlem, Bedford Stuyvesant, and the other Black communities[,] ... who ultimately profits from the drug addiction of Black people" and "that the police are alien hostile troops sent into the Black colonies by the ruling class, not to protect the lives of Black people, but rather to protect the economic interests and the private property of the capitalists and to make certain that Black people don't get out of place.[25]

Though strident and polemical in its language, Tabor's *Capitalism Plus Dope Equals Genocide* offered inescapable critique. First, it foreshadowed New York's Knapp Commission's revelations, two years later, of gross, organized, and systemic corruption (including drug dealing and the protection of kingpins) within the New York City Police Department. It also was analytically prescient, anticipating later analyses of the War on Drugs and mass incarceration in the 1990s and after. Even Tabor's deployment of the term genocide (which, aside from the work's title, appears only once, at the end of the pamphlet: "Dope is a form of genocide in which the victim pays to be killed") was not sui generis but rather drew from a larger international discourse and the thwarted Third-World-identified efforts since the early 1950s (including African Americans and Puerto Ricans in the US) for United Nations recognition of human rights abuses committed by colonial or neocolonial powers such as Britain, France, Belgium, Portugal, and the US as genocidal. For African Americans, the history of such international appeals for intervention on mass murder dates at least as far back as Frederick Douglass and Ida B. Wells. In the post-WWII years, various Black American efforts to enlist the aid of the United Nations to intervene on human rights grounds included those of W. E. B. DuBois and the NAACP's "An Appeal to the World" in 1947, Black Communist attorney William L. Patterson and the Civil Rights Congress's 240-page petition titled *We Charge Genocide: The Historic Petition to the United Nations for Relief From A Crime of the United States Government Against the Negro People* (1951), and of El-Hajj Malik El-Shabazz (Malcolm X) after 1960.[26]

25 Michael "Cetewayo" Tabor, *Capitalism Plus Dope Equal Genocide* (Black Panther Party, 1970).

26 Mary L. Dudziak, *Cold War Civil Rights: Race and the Image of American Democracy* (Princeton University Press, 2000); Carol Anderson, *Eyes Off the Prize: The United Nations and the African American Struggle for Human Rights, 1944–1955* (Cambridge University Press, 2003); Brenda Gayle Plummer, *Window on Freedom: Race, Civil Rights, and Foreign Affairs,*

On the other hand, absent a larger political agenda of community self-determination or an articulated vision of rehabilitation using a language of rights and democratic promise, methadone maintenance therefore appeared to many as a potential weapon, a useful tool of colonial pacification of the American ghetto to be turned against the people whom it was purported to serve. Certainly, skeptics argued, a government mired in an imperialist war in Southeast Asia, and which generally had remained uncritical of human rights violations enacted by state governors in the Deep South and by European allies in African colonies, could not unquestionably be said to be above such abuses against its own population. As I have argued elsewhere, pro-methadone politicians or even physicians did little to allay their fears, preferring to tout its anti-crime virtues than to figure it within the continuing rights revolutions. Further, the most salient innovation presented by methadone maintenance was not its emergence in the pharmacopoeia (that had happened in the 1930s), but its enactment, to use Annemarie Mol's term, of addiction as a metabolic disease, and the medicalization of rehabilitation as the cessation of heroin use in favor of activities deemed socially productive (resumption of educational and vocational pursuits).[27]

Neither premise – mere abstinence nor productive labor in capitalism – seemed an especially adequate response to a view of addiction as *alienation*, the product of the exact social and economic system into which methadone promised to (re)introduce its patients. A 1969 discussion regarding methadone maintenance airing on "Right Now," a local Sunday morning public

---

1945–1988 (University of North Carolina Press, 2003); Manning Marable, *Malcolm X: A Life of Reinvention* (Viking, 2011); Gerald Horne, *Black Revolutionary: William Patterson and the Globalization of the African American Freedom Struggle* (University of Illinois Press, 2013); Civil Rights Congress and William L. Patterson, *We Charge Genocide: The Historic Petition to the United Nations for Relief from a Crime of the United States Government against the Negro People* (New York, 1951).

27 Roberts, "'Rehabilitation' as Boundary Object"; Samuel Kelton Roberts Jr., "The Politics of Stigma and Racialization in the Early Years of Methadone Maintenance Regulation," in *Methadone Treatment for Opioid Use Disorder: Improving Access through Regulatory and Legal Change: Proceedings of a Workshop*, ed. Lisa Bain, Sheena M. Posey Norris, and Clare Stroud (The National Academies Press, 2022), 136–51; Helena Hansen and Samuel Roberts, "Two Tiers of Biomedicalization: Buprenorphine, Methadone and the Biopolitics of Addiction Stigma and Race," in *Critical Perspectives on Addiction*, ed. Julie Netherland (Emerald, 2012), 79–102; Annemarie Mol, *The Body Multiple: Ontology in Medical Practice* (Duke University Press, 2002). See also Mical Raz, "Treating Addiction or Reducing Crime? Methadone Maintenance and Drug Policy under the Nixon Administration," *Journal of Policy History* 29, no. 1 (2017): 58–86.

affairs television program, featured Wallace White, a self-described former addict and a counselor in Harlem's Addicts Rehabilitation Center (one of the earliest African American programs in the country). White's argument, that rehabilitation entailed more than a chemical cure, and rather required deep cognitive reorientation ("the way they [recovering addicts] think and feel about different subjects; all this has to be changed before you can say an addict has been rehabilitated") led him to call methadone nothing more or less than "a slow form of genocide." Coming from an employee of the ARC, one of the city's many treatment organizations in competition with MMT programs, White's assessment was almost predictable. Less so, however, was the ardent agreement from another featured guest, the assistant principal of an East Harlem high school who worried that a large portion of a young generation might wind up "addicted ... to another type of drug. They have to go back sort of more or less for a refill," and hence would never be free of their addiction.[28] Chicago *Defender* columnist Curtis Burrell similarly feared the potential for social control: "methadone and general drug rehabilitation programs offer inescapable racial consequences. ... Today's drug rehabilitation programs could become the New Enslavement. The unexpected form of genocide."[29]

It was not solely a Black critique. The anti-war, pro-Civil Rights, and largely White Medical Committee for Human Rights (MCHR) announced its opposition to methadone.[30] So, too, did the leftist and predominantly White Health Policy Advisory Center (HEATH-PAC), whose members were of the belief that methadone maintenance represented only a quick "medical 'fix'" destined to do no better than the "proliferating treatment programs, ... designed for the most part by white professionals, [that] have little chance of success for great numbers of black and brown addicts."[31] Meanwhile, in Baltimore, a meeting of more than four hundred White and Black professionals and lay workers in 1972 featured round condemnations of methadone maintenance, with one speaker describing methadone as an "agent of chemical fascism."[32]

28 "Methadone a Form of Genocide: Ex-Addict," *New York Amsterdam News*, May 10, 1969.

29 Rev. Curtis E. Burrell Jr., "Black Addiction: A Summary and Overview," *Chicago Daily Defender*, October 21, 1971.

30 William L. Claiborne, "U.S. Methadone Role Scored," *The Washington Post*, May 14, 1972.

31 HEALTH-PAC Workshop on Drug Addiction, Harriet Block, and Lester Wallerstein, "Who Benefits from the American Drug Culture?," *HEALTH-PAC Bulletin*, June 1970.

32 Claiborne, "U.S. Methadone Role Scored."

In the tense late- and post-Civil Rights years, and within the politics of Third Worldist-oriented grassroots health activism and movements for community participation in, and even control of, education, healthcare, and policing, framing methadone maintenance as a form of "genocide" was more than a hyperbolic exaggeration, but rather a register of biopolitics itself. It signaled a sociopolitical analysis looking beyond medicine and medicalization, connecting structural violence and racism to the lack of viable options afforded to Black subjectivity and life itself. It called attention to what medical anthropologist Nancy Scheper Hughes, working from Hannah Arendt, later identified as the ***genocidal continuum***: the series of structurally and epistemically violent policies and practices – "the many ordinary betrayals, the small wars and invisible genocides, already perpetrated against certain classes of sub-citizens" – which usually do not end in genocide but which always precede it. In a similar fashion, historian and political theorist Achille Mbembe would have labeled this variety of politics as one which highlighted the ***necropolitics*** of structural violence, specifically a state's power of "subjugation of life to the power of death."[33]

Historians have not been oblivious to social movements' deployment of genocide as an analytical frame. Historian and sociologist Alondra Nelson has noted of the Black Panther Party's health campaigns that "charges of state-backed genocide through medical neglect and mistreatment" as well as "fatal incidents of police brutality, the unchecked proliferation of drugs in black communities, and attempts to temper procreation through the abusive, compelled[,] sterilization of African American women" constituted not exaggeration but an analytical frame of the plight of Black and Latinx Americans.[34] Similarly, historian and geographer Jena Loyd describes a post-1964 peace and gender rights political language, noting that "Black and Chicana welfare mothers linked their unmet needs to wartime spending, and the Third World Left argued that the U.S. state was responsible for a geography of genocide linking Vietnam and communities of color at home." Student, antiwar, and Black, Brown, and Asian American groups "increasingly used the language of genocide and repression to show the violent continuities between direct police repression, poverty, and state cutbacks [to social services]."[35] As historian Alexandra Stern has noted of the

33 Nancy Scheper-Hughes, "The Genocidal Continuum," in *Power and the Self*, ed. Jeannette Marie Mageo (Cambridge University Press, 2002), 29–47; Achille Mbembe, "Necropolitics," *Public Culture* 15, no. 1 (2003): 11–40; Achille Mbembe, *Necropolitics* (Duke University Press, 2019).

34 Alondra Nelson, *Body and Soul: The Black Panther Party and the Fight against Medical Discrimination* (University of Minnesota Press, 2011), 132–33.

35 Jenna M. Loyd, *Health Rights Are Civil Rights: Peace and Justice Activism in Los Angeles, 1963–1978* (University of Minnesota Press, 2014).

same decades of crisis, reproductive justice activists frequently "condemned practices they associated with racism, sexism, oppression, and exploitation and regularly expressed their moral outrage with terms such as *imperialism*, *fascism*, and *genocide*."[36]

* * *

Of course, calling attention to the uses of genocide discourse as structural critique worthy of serious historical consideration should not imply an *a priori* ethical privilege extended to such points of view. After all, such analyses will vary according to their philosophical and ethical groundings, often conferring value and worthiness differentially. An example external but biopolitically connected to drugs politics are the various controversies in which some Black Americans alleged genocidal intent in the state provision of abortion, tubal ligation, and other birth control services. Formed within an ethnic group whose meaningful survival never was assured (and, indeed, whose disappearance many White physicians and vital statisticians had predicted in the late nineteenth century), Black American political culture might be expected historically to have fostered a strong current of pronatalism. Black elites at the turn of the twentieth century typically rejected the "Negro extinction thesis," but in quasi-eugenic fashion agonized in their conviction that Black lower-class fecundity surpassed that of educated couples.[37] Often masculinist, and certainly patriarchal, political rhetoric of the 1960s and 1970s correctly identified the eugenic, even genocidal, potential of liberalized sterilization laws (tens of thousands of Black, Latina, and Native women of childbearing age were sterilized either coercively or without their knowledge in the 1960s and 1970s), but often turned that recognition into a blanket condemnation of all birth control. It was emblematic of the conundrum of gender politics in many of the era's ethnic rights and nationalist movements, specifically the subordination of women within these movements and their

36 Alexandra Minna Stern, *Eugenic Nation: Faults and Frontiers of Better Breeding in Modern America* (University of California Press, 2005).

37 Michele Mitchell, *Righteous Propagation: African Americans and the Politics of Racial Destiny after Reconstruction* (University of North Carolina Press, 2004); Shantella Yolanda Sherman, "In Search of Purity: Popular Eugenics and Racial Uplift among New Negroes, 1915–1935" (PhD dissertation, University of Nebraska, 2014); Christina Simmons, "African Americans and Sexual Victorianism in the Social Hygiene Movement, 1910–40," *Journal of the History of Sexuality* 4, no. 1 (1993): 51–75; Kelly Miller, "Eugenics of the Negro Race," *The Scientific Monthly* 5, no. 1 (1917): 57–59; Chandler Owen, "Women and Children of the South," *The Birth Control Review* 3, no. 7 (1919): 9; E. Franklin Frazier, "Eugenics and the Race Problem," *Crisis* 31, no. 2 (1925): 91–92.

ideological relegation to domestic roles and "bearers of the race." Hence the pained frustration of Black women who had been, as Toni Cade (Bambara) famously wrote, "browbeaten in the past with the Black Matriarch stick" so badly that they themselves came to believe it or at least to behave as though they did. In answer to the question, "The Pill: Genocide or Liberation?," Cade agreed that "it is a sinister thing for the state to tell anyone not to have a child. And I know it's not for nothing, certainly not for love, that [birth control] clinics have been mushrooming in our communities." However, Black men quick to denounce all birth control as genocidal and counterliberatory conveniently ignored the point that natalist politics did nothing to address the material realities of racism, let alone sexism and heteronormativity.[38] The controversy, which caused difficult to reconcile rifts in Black Power movements as well as mainstream Black political culture, was also a source of tension within the women's movement.[39] Writing in the early 1980s, Angela Davis's assessment, that the White-dominated birth control movement "has seldom succeeded in uniting women of different social backgrounds," found an echo in Imani Woods's complaint against White harm reductionists who similarly disregarded Black political culture and its demands.[40]

Cade was speaking from within the Black women's liberation movement in the 1960s and 1970s. Meanwhile, and as is often the case when a group gains formal rights, many Black political leaders moved from transformative to transactional politics, taking elected or appointed positions in government or organizations partnered with the state. In the case especially of elected officials, it is difficult to ascertain whether reactionary cries of genocide were genuine or a political, even opportunistic, move. As Imani Woods knew well, many of those in the early years of HIV/AIDS who derided harm reduction as genocide were intransigent, even self-serving, in their insistence on abstinence and harsh criminal punishment. The exceptions are relatively few but important. Secular leaders included US Representatives Maxine Waters and John Lewis and New York Mayor David Dinkins. Clergy were more numerous and included Revs. Pernessa Seale, Christine Y. Wiley, Edwin Sanders II, Cecil Williams, and James A. Forbes, Jr.; Bishop Yvette Flunder; Archbishop Carl Bean, and others. Otherwise, Black harm reductionists and HIV activists frequently found themselves confronted by Black civic and elected leaders who rarely if ever considered gay men and people who use drugs as viable

38 Toni Cade, "The Pill: Genocide or Liberation," in *The Black Woman: An Anthology*, ed. Toni Cade (New American Library, 1970), 162–69.

39 Premilla Nadasen, *Welfare Warriors: The Welfare Rights Movement in the United States* (Routledge, 2005); Jennifer Nelson, *Women of Color and the Reproductive Rights Movement* (New York University Press, 2003).

40 Angela Y. Davis, *Women, Race & Class* (Random House, 1981), 202.

constituencies to whom they were accountable.[41] Maligned and criminalized, users were not an organized voting bloc the way unions, churches, civil rights organizations, and parents' groups were. Only when users actively sought treatment (as patients subject to medicalization) did Black (or White) leadership sympathetically view them as anything more than a disappointing drain on precious social services and a threat against whom police protection was made necessary. A similar dynamic held for Black leadership's regard of gay men, with the most liberal generally mustering only ambivalence: in popular church parlance, "hate the sin, but not the sinner," could be heard alternately referring to drug users or gay men.

Another event, a series of hearings on drug decriminalization in September 1988, convened by prominent Black US House Representative Charlie Rangel (Harlem, NY), is illustrative because it shows exactly how deeply enmeshed was the logic of no-tolerance, police action, and incarceration in drug and carceral politics, and the extent to which certain leaders were willing to go in defending that logic for their own ends. The hearing, unambiguously titled "Drug Legalization: Catastrophe for Black Americans," had been occasioned by remarks by Baltimore's Mayor, Kurt Schmoke, who had suggested that judicious decriminalization might prove to be more effective and less expensive than current drug law enforcement. The statement, so far out of the narrow spectrum of drug thinking at the time, immediately garnered for the city's first Black mayor attention from harm reductionists and drug warriors alike. For his part, Rangel, the Chair of the House Select Committee on Narcotics Abuse and Control, availed himself of any opportunity to announce his opposition to "anything approaching the legalization of narcotics," and his opinion that a retreat from no-tolerance would only constitute neglect of America's Black population. The context was critical: since the mid-1960s, an increasing number of large cities like Baltimore had elected Black Americans as mayors. Black political power, however, came only as a result of what many called White flight but which actually was capital flight: the massive shift of economic and political power from urban centers to suburban enclaves. The new Black leadership therefore inherited increasing poverty, declining tax bases, aging housing stock, poor educational systems, lack of job availability, and already frayed medical and public health infrastructures which only barely met the needs of working-class and poor citizens. Reagan-era retrenchment certainly did not help: "in the last 8 years this administration has clearly told you that those are your problems,

41 James Forman, *Locking up Our Own: Crime and Punishment in Black America* (Farrar, Straus and Giroux, 2017); Michael Javen Fortner, *Black Silent Majority: The Rockefeller Drug Laws and the Politics of Punishment* (Harvard University Press, 2015).

not national problems," Rangel intoned. "'We've reduced the Federal taxes, and you have to increase taxes and paddle your own canoe,'" the federal government had effectively told America's mayors. "And that's true whether we're talking about drugs or law enforcement." Almost astoundingly, he did not mention the toll AIDS had taken in those same cities.[42]

As congressional hearings often are, Rangel's was less investigative than exhibitional. As Chair of the Committee, he had the privilege of hand selecting its witnesses, most of whom ardently agreed with his point of view. Black mayors, law enforcement officials, and others serially appeared to condescendingly describe Schmoke as young and misguided, to label illicit drugs "the lethal enemies of our society," and to deride decriminalization and harm reduction as "erroneous and ludicrous" and bordering on "social genocide." Cheered on by Rangel, these voices effectively drowned out those of the three Black mayors who came to speak in favor of drug law reform. Schmoke, Washington, DC's Marion Barry, and Hartford, Connecticut's Carrie Saxon Perry – representing three of the cities with the highest per-capita rates of HIV seroprevalence and infection – each drew the connection between the triangulated syndemic of criminalization, HIV risk and infection, and defunded public health. Yet each left with what only could have been a feeling of disappointment.[43]

* * *

Practitioners of mainstream public health (and sympathetic historians) have frequently attributed African American distrust of their efforts to the legacies of Tuskegee. Some have even argued that popular and inaccurate understandings of Tuskegee have essentially thwarted the best efforts of public health, such as syringe exchange. "The failure to provide adequate treatment options for drug addiction, central to the complaint of African American opponents of needle exchange, most certainly represents tragic neglect and an example of gross inequity," write two scholars reflecting on the controversy in New York. "But not all injustices are the equivalent of

42 Select Committee on Narcotics Abuse and Control, *Drug Legalization: Catastrophe for Black Americans. Hearing before the Select Committee on Narcotics Abuse and Control, U.S. House of Representatives, One Hundredth Congress, Second Session* (US House of Representatives, 1988), 4. See also Charles B. Rangel, "Legalizing Drugs: A 'Dangerous Idea,'" *The Washington Post*, June 11, 1988; Kurt L. Schmoke, "Decriminalizing Drugs: It Just Might Work – and Nothing Else Does," *The Washington Post*, May 15, 1988.

43 Committee on Narcotics Abuse and Control, *Drug Legalization: Catastrophe for Black Americans*, 9.

those represented by Tuskegee."[44] However, this brand of logic misses the point and, more crucially, reflects an unwillingness to deal with the political and intellectual histories of the people with whom regular public health comes into contact. Certainly, the revelation of Tuskegee in 1972 resonated throughout Black America, but mainly as another egregious example confirming what was commonly understood well before then, that Black lives were rather dispensable. Black medical distrust did not begin with Tuskegee, much the same way that allegations of genocide were not *sui generis*, but rather were part of a postwar Black political discourse.

Again, the point is not to identify the heroes and villains of history. Certainly, proponents of methadone, decriminalization, and harm reduction have experienced their own frustrations at political resistance which refused to acknowledge these measures' life-improving potential. Similarly, as many advocates will admit, neither methadone maintenance nor harm reduction have lived up entirely to their full potential, for reasons deriving as much from regulatory and funding limitations as from lack of vision. What federal policies and larger national and global political-economic forces had wrought certainly could not and cannot be undone with just methadone, clean needles, or condoms. The historiographical question is how we can understand resistance and evaluate it on its own terms (and here a popular harm reduction phrase – "meeting people where they are" – certainly applies to the historian's craft). If there is a policy and practice question, it asks what vision of harm reduction addresses the structural vulnerabilities which produce so many (even most) of the harms associated with drug use. The historian will be more qualified to consider the first question than the second. Part of the answer to each, however, is a reframing the categories of "drugs," "risk," "addiction," etc., which are not only messy but often useless in efforts to arrive at more complex and nuanced understandings of the problem itself. At our best, we historians are quite good at deconstructing, unpacking, interrogating, and denaturalizing almost anything the rest of us might take for granted. And a policy orientation which, however briefly, decenters these categories to place them in relationship to other social problems is likely to spur fresh ideas. This was the project undertaken by Imani Woods, whose words began this essay.

44 Amy L. Fairchild and Ronald Bayer, "Uses and Abuses of Tuskegee," *Science* 284, no. 5416 (1999): 919–21.

Chapter Twelve

When Abstinence is Risk: Naloxone's Path to Over-the-Counter Status[1]

Nancy D. Campbell

Abstinence puts opioid users at higher risk for overdose and drug-related death. Abstinence disrupts tolerance and makes users more vulnerable to overdose and overdose death.[2] Tolerance is an adaptation to the effects of high-dose opioids, a neurophysiological state experienced as a reduction in effectiveness of opioids and increased potential to experience the effects of withdrawal. Tolerance serves body and brain as an "allostatic mechanism" of neuroadaptation that protects against the risk of respiratory depression.[3]

When institutions such as drug courts, hospitals, jails, prisons, and treatment programs require abstinence as a condition of treatment, they exacerbate risk of overdose death. When parents, partners, school officials, or

1 The author would like to thank Alice Bell, Nabarun Dasgupta, Maya Doe-Simkins, Alex Kral, Eliza Wheeler, and all those who work to get naloxone to the people who need it most; Michael Hufford at Harm Reduction Therapeutics; and to my full-spectrum support team at the journal *Social History of Alcohol and Drugs*.

2 This finding continues to be borne out; see Brandon del Pozo, Traci C. Green, Morgan Godvin, and Bradley Ray, "The Police Opioid Seizure Temporal Risk (POSTeR) model of increased exposure to fatal overdose," *International Journal of Drug Policy*, 139 (2025): 104789.

3 Catherine M. Cahill, Wendy Walwyn, Anna M.W. Taylor, Amynah A.A. Pradhan, and Christopher J. Evans, "Allostatic Mechanisms of Opioid Tolerance Beyond Desensitization and Downregulation," *Trends in Pharmacological Sciences*, 37, no. 11 (2016): 963–76.

others adopt "zero tolerance" stances, they rarely understand that insisting on abstinence imperils the very people they are trying to protect.

Wider access to naloxone, the opioid antagonist that reverses overdose, is the most effective direct solution to the acute problem of opioid overdose. Increased risk of overdose due to enforced abstinence was first investigated in the context of societal re-entry from Scottish prisons.[4] The biostatistician who led the investigation, Sheila Bird, characterized naloxone as the "direct response to the problem that our studies had quantified."[5] Similar studies followed in the United States.[6] Yet the lesson that abstinence heightens risk of overdose and overdose death is continually forgotten. Naloxone is not enough to counter the ongoing ignorance that surrounds licit and illicit opioid use. The harm reduction movement has worked to overcome this ignorance through naloxone access, overdose prevention education, and evidence produced through community-based research. This chapter considers interactions between organized harm reduction and activist researchers, the federal agencies most directly concerned with this decision (FDA and CDC), and pharmaceutical companies that manufacture and profit from naloxone, in the decade leading up to naloxone's move to being an over-the-counter (OTC) drug.

Overdose prevention educators and naloxone access advocates teach people that abstinence is a practical risk for overdose, for which naloxone is the remedy. Chief among risk factors for overdose and overdose death are "changes in tolerance after a period of low- or non-use."[7] Flying in the face of this established risk factor, abstinence is widely promoted as the necessary first step of recovery. Harm reduction advocates have had to overcome historical patterns of continued refusals to know, to remember, or to recognize the

4 See my discussion of the works of Sheila Bird and Sharon Hutchinson in Nancy D. Campbell, *OD: Naloxone and the Politics of Naloxone* (MIT Press, 2020), 256–66.

5 Quoted in Campbell, *OD*, 259.

6 Ingrid A. Binswanger, Patrick J. Blatchford, P. J., Shane R. Mueller, and M. F. Stern, "Mortality after prison release: Opioid overdose and other causes of death, risk factors, and time trends from 1999 to 2009," *Annals of Internal Medicine* 159, no. 9 (2013): 592–600; Ingrid A. Binswanger, M. F. Stern, R. A. Deyo, Patrick J. Heagerty, A. Cheadle, J. G. Elmore, and T. D. Koepsell, "Release from prison – A high risk of death for former inmates," *New England Journal of Medicine* 356, no. 2 (2011): 157–65; Ingrid A. Binswanger, Patrick J. Blatchford, R. G. Lindsay, and M. F. Stern, "Risk factors for all-cause, overdose and early deaths after release from prison in Washington state," *Drug and Alcohol Dependence* 117, no. 1 (2007): 1–6.

7 See "Summary Report on Naloxone Economic View" (Reagan-Udall Foundation for the Food and Drug administration, 2023), 5.

validity of the concern that abstinence is risk. An epistemology of ignorance[8] haunts the basic recognition that reduced tolerance to opioids places people who use drugs in life-threatening situations. For the past thirty years, participants in the harm reduction movement have focused on overdose prevention. They have trained thousands of people how to position overdose sufferers so that rescue breathing techniques can work, educated people about why and how naloxone works to reverse opioid overdose, and supplied them with naloxone during or after workshops. Long before public health departments got on board with naloxone distribution, harm reduction activists took it into their own hands to train law enforcement and firefighters, teachers and parents. By tracing how the overdose prevention movement promoted the benefits of naloxone – successfully bringing about a reduction in the number of US overdose deaths in 2023[9] – this chapter seeks to overcome a common assumption that abstinence is an unalloyed good that should be promoted at all costs. Abstinence elevates risk of overdose and overdose death, and the costs of promoting it should be calculated accordingly.

Overdose researchers are familiar with widespread failures by partners and family members, law enforcement, policymakers, judges, and other officials to recognize that overdose risk is increased by interruptions of opioid supply from any source. As a recent paper on social, biological, and pharmacological factors that elevate overdose risk after police seizures states:

> Many people find the conclusion that police drug seizures increase overdose risk strongly counterintuitive, considering that governments act to interrupt the supply of illicit drugs to ostensibly reduce risk and save lives. To that end, the presumption is that reducing the quantity of illicit drugs in circulation and interrupting their consumption by people dependent on

8 Anthropological, sociological, and philosophical study of ignorance is flourishing; see Robert Proctor and Londa L. Schiebinger, *Agnotology: The Making and Unmaking of Ignorance* (Stanford University Press, 2008) and Janet Kourany and Martin Carrier, *Science and the Production of Ignorance: When the Quest for Knowledge is Thwarted* (MIT Press, 2020). Science and Technology Studies scholars like myself apply this framework to social movements that get "undone" science done; see Scott Frickel, Sahra Gibbon, Jeff Howard, Joanna Kempner, Gwen Ottinger, and David J. Hess, "Undone Science: Charting Social Movement and Civil Society Challenges to Research Agenda Setting," *Science, Technology & Human Values* 35, no. 4 (2010):444–73. This chapter applies this conceptual framework to harm reduction, overdose prevention, and naloxone access movements, which work to overcome socially produced ignorance about opioid overdose in order to produce new knowledge practices.

9 Matthew F. Garnett and Arialdi M. Miniño, "Drug overdose deaths in the United States, 2003–2023," *NCHS Data Brief* 522 (National Center for Health Statistics, 2024).

> opioids is believed to reduce risk. But at least in the proximate sense, the evidence does not bear this presumption out.[10]

Supply interruption can be deadly. As protective factors like pharmacological tolerance decline, naloxone is a crucial social, biological, and pharmacological remedy for those voluntarily or involuntarily abstaining from opioids. For this reason, the FDA officially "switched" naloxone from a prescription-only drug to an OTC drug in March 2023.

As a "pharmaceutical object,"[11] naloxone frays the seams between risks and benefits of legal and illegal substances and the moral and material concerns associated with manufacturing, distributing, acquiring, and administering them. Refined from legally produced morphine base (thebaine), naloxone acts as a short-term opioid antagonist and is considered an essential medicine. Naloxone has such strong affinity for opioid receptors that it can reverse respiratory depression consequent to opioid overdose. Despite this extraordinary benefit coupled with no potential for abuse,[12] naloxone was controlled as a prescription-only drug from its approval for opioid overdose reversal on April 13, 1971, until March 29, 2023. This chapter tells the story of naloxone's OTC switch, centering the social movement that catalyzed its wider distribution, and asking why it took so long given naloxone's safety profile as a life-saving substance.

The Long and Winding Road to OTC Naloxone

Endo, the Long Island-based company that developed Narcan, considered naloxone to lack consumer appeal. When intravenous naloxone was approved by the FDA in 1971, Endo's name for it was Envizio, a liquid injectable naloxone product supplied mainly to medical markets.[13] Endo tried other formulations and uses, briefly supplying free naloxone pills to researchers searching for methadone alternatives at New York Medical College, Yale University Medical School, and the Maryland State Psychiatric

10 del Pozo, Green, Godvin, and Ray, "The Police Opioid Seizure Temporal Risk (POSTeR) model."

11 He Bian, *Know Your Remedies: Pharmacy and Culture in Early Modern China* (Princeton University Press, 2020).

12 Donald R. Jasinski, William R. Martin, and Charles A. Haertzen, "The human pharmacology and abuse potential of N-allylnoroxymorphone (naloxone)," *Journal of Pharmacology and Experimental Therapeutics* 157, no. 2 (1967): 420–26.

13 See A. Benjamin Srivastava and Mark S. Gold, "Naltrexone: A History and Future Directions," *Cerebrum* (2018): 13–18.

Research Center in the late 1960s.[14] When the New York State Narcotic Addiction Control Center (NACC) attempted to purchase naloxone pills in bulk, DuPont, which acquired Endo as a wholly-owned subsidiary in 1969, feared association with "addiction" and implied that its new property, naloxone, was "raising false hope among addicts."[15] DuPont raised alarm about a potential shortage of thebaine, the "starting material" for naloxone production.[16] Although no thebaine shortage materialized, oral naloxone was too short-acting to deter heroin users from relapse. Relapse prevention studies continued with naloxone's close kin nalorphine and naltrexone, and partial agonist/antagonists such as buprenorphine and cyclazocine.[17]

As emergency medicine expanded in the 1970s, naloxone gradually displaced its predecessor, nalorphine, from emergency and clinical settings.[18] Injectable naloxone was an affordable solution packaged in small glass vials that went generic in the 1980s. Not until harm reduction activists in the mid-1990s reconstructed intramuscular injection of generic naloxone as a life-saving miracle did innovation in naloxone formulation or route of administration unfold. Since then, naloxone access advocates have catalyzed a conversation about naloxone's uneven availability – free to some, costly to others, surveilled, policed, and purveyed as if it was itself addictive. Harm reductionists persuaded and trained first responders to carry naloxone beginning in the early 2010s after a global vanguard started distributing it in the late 1990s and early 2000s. Not until 2012 did the FDA convene scientific workshops on naloxone. Five years after the first, discussed below, the FDA took unusual steps to incentivize development of lower-cost, OTC naloxone by conducting its own Drug Fact Label (DFL) study (this first step towards FDA approval is typically conducted by pharmaceutical companies aspiring to market products for specific indications). Once the FDA labelling study was complete, pharmaceutical companies took that as a green light to proceed with the switch. This chapter recounts naloxone's migration to OTC status.

Like the opioids it "antidotes," naloxone has been reframed in terms of risk, harm, and benefit by various constituencies that sought to confine or "liberate" it from the constraints that had kept it confined to emergency

14 Joseph Lelyveld, "DuPont, in Reversal, Restores Drug to Addiction Researchers," *New York Times*, July 14, 1970, 41.

15 Lelyveld, "DuPont, in Reversal, Restores Drug to Addiction Researchers."

16 Lelyveld, "DuPont, in Reversal, Restores Drug to Addiction Researchers."

17 Author's interviews with Louis Harris, Jerome H. Jaffe, and Herbert Kleber; Nancy D. Campbell and Anne M. Lovell, "The History of the Development of Buprenorphine as an Addiction Therapeutics," *Annals of the New York Academy of Science* 1248 (2012): 124–39.

18 For a fuller account of nalorphine's career, see Campbell, *OD*.

medicine and anesthesiology for decades.[19] Harm reduction activists and advocates sought to gain authority, credibility, and epistemic status deriving from various sources of expertise. Those acting in such spaces have put forward "demedicalized" or "empowerment" models, but they are faced with potential conscription into biomedical models by words like "risk," "benefit," and, increasingly, "harm," which are central to the biomedical frameworks we live by. Historians need not be conscripted into the assumptions made by those who wield these terms as power tools; we are captured by neither FDA nor Big Pharma as we document the actions of industry, industry regulators, researchers, advocates, and activists. Distinctions between drugs and medicines have been shown to be historically contingent, socially constructed, and assimilated to the conceptual practices of power; drugs are medicines, and medicines are drugs.[20]

First out of the OTC gate in 2023, Emergent BioSolutions was approved to market the first *nonprescription* naloxone hydrochloride nasal spray. Five years prior, Emergent had acquired Adapt Pharma, which had issued the first intranasal product under the (old) name Narcan in 2016. The convenient plastic applicator pictured in Figure 1 delivers 4 mg of naloxone intranasally – the same dose as the Narcan product approved in 1971 as an injectable liquid.

Despite its journey to drugstore shelves succeeding in early 2023, Narcan remained relatively unaffordable. A second novelty then appeared in the pharmaceutical marketplace – nonprofit drug development. Harm Reduction Therapeutics began shipping low-cost, OTC two-pack intranasal naloxone at a dosage of 3 mg called RiVive in January 2023 (See Figure 2). The 3 mg reduced dose was the product of long-term negotiations with harm reduction activists and naloxone access advocates, who considered higher doses "overkill," causing an unpleasantly abrupt waking that some experience as punitive. This chapter highlights the multiplicity of naloxones and replies to a risk paradox: when opioid users abstain, tolerance declines and risk of drug-related death increases.

The next section considers naloxone's anticipatory appeal and situates its vaunted status as a life-saving "miracle drug" within the mire of its decade-long development and movement into the regulatory space of "Rx-to-OTC switches." This chapter concludes with reflections on shared responsibilities for preventing preventable deaths from opioid overdose and argues that the well-documented dangers of abstinence have been ignored for too long.

19 Eliza Wheeler, "Joint Meeting of the Anesthetic and Analgesic Drug Products Advisory Committee and the Drug Safety and Risk Management Advisory Committee Meeting," December 17–18, 2018, 27.

20 No one has emphasized this point more dramatically than David Herzberg, *White Market Drugs: Big Pharma and the Hidden History of Addiction in America* (University of Chicago Press, 2020).

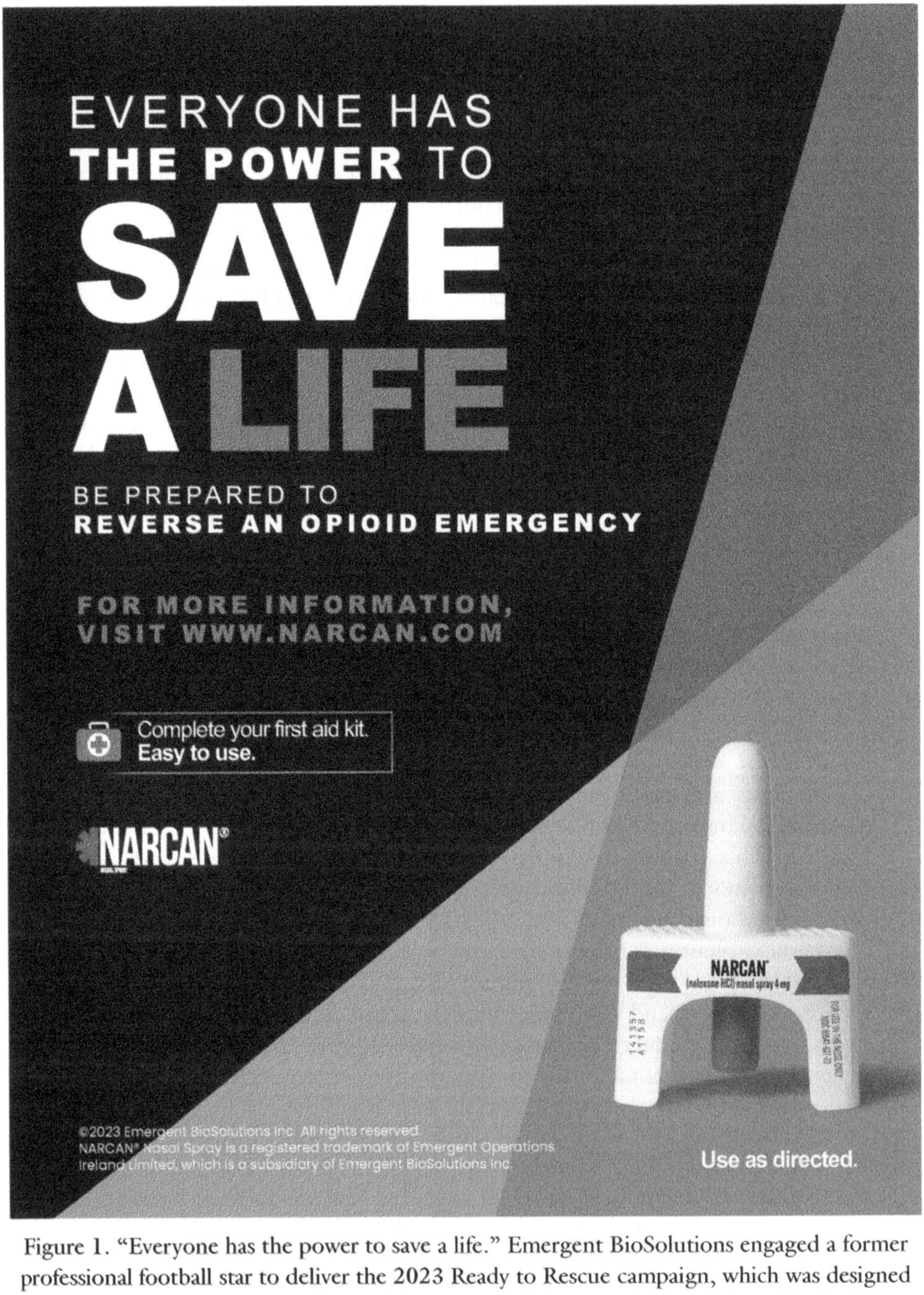

Figure 1. "Everyone has the power to save a life." Emergent BioSolutions engaged a former professional football star to deliver the 2023 Ready to Rescue campaign, which was designed to raise awareness about student athletes' vulnerability to opioid overdose. Used with permission of Emergent BioSolutions Inc.

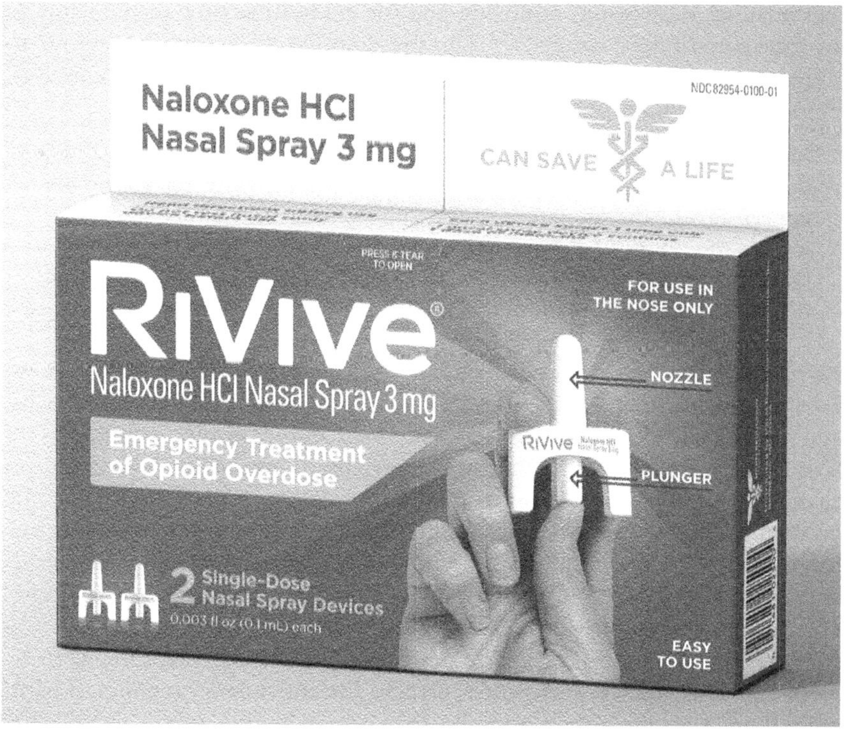

Figure 2. "No company, entity, or individual will profit from sales of RiViveTM." Harm Reduction Therapeutics website at https://www.harmreductiontherapeutics.org/. Used with permission of Harm Reduction Therapeutics.

Vigilance Materialized: Naloxone's Anticipatory Appeal

Naloxone became central to new forms of "pharmaceutical personhood,"[21] based not in consumption, but in an ethos of vigilance that encourages keeping naloxone close – near to hand, carrying it along, leaving it behind for someone to find, taking it home, living with it. The anticipatory practices of overdose prevention – like all preventive regimes based in anticipatory acts – cultivate a preparatory mode. Adams, Murphy, and Clarke characterize anticipatory regimes as "speculative and reactive, in 'preparation for' the event and the trauma as if it were already here, rather than offering 'prevention of' it so that it never happens. ... Anticipation authorizes preemptive actions in the present forced by a purported urgency in the future,

21 Emily Martin, "The Pharmaceutical Person," *BioSocieties* 1, no. 3 (2006): 273–87.

legitimating, destroying, removing and/or eradicating now in the name of an anticipated future danger."[22] This pre-emptive ethos appeals not only to those who anticipate that they might someday need naloxone themselves, but to those who anticipate needing it for others in the future:

> Management of the future becomes a pre-occupation of the present through the obligatory passage-point of "possibility." Possibility is no longer set against the limitation of the "impossible," but rather simply permeates the zones of danger that circulate in and through forecasts as a managerial effect. It is possible, so the injunction goes, to manage the anticipated. Vigilance is requisite.[23]

Naloxone is vigilance materialized. Its anticipatory appeal is vested in an evocative future anterior relationship to potential risks, actual harms, threats, and benefits both existential and material, and "affective economies of fear, hope, salvation and precariousness oriented temporally toward futures already made 'real' in the present."[24] OTC naloxone's affective economy grew from activists' social justice claims, which reached towards "liberatory" futures when harm reduction would be widely available and knowledge exercised not in service of bureaucratically managing the future but by empowering drug users to care for themselves and each other.

Naloxone is an artifact with an anticipatory politics – you carry it to be prepared. This ethos has become central to the anticipatory regimes of harm reduction. The affective economies of harm reduction rearticulated what was possible for whom, widening the scope of managerial bioethical and regulatory regimes, which dilute or damp down attempts to apply the critical pressure of social justice and human rights to regulatory modes. This chapter argues that efforts to create different formulations and distribution patterns shifted the affective ethos from threat, risk, and harm to the benefits of valuation and affirmation. Naloxone's peculiar material aspects – rapid bioavailability and short-lived effects – depend on formulation, route of administration, context of use, and patterns of consumption. Its affinity for opioid receptors, the property through which naloxone works to restore breathing, and its short half-life by comparison to the opioid agonists it antagonizes – call forth anxious attentiveness. The energy around reformulating dosage or route of administration responds to the well-documented phenomenon

22 Vincanne Adams, Michelle Murphy, and Adele E. Clarke, "Anticipation: Technoscience, Life, Affect, Temporality," *Subjectivity* 28 (2009): 258.

23 Adams, Murphy, and Clarke, "Anticipation," 259.

24 Adams, Murphy, and Clarke, "Anticipation," 260.

of over-antagonism,[25] and brought on increased regulatory scrutiny in the context of the evidence-based biomedicalization of everything. Even telling the story of naloxone's path to OTC status requires tacking back and forth between a regulatory story and a social movement story, and between moral, medical, and material concerns.

"The Meeting We Were Not Invited To": Casting Naloxone as an Over-The-Counter Drug

Moral and material concerns delayed the possibility of naloxone going OTC for more than a decade. When harm reduction activists started to distribute naloxone, it was available only in injectable form. After a highly publicized set of overdose events in Boston in the early 2000s, EMTs started assembling "off-label" intranasal spray devices, using atomizers to administer other drugs for naloxone.[26] Long before FDA approval of intranasal naloxone – which did not come until 2014 – the City of Boston and Commonwealth of Massachusetts rolled out an intranasal naloxone distribution program.[27] As overdose calls ticked up and overdose became a public health crisis, Advanced Life Support (ALS) trucks equipped with paramedics became costly and Basic Life Support (BLS) personnel were not allowed to administer drugs by injection. Non-approved intranasal naloxone was not a perfect solution to this problem – it took time and know-how to assemble the nasal atomizer used to administer other life-saving drugs. Harm reduction advocates began to assemble kits containing nasal atomizers and naloxone vials for distribution by harm reduction programs.

Community-based naloxone distribution programs in Massachusetts "incentivized people to come back and tell us what had happened. After the first three months, we didn't need to do that because the uptake was really rapid. It started out that we were only offering it once a week when Andy [Epstein] could be there because she was the nurse. She quickly realized that wasn't going to work because her time was expensive and people were coming all the time. The word spread like wildfire. People were asking:

25 Joanne Neale and John Strang, "Naloxone: Does over-antagonism matter? Evidence of iatrogenic harm after emergency treatment of heroin/opioid overdose," *Addiction* 110, no. 10 (2015): 1644–52.

26 See Maya Doe-Simkins, Alexander Y. Walley, Andy Epstein, and Peter Moyer, "Saved by the nose: bystander-administered intranasal naloxone hydrochloride for opioid overdose," *American Journal of Public Health* 99, no. 5 (2009): 788–91.

27 Author's interview with Maya Doe Simkins, September 27, 2013.

'Where can I get that Narcan?'"[28] From 2007 to 2010, Massachusetts mapped where overdoses occurred and expanded naloxone access statewide, using the off-label, non-FDA-approved, hand-assembled intranasal setup. Rather than wait for FDA approval of a re-designed intranasal technology, Massachusetts invested in social infrastructure and bricolage – on-site assembly of nasal naloxone kits from preassembled parts.

Innovations in naloxone's formulation or delivery mechanism mainly responded to concerns that people who were not trained as medical professionals might be called upon to prepare and administer naloxone; they might be scared or nervous.[29] Expertise with injection equipment is routine for some, but not all, drug users and associates.[30] The FDA went on to approve several intranasal innovations – but not until 2014 – so the City of Boston and the Commonwealth of Massachusetts continued mass distribution (as they do at the time of writing). Companies used R&D investment in the intranasal applicator, however, to drive prices up; the intranasal product has always been more expensive than generic injectable naloxone. One of the most notorious examples of this era was the priciest naloxone product ever made, kaléo, Inc.'s "tell-me-how-to-use it drug," Evzio (a name that echoed Endo's original name, Envizio). Virginia-based pharmaceutical manufacturer, kaléo, obtained FDA approval on April 3, 2014, to market an intranasal naloxone twin-pack retailing for more than $4,000. The product provided verbal instructions similar to the "talking" AEDs on the commercial market. Since discontinued due to public and Congressional outrage, Evzio stands as a prime example of predatory pharmaceutical pricing and pharmacy misconduct, including fraudulent and false prior authorization requests.[31] Joining price-gouging Epi-Pen manufacturer Mylan, Inc., and Martin Shkreli's steep price increases and restricted distribution scheme for Daraprim (prescribed for malaria and parasite infections in immunocompromised people with AIDS and cancer),[32] the unaffordability of the elaborate

28 Author's interview with Doe-Simkins, 2013.

29 The problem of how to organize community distribution of an injectable prescription drug is described in depth in Campbell, *OD*.

30 Sarah Brothers, Alex H. Kral, Lynn Wenger, Kelsey Simpson, and Ricky N. Bluthenthal, "Assisted injection provider practices and motivations in Los Angeles and San Francisco California 2016–18," *International Journal of Drug Policy* 92 (2021): 103052.

31 According to a US Department of Justice press release on November 9, 2021, "Kaléo Inc. Agrees to Pay $12.7 Million to Resolve Allegations of False Claims for Anti-Overdose Drug," at https://www.justice.gov/opa/pr/kal-o-inc-agrees-pay-127-million-resolve-allegations-false-claims-anti-overdose-drug.

32 Michael A. Carrier, Nicole L. Levidow, and Aaron S. Kesselheim, "Using Antitrust Law to Challenge Turing's Daraprim Price Increase," *Berkeley Technology Law Journal* 31 (2016): 1379.

device was linked in the public mind to astronomical price increases in the Epi-Pen auto-injector subsequent to its 2016 redesign to prevent accidental needlesticks. Touting improved safety as "innovation" rather than harm reduction, Mylan CEO Heather Bresch defended the company's R&D and awareness campaigns – and was widely derided in the face of her testimony before the House Committee on Oversight and Government Reform.[33] As clamor for OTC naloxone grew louder, naloxone access advocates banded together to create more affordable ways to get the generic injectable out to people who had fewer qualms about injection. The industry pursued intranasal naloxone, sensing market expansion due to public concern about the increase in opioid overdose deaths.

During the 2012 hearings we now turn to, there was no FDA-approved intranasal naloxone on the market. That year, neuropharmacologist Phil Skolnick, then director of the National Institute on Drug Abuse's Division of Therapeutics and Medical Consequences (DTMC), joined with Lightlake Therapeutics to develop the intranasal applicator currently in common circulation. This two-pronged plastic applicator had a central plunger and was approved in late 2015 and launched in early 2016 when the company name changed to Opiant.[34] But naloxone did not go OTC until March 2023 despite harm reduction activists and naloxone access advocates broaching this idea. Few were present at the FDA Center for Drug Evaluation and Research (CDER)'s first hearing about OTC naloxone on March 23, 2012 – because "none of us were invited," as recalled by Prevention Point Pittsburgh's Alice Bell in a 2017 interview.[35] The first 2012 meeting considered an array of possible OTC candidates, including naloxone and oral contraceptives.[36] The Harm Reduction Coalition was represented by counsel Whitney O'Neill Englander, a survivor of a naloxone-reversed opioid overdose. Another social

33 Toni Clarke, "U.S. lawmakers blast Mylan CEO over 'sickening' EpiPen price hikes," Reuters, September 21, 2016, https://www.reuters.com/article/idUSKCN11R2OG/.

34 On the history of the partnership with NIDA, see "Lightlake Therapeutics Inc. Files Investigational NDA For Naloxone Nasal Spray For Reversing Opioid Overdose," July 23, 2014, at https://www.drugs.com/nda/naloxone_140723.html. On the approval, see "FDA Approves Narcan (naloxone) Nasal Spray to Treat Opioid Overdose," November 18, 2015, at https://www.drugs.com/newdrugs/fda-approves-narcan-naloxone-nasal-opioid-overdose-4300.html.

35 Author's interview with Alice Bell, May 3, 2017.

36 Docket No. FDA–2012–N–0171. Public Hearing – March 23, 2012a. "Using Innovative Technologies and other Conditions of Safe Use to Expand Which Drug Products Can Be Considered Nonprescription."

movement-oriented coalition, the Oral Contraceptives Over-the-Counter Working Group, presented the venerable track record of oral contraceptives as among the "best studied and safest medications that are on the market today," noting that their drug was "not addictive, unfortunately."[37]

At this first FDA hearing on OTC drug candidates, Englander explained essentially what activists had been doing: "if someone ... were to get a prescription from their doctor to get naloxone right now for the nasal, they would literally have to get a prescription for the naloxone and for the nasal adapter and it would have to be bought separately and put together." Despite the intramuscular injection and off-label intranasal kits activists had by this point been assembling for years, FDA held out for an intranasal product. Englander noted that "what we're hearing from the folks at FDA here are that they're very interested in laying down the pathways for intranasal naloxone. ... So I would agree that the injection form would not be the best option for an over-the-counter."

Speakers at the March 2012 hearings portrayed Rx-to-OTC switches as exceedingly complex "struggles," or even "battles," characterizing OTC switches as infeasible, unpredictable, and unmanageable unless participants were equipped with specialized expertise. They argued that "every effort should be made to ensure that the process for an OTC switch is as predictable and manageable as possible and that the agency be flexible in considering creative approaches to the design and implementation of special conditions of use."[38]

Although naloxone access activists and harm reduction advocates were largely cut out of the initial FDA hearing, they followed the process closely. Nabarun Dasgupta, a North Carolina "pharmacoepidemiologist" alert for opportunities to move naloxone out of prescription-only status, communicated weekly with harm reduction comrades via nationally coordinated NOPE calls, through which they actively connected for years to share information and build relationships prior to converting to a more passive Google group.[39] Bell credited Dasgupta with catalyzing the presence at the second FDA hearing later that spring:

> Actually, Nab [Dasgupta] had heard [the April 2012 FDA meeting] was going to be announced and he said: "What we need to do is, as soon as they announce it, we all need to call to ask to give community comment." So a bunch of us did that. At that point, there really weren't [many] states

37 FDA, 2012a, Daniel Grossman, 41–42.

38 FDA–2012–N–0171, 2012a, 10. Comment by David Bradford, PEGUS Research and adjunct faculty at the University of Utah School of Medicine.

39 Author's 2013–2018 interviews with Alice Bell, Dan Bigg, Nabarun Dasgupta, Maya Doe-Simkins, Roxanne Saucier.

> that had passed laws around naloxone. ... I remember what I talked about was, we've been giving out naloxone since 2005 and I get calls all the time from parents who say: "I just heard about this [naloxone]. Do you mean to tell me that if I had had this in my medicine cabinet, my kid might be alive today?" I said to the FDA: "I'd like to have something to tell them, besides, 'We actually can't give you naloxone because we're only allowed to prescribe naloxone to people who are themselves at risk.'"[40]

Harm reduction activists and naloxone access advocates showed up in force at the FDA's second hearing on the "Role of Naloxone in Opioid Overdose Fatality Prevention" on April 12, 2012.[41] They were met with heightened security upon entrance. Peter Lurie, special adviser in the FDA Office of Policy and Planning, portrayed pharmaceutical opioid overdose deaths as a huge problem that outstripped deaths from all illegal drugs combined. In solidarity, Lurie left his FDA badge with security so he would be "stuck" with the activists.[42] His purpose was to "help us collectively make the best use of naloxone for the public health."[43] Robert Rappaport, then director of the FDA division on analgesic, anesthetic, and addiction drug products, sought to "establish whether allowing naloxone to become more widely available for use by nonmedical personnel in treating these overdoses is one mechanism that should be considered as a potential intervention."[44] Naloxone's uneven availability was noted in the "interest of some areas in intranasal naloxone to bring home,"[45] because death rates were higher where it was unavailable due to "funding and resource shortages, both for prevention efforts and for treatment interventions."[46] The state of knowledge

40 Author's interview with Bell, 2017, 16. In the early days of naloxone distribution, kit assembly relied on volunteers and imparted social solidarity. NOPE calls enabled harm reduction activists to gather, swap strategies, and build relationships.

41 Co-sponsored by the FDA Center for Drug Evaluation and Research, Office of the Assistant Secretary for Health, National Institutes on Drug Abuse, Centers for Disease Control and Prevention, "Role of Naloxone in Opioid Overdose Fatality Prevention," April 12, 2012b.

42 FDA, "Role of Naloxone in Opioid Overdose Fatality Prevention," 13, lines 5–9.

43 FDA, "Role of Naloxone in Opioid Overdose Fatality Prevention," 14, lines 17–20.

44 FDA, "Role of Naloxone in Opioid Overdose Fatality Prevention," 15, lines 11–16.

45 FDA, "Role of Naloxone in Opioid Overdose Fatality Prevention," 33.

46 FDA, "Role of Naloxone in Opioid Overdose Fatality Prevention," 46, lines 11–16.

about naloxone was underdeveloped enough at this late date that dosage and effects had to be discussed in detail. Yet by this point, harm reduction activists and naloxone access advocates had been obtaining, distributing, using, and educating community members how to use naloxone to prevent opioid overdose deaths for over a decade. Their level of technical expertise was high, they were frustrated at FDA foot-dragging – and, in 2012, there was no approved intranasal product when a national naloxone shortage constricted access alongside continuing uncertainty about legal frameworks enabling it.

The FDA considered activist presence simply a signal of stakeholder diversity, and confined harm reductionists to a public comment period late in the proceedings. Among other stakeholders, the "public" included parents, mainly mothers, who had lost children to overdose. Public comment was structured into four six-person panels, giving each person two minutes to speak – a brief period literally marked by a traffic light that turned green, yellow, and red to signal the time remaining. The first panel was composed of Temple Law School's Leo Beletsky; Alice Bell; Dan Bigg; Robert Childs of the North Carolina Harm Reduction Coalition and cofounder with Dasgupta of Project Lazarus; parent Pam Lynch; and Susan Gregory, a parent from Families Against Narcotics in Sterling Heights, Michigan, whose son died of a heroin overdose in the presence of two other individuals. Gregory stated that she "didn't know about naloxone then. What if the addicts with my son had been trained to save his life or not afraid of being prosecuted? … Why wasn't I told about naloxone? If my son was a diabetic or allergic to bees, I'd be prepared with the right medication. We have defibrillators on hand everywhere to save lives. To me, any risk of using naloxone, of which I can't see, is very minimal compared to death."[47] The risk-benefit calculus mobilized by naloxone access advocates was that of minimal risk relative to the most maximal risk of all – death.

Dasgupta urged the FDA to take aggressive action against pharmaceutical manufacturing monopolies, which he cast as "unreliable and unable to even tell the public when naloxone will be regularly available in the United States again."[48] Dasgupta saw his role as "translat[ing] between the street-level, human side and the cold, hard numbers."[49] Also effective at the April 2012 hearing were parents such as Marianna Kate Duncan, whose son had died "surrounded by friends that were not using heroin and had no idea how to deal with an overdose. By the time they recognized he was having respiratory distress and could not be resuscitated, they called 911. Unfortunately, the rescue came too late. Nick suffered brain death and was removed from life support four days later. … Nick did not have to die from an overdose.

47 FDA, "Role of Naloxone in Opioid Overdose Fatality Prevention," 264.

48 FDA, "Role of Naloxone in Opioid Overdose Fatality Prevention," 267–68.

49 Author's interview with Nabarun Dasgupta, October 11, 2013, 4.

Had these friends been provided with information about overdose prevention, recognition and treatment, or had they had access to naloxone, Nick would still be with us today."[50]

This kind of future anterior imagination in which a person who has died could have remained alive *if* naloxone had been present, *if* persons present had known how to use naloxone, *if* the person had suffered from any other chronic condition was often encountered at this hearing. Parent Marilee Murphy Odenhal of Freeport, Illinois, explained:

> The FDA considers matters in scientific terms. Well, scientific fact is that naloxone could have saved Ian's life. I live with the certain knowledge that had my son suffered from cancer, doctors would have exhausted their skills and tried every possible drug to save his life. But no doctor ever mentioned naloxone to me. I never even heard the word until four months after Ian's death, and that from harm reductionist. Why naloxone hasn't been touted on every media outlet and shouted from every rooftop, I will never understand. It makes me livid. I have the rest of my life to live without Ian, and I cannot describe that kind of loss to you.[51]

A fissure between science and society expressed at these hearings opened between those who know or should know, those who do not know but should have known, and those who were dead but should be alive. Joanne Peterson of Learn to Cope, a Massachusetts parent organization, lamented lack of federal funding for naloxone because "it doesn't seem to fit anywhere."

Despite a decade and a half of activism, harm reduction infrastructure "fit" in only a few places in 2012. Representing the DOPE Project of San Francisco, which had been distributing naloxone since 2003, Eliza Wheeler had "literally heard hundreds of stories of people using naloxone to save someone's life. I myself have used it four times, and I'm here to tell you that it's not rocket science and that those four people are still alive today." She contrasted the "intensely powerful experience" of saving lives to the disheartening nature of

> all of the criticisms and concerns about what we do. What's happening here today is clearly a shift in that which I am grateful for, and thank you. But, frankly, I'm also really sick of hearing about how there's not evidence that this can work and that people can't recognize an overdose, they can't use naloxone, they can't put it together, they don't know how to use a needle, it might not be safe, it might increase or encourage their drug use, it sends the wrong message, they won't call 911. It gets a little tiresome to keep having to hear this when we see the evidence in front of us every day.[52]

50 FDA, "Role of Naloxone in Opioid Overdose Fatality Prevention," 272–73.
51 FDA, "Role of Naloxone in Opioid Overdose Fatality Prevention," 282–83.
52 FDA, "Role of Naloxone in Opioid Overdose Fatality Prevention," 291–92.

By 2012, naloxone access activists were distributing both vials to be loaded into syringes (an activity at which most intravenous drug users are adept) and "off-label" intranasal naloxone. Although there was reason to explore the efficacy of intranasal administration – the vials were finicky and it took time to load them into syringes or to assemble the off-label intranasal kits – there was also question about different routes of administration. Did intramuscular injection work as well as intravenous injection? Early investigations by Australian "overdose contrarians" Shane Darke and Johan Duflou cleverly measured presence or absence of a heroin metabolite, 6 monoacetyl morphine (6MAM), and determined the temporal window within which naloxone could have been administered and death averted.[53] Intravenous naloxone was well documented, but subcutaneous/intramuscular injection and intranasal routes remained to be researched. Hedging their bets, US naloxone access advocates assembled kits that did both (Figure 3).

Need for intravenous injection was a chief reason that naloxone was limited to the category of prescription-only medicine. If researchers could show that intramuscular or intranasal administration carried the same or similar benefits as intravenous injection for kick-starting breathing, these other routes would open. Developmental delays stymied the intranasal formulation despite its clear benefits such as reducing risks of injection like needlestick injuries and/or blood-borne virus transmission.

Evolution and Innovation in the Naloxone Spray Market

Emergency medical personnel working with harm reduction activists "jerry-rigged" a non-FDA approved intranasal naloxone delivery system by assembling a prefilled naloxone syringe into a "needleless" nasal atomizer device used for other drugs. As outlined above, these practices demonstrated that naloxone could be successfully administered through the nose *before* innovation of a nasal applicator specific to it.[54] FDA did not approve a branded intranasal naloxone until 2014, when it approved the Amphastar device pictured in Figure 4. The intranasal device that most current readers picture was not approved until April 19, 2019, for administration by "people

53 Shane Darke and Johan Duflou, "The toxicology of heroin-related death: estimating survival times," *Addiction* 111, no. 9 (2016): 1607–13.

54 Amphastar Pharmaceuticals manufactured injectable, intranasal, and inhalation products, and produced prefilled Luer Lock syringes with generic naloxone hydrochloride that could be paired with an atomizer device for intranasal delivery. See https://www.mass.gov/service-details/naloxone-facts-and-formulations.

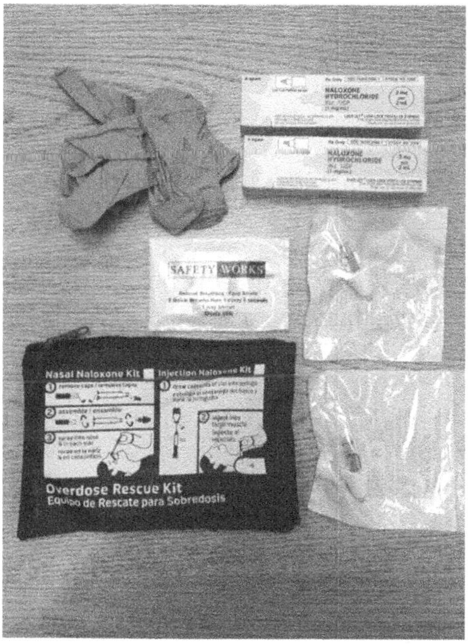

Figure 3. Naloxone kit illustrating constituent parts for both nasal and injection routes of administration. Harrisburg, Pennsylvania. 2017. Photograph by the author.

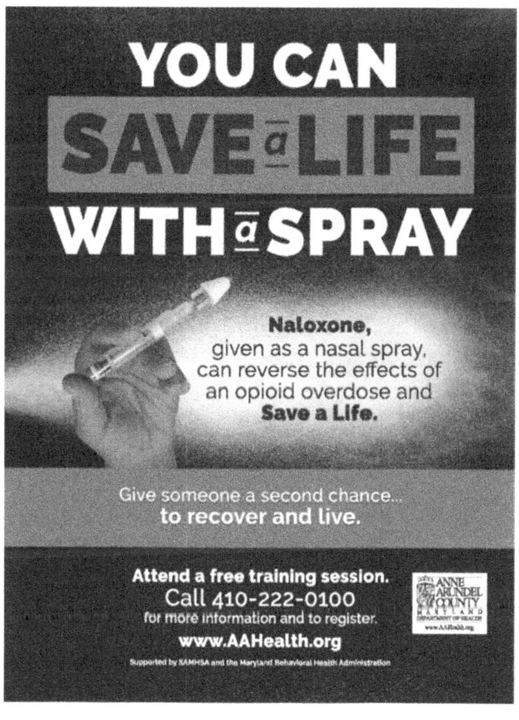
YOU CAN
SAVE a LIFE
WITH a SPRAY
Naloxone,
given as a nasal spray,
can reverse the effects of
an opioid overdose and
Save a Life.
Give someone a second chance...
to recover and live.
Attend a free training session.
Call 410-222-0100
for more information and to register.
www.AAHealth.org
Supported by SAMHSA and the Maryland Behavioral Health Administration
ANNE ARUNDEL COUNTY
MARYLAND
DEPARTMENT OF HEALTH

Figure 4. Amphastar's first FDA-approved intranasal naloxone delivery syringe. Used with permission of Amphastar Pharmaceuticals, Inc.

without formal medical training."[55] In the interim, harm reductionists had plenty of "people without medical training" administering naloxone, saving lives both counted and uncounted, and documenting these saves. A striking feature of naloxone's risk/benefit history was this ongoing denial and downright amnesia that it had worked – and was working outside medical settings – since the late 1990s. Widely distributed by harm reduction outlets and tracked by associated researchers, naloxone clearly worked for first responders, including firefighters and law enforcement, as well as members of the general public, parents and partners, and drug users themselves.

Narcan's rebranding as an intranasally administered rescue medication built on decades of use in community settings and almost fifty years in emergency settings. It would have surprised Nancy Caroline, author of *Emergency Care in the Streets* (originally published in 1979, now in its ninth edition), to hear that Narcan was just approved in 2014. Injectable naloxone was called Narcan when Pittsburgh physician Caroline first wrote her advice to paramedics to inject it "VERY SLOWLY" and "TITRATE the Narcan to the patient's respirations."[56] When Dan Bigg initially obtained the generic, injectable liquid used at the Chicago Recovery Alliance and set up a national clearinghouse for the product, it had been off-patent for years – yet it was still referred to as Narcan, just as generic tissues are referred to as Kleenex. Drug users casually referred to having been "narcanned," brought back from the dead. Today, however, only the intranasal device, Narcan, now made by Emergent BioSolutions, which bought Adapt Pharma, may technically be referred to as Narcan. The shift to intranasal administration coincided with naloxone's appearance in public health departments and extensive promotional campaigns such as those on New York City subways.

Moral Uptake and Moral Hazard

Unlike the 2012 hearings, the "Who's Who" of naloxone access advocacy did not have to storm the gates of the next national meeting, titled "Exploring Naloxone Uptake and Use," and co-sponsored by NIDA, SAMHSA, CDC, and FDA on July 1–2, 2015. The latter was on the cusp of approving

55 As Scott Weiner observed in "Should you carry the overdose rescue drug naloxone?," the US Surgeon General Jerome Adams' advisory letter on intranasal naloxone was the first advisory letter since a March 11, 2005, advisory on alcohol use during pregnancy. See this May 4, 2018 post, updated on April 23, 2019, upon approval of a generic intranasal spray formulation: https://www.health.harvard.edu/blog/should-you-carry-the-opioid-overdose-rescue-drug-naloxone-2018050413773.

56 Nancy L. Caroline, *Emergency Care in the Streets* (Little, Brown, 1979), 351.

intranasal naloxone products from Adapt Pharma and Invidior. In arguing for making naloxone OTC, community-based organizations pointed to their perennial lack of "medical/legal infrastructure (e.g., [having] a prescriber who is willing to work with them)." Roxanne Saucier spoke with the authority of international experience working to build harm reduction programs in China, Korea, Russia, Thailand, and Vietnam. Leo Beletsky cast OTC naloxone as part of a comprehensive legal strategy that included reforms to Good Samaritan laws. Physician Ingrid Binswanger noted that naloxone would be "analogous to other prescriptions I write, such as epinephrine for individuals with a history of anaphylaxis or glucagon for diabetics. It's basically giving a prescription to someone who may use it on someone else who needs it. And then it would encourage physician patient discussion about the true risks of overdose, and I think that might be the most useful part of having the naloxone to give in primary care." The notion that physicians could give away samples or co-prescribe to anyone prescribed high-dose opioids sparked conversations about insurance coverage. Human Rights Watch attorney Megan McLemore urged the FDA to authorize all extant naloxone formulations OTC, noting that "most people who are dying are outside the medical and insurance model" and applauding the "efforts of the FDA to prepare every step for a manufacturer to come forward, including doing the label research for them, but the fact is that none have done so to date."[57]

Renegotiating the terms of an implied social contract that is wider than naloxone, the harm reduction and overdose prevention movement adopted health equity and human rights goals. As a form of symbolic political capital, naloxone is "power in a bottle," the embodiment of a "miracle medicine," and community-based distribution a social movement for human rights. But phantasms of risk also pervade naloxone's risk-benefit history. The movement to change naloxone's status as a Prescription Only Medicine would make community distribution legal and gain recognition for the reality that the person to whom naloxone is prescribed is likely not the person to whom it is administered. Intranasal naloxone got trapped in a regulatory hell in part because cultural productions continue to condition decision-making in clinical, regulatory, and public policy domains. In "Life Is Hell After Narcan, Heroin's Miracle Cure," a photo illustration created by *The Daily Beast* that ran above an article by Christopher Moraff on March 22, 2016, media consumers were characterized as "hooked" on a miracle drug that magically reversed opioid overdose – but made their lives "hell" afterwards. The alchemy of this antidote was compared to the Promethean nature of the technology of fire and accompanied by allusions to a moral economy in which the life you save may not be worth saving because of the ensuing

57 FDA, "Role of Naloxone in Opioid Overdose Fatality Prevention," 74–75.

"hell." The foregrounded hand holding the naloxone applicator was clearly white, mottled, with chipped and ill-kept nails – details less foregrounded than the sleek, pure white plastic of the intranasal naloxone delivery device it is holding. The naloxone applicator clearly resembled the Amphastar device pictured in Figure 4 but its only identifiable markings established it as an accurately measured dose delivery system – the illustration showed scientific precision about to be engulfed in the metaphorical flames of the heroin user's hell.

On October 5, 2016, the FDA hosted a joint meeting of the Anesthetic and Analgesic Drug Products Advisory Committee and the Drug Safety and Risk Management Advisory Committee titled "FDA Advisory Committee on the Most Appropriate Dose or Doses of Naloxone to Reverse the Effects of Life-threatening Opioid Overdose in the Community Settings." Adapt Pharma, then the manufacturer of the intranasal Narcan approved in late 2015, discussed the need for a "common threshold for naloxone onset and exposure to apply for all formulations and routes of administration that approximates 2mg naloxone administered by injection (the high end of the established safe and effective initial dose range), rather than 0.4mg (the low end of the initial dose range)."[58] This would reduce competition from a "non FDA-approved Improvised Nasal Naloxone Kit [*sic*]," for which Adapt maintained the "pharmacokinetic properties" had not been published. FDA acknowledged that there were effective reversals with the improvised kit, but such evidence had not yet been "quantitated."

Touting naloxone's favorable risk/benefit profile but contravening naloxone access advocates preference for lower dose products more acceptable to the user community, Adapt Pharma advocated moving towards the upper end of the dosage range, citing fentanyl's ubiquity in the US opioid and stimulant supply and resulting increases in drug-related deaths.[59] On July 11, 2016, Adapt filed a Citizen Petition requesting the FDA to set guidelines for a fixed, optimal, effective dose and pharmacokinetics of *any* product containing naloxone, for use by *anyone* – a move that can only be interpreted as an attempt to safeguard their product market. By the next month, Adapt Pharma Narcan Nasal Spray had become the leading naloxone product on the US market. Adapt's advocacy of higher-dose naloxone ran counter to the harm reduction movement, which advocates titration and gentler waking along the lines advocated so long ago by Nancy Caroline and up-to-date

58 Adapt, presentation given in September 2016, 3–4.

59 In *Deaths of Despair and the Future of Capitalism* (Princeton University Press, 2020), Anne Case and Angus Deaton argue that fentanyl is entirely responsible for the increase in African American overdose deaths since 2013.

practice, rather than abrupt precipitated withdrawal.[60] While Adapt acknowledged titration as desirable in clinical practice, the company argued that in community settings,

> the goal for ALL community use naloxone products should be to safely, rapidly and readily achieve a consistently adequate initial naloxone exposure to bridge to the arrival of medical care. To avoid confusion in the community setting and recognizing the multiple unknown factors that impact an adequate dose, the Sponsor believes that one common threshold of onset and exposure should apply to all naloxone products intended for community use.

By 2016, all naloxone manufacturers had increased prices to the point that community-based distribution was slowing. Although licensed and approved intranasal kits could be purchased, the non-FDA approved kits still circulated along with the glass vials containing injectable form of naloxone. Naloxone was in the process of a paradoxically expansive containment.

Phantasms of risk hampered naloxone by alloying it with the risks of the opioids it antidotes. No one gets "hooked" on naloxone, yet headlines like "Getting Patients Hooked On an Opioid Overdose Antidote, Then Raising the Price" appeared.[61] Risks incurred by opioid users spurred competition as pharmaceutical manufacturers realized that the annual "naloxone spray market" was expected to reach two billion dollars by 2028.[62] This widened the margin for Teva Pharmaceuticals, the Israeli generics manufacturer, and Emergent BioSolutions, which acquired Narcan Nasal Spray (naloxone hydrochloride HCI) by purchasing Adapt in 2018, to enter a lucrative market as the number of consumers who would need naloxone was expected to

60 Paige M. Lemen, Daniel P. Garrett, Erin Thompson, Megan Aho, Christina Vasquez, and Ju Nyeong Park, "High-dose naloxone formulations are not as essential as we thought," *Harm Reduction Journal* 21, no. 1 (2024): 93.

61 Shefali Luthra, "Getting Patients Hooked On an Opioid Overdose Antidote, Then Raising the Price," *Washington Post*, January 30, 2017.

62 Ravi Gupta, Nilay D. Shah, and Joseph S. Ross, "The Rising Price of Naloxone – Risks to Efforts to Stem Overdose Deaths," *New England Journal of Medicine* 375 (2016): 2213–15; Harrison Jacobs, "Price of Naloxone Skyrocketing," *Business Insider*, August 1, 2016, http://www.businessinsider.com/price-of-naloxone-narcan-skyrocketing-2016-7; Sarah Karlin-Smith, "Price Spikes for Life-Saving Drug," *Politico*, May 16, 2016, http://www.politico.com/story/2016/05/drug-prices-addiction-223192; Melody Peterson, "As Need Grows for Painkiller Overdose Treatment, Companies Raise Prices," *Los Angeles Times*, July 17, 2016, http://www.latimes.com/business/la-fi-naloxone-sales-20160707-snap-story.html.

Table 1. “A Second Chance: Overdose Prevention, Naloxone, and Human Rights in the United States,” Human Rights Watch, April 2017, 37. The price of 0.4 mg/ml of injectable naloxone manufactured by Hospira prior to 2005 was less than one dollar. Creative Commons.

Naloxone Product	Manufacturer	Previous Available Price (yr)	Current Price (2016)
Injectable or intranasal 1 mg/1 ml vial (2ml) (mucosal atomizer device separate)	Amphastar	$20.34 (2009)	$39.60
Injectable 0.4 mg/1 ml vial (10 ml)	Hospira	$62.29 (2012)	$142.49
Injectable 0.4 mg/1 ml vial (1 ml)	Mylan	$23.72 (2014)	$23.72
Injectable 0.4 mg/1 ml vial (1 ml)	West-Ward	$20.40 (2015)	$20.40
Auto-injector, two pack of single-use prefilled auto-injectors (Evzio)147	Kaleo (approved 2014)	$690.00 (2014)	$4,500.00
Nasal spray, two pack of single-use intranasal devices (Narcan)	Adapt (approved 2015)	$150.00 (2015)	$150.00

expand.[63] Intranasal naloxone products appealed to a middle-class medical consumer market – the kind of consumers who had home medicine cabinets and health insurance to pay for naloxone priced so far above market that it might as well have been sold on the moon. Responding to astronomical prices, health equity activists and harm reduction advocates touted the benefits of good old-fashioned, low priced, liquid, injectable naloxone. The FDA independently took a different route to incentivize OTC naloxone sprays.

From Regulatory Hell to the Proactive Regulatory Space of the Switch: Rx-to-OTC

The FDA took the unusual – indeed, unique – step of calling for proposals for OTC naloxone in January 2017.[64] For the first time in its history, the regulatory agency designed, tested, and validated its *own* schematic Drug Fact Label (DFL). This first step would have to be taken *if* a pharmaceutical company should happen to develop an OTC naloxone and *if* the agency should happen to approve it as an OTC drug. Commissioner Scott Gottlieb stated: "This is the first time the FDA has proactively developed and tested a DFL for a drug to support development of an OTC product. ... One of the key components for OTC availability is now in place. In short, we've crafted model labeling that sponsors can use to obtain approval for OTC naloxone and increase its access. This action was part of our broader commitment to addressing the opioid crisis."[65]

63 See https://www.marketexpert24.com/2019/11/06/naloxone-spray-market-growing-with-new-healthcare-innovations-with-major-key-players-teva-pharmaceutical-industries-ltd-emergent-biosolutions-inc/; and Janet Burns, "Overdose Training In Jail Gets Naloxone To Where It's Needed Most, Data Show," October 31, 2019, https://www.forbes.com/sites/janetwburns/2019/10/31/overdose-training-in-jail-gets-naloxone-to-where-its-needed-most-data-show/#4611cd9d3513.

64 Janet Woodcock, long-time Director of the Center for Drug Evaluation and Research (CDER) and Acting Director of CDER's newly formed Office of Pharmaceutical Quality (OPQ) at the FDA, issued this invitation alongside Theresa (Terri) Michelle, who directs the FDA division in charge of OTC product review, the Division of Nonprescription Clinical Evaluation (DNCE) in the Office of Drug Evaluation (ODE). See: https://www.focr.org/news/stat-new-janet-fda-turns-quiet-problem-solver-who-brings-expertise-%E2%80%94-and-little-controversy.

65 https://www.fda.gov/news-events/press-announcements/statement-fda-commissioner-scott-gottlieb-md-unprecedented-new-efforts-support-development-over.

Lauding its own proactivity, the FDA encouraged innovation in the OTC naloxone arena – a good twenty years after harm reduction activists and human rights advocates started calling for it. Rx-to-OTC switches rely on anticipatory science and imaginative enactments – firms must show what happens when physicians are removed from self-treatment. Designing "credible simulations" from which physicians are removed cannot be experimental, according to David Bradford of PEGUS Research, which had been conducting actual use trials for twenty years:

> Key elements of subject behavior in an actual use trial cannot be controlled by protocol, so a complex assessment of subject's self-directed decisions and behaviors must be made. The task is made more difficult by the varying degree of subject understanding of both the task itself and the questions we ask about their choices. All this is done with a very heterogeneous sample of subjects whose cognitive ability, familiarity with the drug and the indication being treated, general cognitive and reading ability, and disposition toward self-treatment range across a wide spectrum. We'd argue that compared to that complexity, the interpretation of the results of an experimental trial is a walk in the park.[66]

The difficulties of observational trials of actual use that mimic real-world conditions were laid squarely at the feet of the human subjects enrolled in them in the 2012 FDA hearings: "Ultimately the regulatory decision about approval of a drug for OTC sale hinges on whether subjects select and use the drug properly."[67] "Degrees of artificiality" of such studies and lack of imagination for the conditions of actual use have much to do with why certain Rx-to-OTC switches fail.[68] Community distribution of take-home naloxone had amassed an evidence base and a track record of subjects using naloxone to save one another's lives – arguably, these "actual use studies" could have been taken into account without need for imagination or artifice. There was an opportunity to build upon decades of work by harm reduction activists and public health advocates.

The actual social, political, and economic contexts to which FDA was responding with its 2017 call resulted from decades of work by activists to tip the public ledger towards lower-cost naloxone. Instead of simply designating or declaring it OTC – an action that many activists and advocates believed was within the FDA's power – the regulator instead conducted a DFL study to encourage companies to innovate in this space. One of the architects of naloxone's OTC switch, John Pinney of Pinney Associates, described

66 FDA, "Role of Naloxone in Opioid Overdose Fatality Prevention," 8.

67 FDA, "Role of Naloxone in Opioid Overdose Fatality Prevention," 8.

68 FDA, "Role of Naloxone in Opioid Overdose Fatality Prevention," 12.

becoming aware that the FDA had conducted its own labeling study at a regulatory scientific quality conference he attended in 2017 with Michael Hufford of Harm Reduction Therapeutics. Pinney's consulting group was working in what he described as a "lukewarm" way with kaléo, Inc. As the naloxone spray market formed up, the "OTC switch space" opened.

Naloxone is but one exhibit in a spacious gallery including everything from vaginal cream for yeast infections to Plan B emergency contraception. Several narrative frames have been essential for building scientific and policy consensus on the risks and benefits of wider distribution of naloxone. Imaginative framings of risk, benefit, harm, and anti-harm pervade the Rx-to-OTC space, which brims with talk of creativity and innovation (although disappointment dogs triumphal accounts of successful switches). Relevant actors are drug developers with technical and commercial expertise in the regulatory domain known as the "OTC switch space" – as illustrated by this text on the "art" of the switch:

> Since 2013, there have been six successful Rx-to-OTC switches – and a plethora of high-profile switch failures and disappointing results. Successful switches are as much an art as a science, and it has become increasingly apparent that switch teams must revise their best practices if they are to effectively lead an Rx product through the switch to OTC. Our speaking faculty, representing Bayer, Pfizer, Johnson & Johnson, Sanofi, Galderma, and many other organizations, will help you to:
>
> - Grasp the fundamentals of the switch process
> - Review successful case studies and strategies
> - Innovate with OTC packaging and label writing
> - Stay up to date with regulatory challenges and initiatives
> - Brainstorm new marketing and branding strategies[69]

Readers would be forgiven for assuming that the Rx-to-OTC switch space is one of innovation and not continual repurposing of drugs already on the market, given the consistency with which signifiers of creativity and novelty are paired with the term "switch" in this rhetorical space.[70] Reading public documents that urge naloxone's move from prescription-only to OTC

69 From ExL Pharma's third annual Full Life Cycle Switch Event, the RX-to-OTC Switch Summit, held in 2016, see this flyer: http://info.exlevents.com/rs/195-NER-971/images/C808_Cruz.pdf.

70 Lorraine Code, *Rhetorical Spaces: Essays on (Gendered) Locations* (Routledge, 1995).

status, this regulatory space was retrograde in relation to the proactive social imaginaries of movement actors seeking to democratize naloxone.

Naloxone's trip through the agonistic zone of regulatory hell ultimately propelled it through the "Rx-to-OTC switch space" and into OTC status. Regulatory arenas are rhetorical spaces where epistemic authority is constituted, reproduced, and maintained; such spaces can be quite vicious and defensive. The OTC switch space is rhetorically constructed as a gladiatorial arena to such an extent that Edwin Hemwall of Merck Consumer Care, a "veteran" of a decade-long campaign to switch the statin Mevacor to OTC status, claimed to have the "scars to show for it. But maybe if there's such a thing as a switch purple heart, I might also have one of those."[71] Perhaps the harm reduction activists and naloxone access advocates have earned "switch purple hearts," too.

Movement Versus Model: The Affective Economies of Naloxone in 2018

Naloxone was remodeled by harm reduction activists, drug policy reformers, and researcher-advocates attracted to the task of producing evidence for its efficacy. Overdose prevention was to take place through community distribution modeled on mutual aid, social movement direct action, and needle and syringe exchange. These "evidence-based activists"[72] built novel social infrastructure and public policy to wrest naloxone from the medical enclave and put it in the hands of those who needed it most – drug users themselves. Drug users were most likely to witness and attend to an overdose, a realization widely credited to Dan Bigg of the Chicago Recovery Alliance, as was made emphatically clear by Eliza Wheeler, the opening witness on the second day of the 2018 FDA Advisory Committee, a meeting convened months after Bigg's untimely death that August:

> None of us would be here today, including industry who are developing products related to naloxone, to the community, without this person. My colleagues mentioned him yesterday. This is Dan Bigg. He founded the Chicago Recovery Alliance, and he was the first person in the world to distribute naloxone to the community. Naloxone was first distributed to the community, specifically people who use drugs, off of this van in Chicago

71 FDA, "Role of Naloxone in Opioid Overdose Fatality Prevention," 7, 80.

72 These are among the many "protagonists" I interviewed for Campbell, *OD*, and they include researchers such as Phil Coffin, Nabarun DasGupta, Traci Green, Alex Kral, Sharon Stancliff, Alexander Walley, and Maya Doe-Simkins, who self-identified as a "reluctant researcher."

starting in 1996. Prior to that, naloxone had been used for about 25 years in hospital and in pre-hospital settings.[73]

Wheeler's slides and speech portrayed harm reductionists' efforts as a movement resistant to medicalization aimed at "liberating" naloxone from its captors. She indicated that by the time of the 2012 hearings, the CDC had listed 188 active naloxone distribution programs operating in the United States, each based on the "model we know works" – community-based distribution of naloxone "directly to people who use drugs and their community by people who are trusted in the community with low threshold/low barrier program models."[74] The harm reduction "model" was never meant to be a "medical model," she continued, questioning the premises of the 2018 hearing – the idea that there ought to be co-prescription of naloxone for patients prescribed high-dose opioids, and the idea that pharmacies ought to serve as distribution points. Instead, she offered a "demedicalized" approach to naloxone that neither accepted drug use as "disorder" or "disease," nor pathologized it.

The community distribution model mattered to the movement – just as it had once mattered to the HIV/AIDS movement, which had paved the way with the FDA and CDC, opening both agencies to be more inclusive of community participation and more attentive to health social movements.[75] Wheeler, Doe Simkins, and others created the Opioid Safety and Naloxone Network (OSNN) Buyers Club, a purchasing group strategically designed to ensure that medical professionals are not sole gatekeepers of naloxone. Today called Remedy Alliance/For The People, OSNN formed following a summit at Temple University law school in 2008.[76] Remedy Alliance/For The People grew out of naloxone distribution centered at Chicago Recovery Alliance. Novel community distribution schemes were based on cannabis grower's and buyer's clubs mobilized in the early days of HIV and AIDS.[77] They depend on corporate largesse given high pharmaceutical prices. Direct Relief, the Pfizer Foundation-centered humanitarian aid program for rural

73 Joint Meeting, December 17–18, 2018, 27.

74 Joint Meeting, December 17–18, 2018, 30; Eliza Wheeler, T. Stephen Jones, Michael K. Gilbert, and Peter J. Davidson, "Opioid Overdose Prevention Programs Providing Naloxone to Laypersons – United States," *MMWR* 64, no. 23 (2014): 631–35.

75 Steven Epstein, *Impure Science: AIDS, Activism, and the Politics of Knowledge* (University of California Press, 1996); Steven Epstein, *Inclusion: The Politics of Difference in Medical Research* (University of Chicago Press, 2007).

76 See https://remedyallianceftp.org/pages/our-story.

77 Wendy Chapkis and Richard J. Webb, *Dying to Get High: Marijuana as Medicine* (New York University Press, 2008).

naloxone delivery, works via a disaster relief model that relies on at-will donations of naloxone, re-couching this "pharmaceutical object" within the very biomedical model that harm reduction evolved to counter. Direct Relief has been a licensed "wholesale pharmacy to secure prescription medicines for use abroad" since 1962 (naloxone was added much later), following "strict internal protocols regarding the suitability of types of products, inventory controls, and the qualifications of trained health professionals on the receiving end of aid shipments. This focus also established strong ties to U.S. healthcare companies, which have long supported our efforts with donations of high-value pharmaceutical and other medical resources allocated through our assistance program."[78] Humanitarian aid bridges gaps in the hollowed out spaces between failing states and needy subjects.[79] Humanitarian aid organizations get essential medicine to rural areas of the United States – indicating the utter failure of the biomedical model to address health disparities and inequities at work in the opioid arena. People who do not have health insurance do not seek healthcare unless they absolutely must. The biomedical model introduces the problems of uneven availability, narrowed options, poor reach, bureaucratic red tape, and, above all, high levels of distrust and social distance between "clients" and "providers."

An early example of the impetus to set aside medical gatekeeping came from physicians, nurses, medical students, and other healthcare providers within the harm reduction movement itself. Alexander Walley, a Boston medical doctor allied with Massachusetts naloxone access activists, argued to get doctors out of the picture so that community health workers could "access populations at highest risk" who did not enjoy a "traditional doctor-patient relationship."[80] Attempts to get pharmacy (and prescribing physicians) out of pharmaceuticals was a clearer path in the case of cannabis buyer's clubs, where activists were growing the plants on which "products" were based. Naloxone, however, like the other non-synthetic opioids it antidotes, is derived from thebaine, a highly controlled pharmaceutical object that would be impractical and illegal to home brew. Instead, Wheeler explained, "we limit the buyer's club to nongovernment community-based organizations who are distributing naloxone directly to people who use drugs. We distributed 506,000 doses last year and 20,845 doses year to date as of last

78 See the organization's website at: https://www.directrelief.org/about/history/.

79 Michael Mascarenhas, *New Humanitarianism and the Crisis of Charity: Good Intentions on the Road to Help* (Indiana University Press, 2017); Rosalind P. Petchesky, *Global Prescriptions: Gendering Health and Human Rights* (Zed Books, 2003).

80 FDA, "Role of Naloxone in Opioid Overdose Fatality Prevention," 108.

Tuesday. In 2018, we're going to likely hit just under a million this year."[81] Although her San Francisco program distributed a "cumbersome" nasal formulation (the atomizer had to be hand-assembled for use with liquid naloxone for intramuscular injection as described above), Wheeler assumed injectable naloxone as the standard of care and emphasized a social model of overdose education "conceived of and first implemented by people who use drugs, allies, and practitioners of harm reduction as part of a radical public health movement based on those principles that you see there."[82]

Harm reduction is unique in connecting pragmatic actions not with identity, but with expertise resulting from lived experience of drug use, drug user advocacy, and overdose prevention. Wheeler exhorted the advisory group to "[s]eek our technical assistance and guidance. People who use drugs and other harm reduction experts, researchers, and policymakers are the innovators of this intervention and are the experts. Compensate us for our expertise and ensure that people with lived experience and people who use drugs are involved in decision-making about their own lives."[83] Naloxone advocacy works through a lateral "empowerment model" that centers drug users' concrete knowledge, technical expertise, and knowledge of vernacular pharmacology. The movement has been far more effective for attending to drug user health than the abstract, hierarchical "medical model" that rests upon the regulatory regimes enacted by the FDA, the drug control apparatus underpinned by the DEA, and the disregard for and undermining of nonmedical expertise.

Pharmaceutical manufacturers, packagers, and distributors are unlikely to see profit in low-cost naloxone; they donate free or low-cost naloxone while keeping prices to consumers high. Funded by the San Francisco City Public Health Department, Wheeler's program was obtaining naloxone for a dollar a vial at the time of the 2018 advisory meeting. Programs throughout the country relied on the CRA's standing orders; indeed, the CRA essentially ran a national naloxone clearinghouse, in addition to its own mobile delivery services, for years before Remedy Alliance was formalized. The seeming failure of the federal government to ensure naloxone access led to its patchwork of availability, and contortions "worthy of Cirque du Soleil" by industry

81 Joint Meeting, December 17–18, 2018, 32.

82 Joint Meeting, December 17–18, 2018, 39. Political theorist Nancy Fraser has called this a "politics of recognition," an interpretive bid for the primacy of identity shaped in the process of activity within the context of political struggles and safeguarding against reification and/or displacement of recognition over the politics of redistribution. See Nancy Fraser, "Rethinking Recognition," *New Left Review* 3 (May/June 2000): https://newleftreview.org/issues/ii3/articles/nancy-fraser-rethinking-recognition.

83 Joint Meeting, December 17–18, 2018, 37.

representatives justifying keeping prices out of reach for the community-based organizations who to this day move most of the naloxone in the United States.[84] Such acrobatics were pointed out by Michael Hufford, co-founder of the not-for-profit pharmaceutical company, Harm Reduction Therapeutics, which aimed to lower the cost of naloxone for public-facing school districts, first responders, public health departments, and community-based programs served by the Remedy Alliance. While long-running controversies over dosage, formulation, and route or method of administration may sound like "merely" technical matters, they illustrate how sociotechnical matters of concern structure the conditions of possibility for harm reduction practice.

Conclusion

Accrual of authority, credibility, and epistemic status deriving from expertise is the goal of those acting agentically in such spaces. Words like "risk," "benefit," and, increasingly, "harm," exert an undertow of conscription into medical models central to the biomedical frameworks we lived by during the period when harm reduction actants put forward "demedicalized" models aiming to "empower" those who carried naloxone and knew how to use it. For them, naloxone was neither medicine nor drug – the distinction of this "rescue remedy" was its capacious flexibility relative to the brittle distinctions between medicines and drugs. Naloxone access actants expanded the space, multiplying the meanings, contexts, and spaces for interpretive flexibility and playful pluralities. Harm reduction activists accomplished widened access to naloxone through an array of strategies and tactics used to expand their cultural reach. OTC was one such strategy; others such as the "safe supply" movement and overdose prevention centers were others by which harm reduction has evolved. Perhaps harm reduction will take on the protective coloration of medicine or retreat underground again in the face of the remodeling of the FDA and the CDC during Trump's second administration and the assault upon the administrative, regulatory state. What historians can predict is that much of the work of access advocates will be forgotten – this chapter is written against that predictable amnesia. The relative normalization of naloxone access by the 2020s is in danger of being forgotten as it becomes less available with cuts to federal funding, reprioritization at the state level, and tightened reins on harm reduction and drug treatment services.

An ethos of future anterior forgetting pervades constructions of risk and benefit in relation to naloxone and to the opioids it antagonizes. Most

84 Author's interview with Michael Hufford, 2020.

repeatedly forgotten are the robust findings that abstinence is itself a risk factor for overdose death. The risks associated with abstinence fly in the face of conventional wisdom that abstinence is the essential first step towards successful treatment and recovery from opioid use disorder. Drug users will still die largely preventable deaths until we recognize that abstinence is a risk, and ... we have drugs and medicines for that!

In tracing how changes of state and status were accomplished in the regulatory spaces that govern Rx-to-OTC switches, this chapter has documented how an anticipatory regime allowed speculative forecasts and constructs of moral hazard to displace actual harms, including deaths. The affective states of anticipatory regimes continually reoriented historical actors and reanimated the material trajectory of an actant like naloxone.[85] Harm reduction movements confronted a space in which attention to documented harms – even death – was displaced by phantasmatic speculations about risks that then had to be painstakingly demonstrated *not* to occur. The anticipatory regimes into which naloxone has been conscripted rest upon phantasmatic assumptions such as notions that naloxone's very presence is a "moral hazard" or that having it on hand encourages drug users to take more risks. Researchers working with access advocates then had to design studies to demonstrate that these phantasmatic risks do *not* occur. Similarly, the idea that naloxone is itself "addictive" is a phantasmatic risk. Such demands to disprove things that are not actually happening have required creative biostatisticians and researchers who can envision how to accomplish studies that demonstrate that these phantasmatic risks are not heightened, while also demonstrating that deaths have been prevented by community members' or bystanders' use of naloxone to save lives. Yet the risks of abstinence remain counterintuitive to such a degree that they are discounted as if the actual risks of abstinence are not actual risks. Abstinence is the most concrete risk for overdose and overdose death – as tolerance declines and relapse becomes likely, risk is not phantasmatic.

Anticipatory regimes deal in risky dynamics. The FDA traffics in anticipatory regimes, calibrating what might happen if a consumer product was regulated more or less restrictively; if physicians or pharmacists were not engaged in patient education, would consumers correctly diagnose the situation, comprehend the label, select correct dosage, and use the product safely and appropriately? If it is not the "consumer" who diagnoses and administers naloxone, but someone else who must act – a "witness," "bystander," or "observer," how will that person know that an overdose is occurring or that naloxone is an appropriate response? How long will it take them to judge the situation as one of appropriate use? While such concerns do not differ completely the slippage between "self care" and purchase involved in other

85 Adams, Murphy, and Clarke, "Anticipation," 247.

OTC products, it is fair to say that potentially saving a life through overdose reversal differs from self-treating a yeast infection or headache.

Anticipatory regimes also got connected to the hype of "innovation," which typically signals the presence of novelty. Naloxone was an old drug by the time it became a pharmaceutical object of contention. This chapter was written after the fiftieth anniversary of its FDA approval for overdose reversal; after naloxone access activists and advocates had convinced public health departments, firefighters, and law enforcement to carry it; and after they had developed programs to educate community members about it, and to distribute it. Consumers, governments, and regulators found intranasal administration more palatable. Public purchasers were willing to pay for the convenience of the intranasal product – but as need increased, naloxone became so unaffordable that people began referring to it as "paying through the nose." The politics of palatability infuriated and exhausted US harm reduction activists who had witnessed both injectable naloxone and the cobbled together intranasal kits working to save lives. Why should technology matter in the face of saving lives?

Risk, too, is cobbled together, an assemblage composed of lack of innovation, lack of healthcare access, and lack of political will to overcome regulatory barriers to distribute a lifesaving medication – in this case compounded by the "undone science" of overdose.[86] Where there is undone science, there is epistemic conflict over who should bear the costs of innovation. In the case of naloxone, who should bear the costs of accumulating an evidence base to document the bioavailability of intranasal naloxone once Massachusetts EMTs and activists had established proof of concept using their cobbled together system? Who should have borne the costs of determining the public health effectiveness of community-wide distribution? Who should have borne the costs of widening implementation of this public health intervention? Perhaps those who advocate abstinence should bear some responsibility for re-educating the public about the risks they are encouraging drug users to run.

Arguably the developmental and regulatory delays recounted in this chapter cost lives, enhanced risk, and delayed life-saving access to naloxone. US harm reduction activists have spent their lives hurdling law, policy, and regulatory challenges in each of the fifty US state governments. In the overdose death prevention domain, risks are an actuarial, "many-headed monster,"[87] but risk remains abstract, conceptual, and potential in the face of empirically well-documented harms like death tolls, which are taken to express

86 Campbell, *OD*.

87 Matthew D. Adler, "Risk, Death and Harm: The Normative Foundations of Risk Regulation," *Minnesota Law Review* 87 (2003): 1293–445.

the realities of cold, hard facts. As we participate in the intertwined cultural work of risk and remembrance, we must remember how what we remember and what we forget is entangled with whose risks count, what we count, and how we count.[88] Risk is actuarial, but it is remembered in the abstract and imagined future anterior tense – there was a time when, if we'd known the risk, we would have kept naloxone on hand and perhaps we would not have insisted upon abstinence. Keeping harms like overdose deaths present, visible, and culturally central works against the future forgetting to which we are encouraged by risk-regulating agencies. Legal scholar Matthew Adler points out that such agencies "*do* have substantial statutory discretion to take account of the racial or socioeconomic pattern of death"[89] – they *choose* not to do so. Similarly, when abstinence is promoted as a social good, it is a choice to forget that abstinence also incurs risk. If only we had known the risks that we were running, we could have chosen to keep someone alive rather than letting them die. That is the promise of naloxone and the keepers of its flame.

88 I owe this insight to Jacqueline Wernemont, *Numbered Lives: Life and Death in Quantum Media* (MIT Press, 2018), 81.

89 Adler, "Risk, Death and Harm," 1425.

Part Five

Consumer Paradigms of Risk and Benefit

Chapter Thirteen

"A Healthy Reactive Tendency": Risks and Benefits of Cannabis and User Agency in the 1930s[1]

Bob Beach

In July 1939, Walter Bromberg, a psychiatrist working at Bellevue Hospital in New York, published the third in a series of articles on cannabis and its psychiatric effect on users. His conclusions challenged prevailing assumptions about the drug's effects that drove nationwide efforts to control cannabis, culminating in the passage of federal regulatory legislation in 1937.[2] The studies generally ignore or downplay the agency of individual patients, concerned more with the often violent effects of acute intoxication.[3] For one of them, "Case 23," a twenty-year-old Black man admitted in October 1936, Bromberg made the following observation:

1 I'd like to thank the editors and reviewers who helped me fine-tune my argument here and gave me important new perspectives on my evidence. Appreciation to the staff at the Special Collections Library at Penn State who provided helpful assistance with Anslinger's papers at the earliest stages of my research. The staff at NARA II also helped me to navigate Record Group 0170. Finally, thanks to Richard Hamm for his eternal patience and guidance through my research!

2 United States, *Marihuana Tax Act of 1937*, Public Law 75-238, 75th Congress, 1st Session, 50 Stat. 551 (August 2, 1937).

3 Walter Bromberg, "Marihuana Intoxication," *American Journal of Psychiatry* 91 (1934): 301–13; Walter Bromberg, "The Effects of Marihuana," in *Proceedings of the Association for Research in Nervous and Mental Disease* (Williams & Wilkins Company, 1938), 180–89; Walter Bromberg, "Marihuana: A Psychiatric Study," *Journal of the American Medical Association* 113, no. 1 (1939): 4–12.

> The patient in whom a functional psychosis is developing strives to overcome the unconsciously perceived difficulties. In this sense the use of marihuana represents a healthy reactive tendency, even though the mechanism may be unknown to the patient. Case 23 illustrates this problem. A boy who had made a successful adjustment on a moderate level of social attainment began to show schizoid behavior shortly after beginning to use marihuana. The process continued to a psychotic state. What role did the drug play? Could the psychosis have begun without the drug? Was the use of cannabis the patient's attempt to cure his developing psychosis? These are problems needing careful judgement and study and wide clinical experience.[4]

The vast majority of Bromberg's work involved patients who either self-admitted during a crisis or were brought to Bellevue by police out of concern for public safety. Bromberg's analysis of the risks of cannabis did challenge the exaggerated claims made in the press about the drug's effects but stopped short of suggesting the drug had legitimate use, attributing patient use instead to latent psychological, personality, or indeed racial "flaws." For Case 23, however, Bromberg suggested that the patient made a conscious, though perhaps uninformed, decision to use cannabis for its benefits against some unknown affliction. He had used cannabis for a long time and had cannabis-related incidents in the past, but for whatever reason Bromberg seemed curious about the patient's continued use early on, prior to any overt negative effects. No other comment appears about the man's motives so his reasons for continuing early on, the accuracy of his self-diagnosis (or whether it was made at all), or whether his use of cannabis was beneficial in any way are nebulous. However, Bromberg's suggestion has significant implications for the study of cannabis users during the 1930s in the United States.

This essay examines the first-hand articulation of cannabis users' assessment of the risks and benefits of cannabis use and argues that some cannabis users chose cannabis for a specific health-related reasons and articulated their navigation of the risks (health risks, but also legal risks) and the benefits of using cannabis in the context of pursuing explicitly healthful outcomes. By centering the analysis on the voices of users and assessing their justifications on their own terms, I argue that cannabis users challenged the prevailing assumptions about both the medical utility of cannabis, and the risks associated with its use.

Conclusions about the risks and benefits of cannabis had evolved into consensus in the medical, legal, and law enforcement communities for decades by the time of Bromberg's commentary on Case 23. Adam Rathge has convincingly laid out the trajectory of the medical view of cannabis. In

4 Bromberg, "Marihuana: A Psychiatric Study," 9.

the mid-nineteenth century, practitioners touted the promise of medicinal cannabis, as they did with many other psychoactive substances at the time, as a potential cure for a diverse range of physical ailments. Over time, problems with accurate dosing, consistent effects, and the unpleasant effects of acute cannabis intoxication doomed cannabis as a reliable medicinal application well before states and the federal government sought strict regulations in the 1930s.[5] At the same time, the process of establishing clinically standard assessments of risk and benefit was in the midst of developing in the thirties. As such, the disconnect between professional and popular medical knowledge was less distinct than it would become under more tightly regulated experimental conditions.[6] Additionally, the emergence of self-help medicine in the early twentieth century reinvigorated a more popular understanding of medicine even as the medical infrastructure increasingly became dismissive, and even hostile, to those opinions.[7] Nevertheless, these popular opinions remained viable options for some, leading some to decide to start using cannabis for explicitly medical reasons, despite the risks of experiencing a psychotic episode, and during the 1930s, under increased risk of legal penalties attached to its sale, distribution, and use.[8]

The evidence is scattered over the archival record. Newspaper evidence provides an intriguing, although limited, window into user perspectives. Reporting on court cases where defendants make claims of self-medication as a defense for violations of cannabis control regulations, however, does

5 Adam R. Rathge, "Cannabis Cures: American Medicine, Mexican Marijuana, and the Origins of the War on Weed, 1840–1937" (PhD dissertation, Boston College, 2017).

6 Bennett Holman, "Humbug, the Council of Pharmacy and Chemistry, and the Origin of 'The Blind Test' of Therapeutic Efficacy," in *Uncertainty in Pharmacology: Epistemology, Methods, and Decisions*, ed. Adam LaCaze and Barbara Osimani (Springer Nature, 2020), 397–416; Joseph M. Gabriel, "The Testing of Sanocrysin: Science, Profit, and Innovation in Clinical Trial Design, 1926–31," *Journal of the History of Medicine and Allied Sciences* 69, no. 4 (2014): 604–32; Charles E. Rosenberg, "The Therapeutic Revolution: Medicine, Meaning, and Social Change in Nineteenth-Century America," *Perspectives in Biology and Medicine* 20, no. 4 (1977): 485–506; Morris J. Vogel and Charles E. Rosenberg, eds., *The Therapeutic Revolution: Essays in the Social History of American Medicine*, 3rd ed. (University of Pennsylvania Press, 2016).

7 Nancy Tomes, "Merchants of Health: Medicine and Consumer Culture in the United States, 1900–1940," *The Journal of American History* 88, no. 2 (2001): 519–47.

8 Bradley Borogerdi, *Commodifying Cannabis: A Cultural History of a Complex Plant in the Atlantic World* (Lexington Books, 2021); Rathge, "Cannabis Cures"; Nick Johnson, *Grass Roots: A History of Cannabis in the American West* (Oregon State University Press, 2017).

provide some larger context for the analysis of more direct and informal examination of users under institutional supervision in various contexts. US servicemembers were studied in the Panama Canal Zone to determine the effect of cannabis use on insubordination and a series of suicides on a military base. The federal government, specifically the Federal Bureau of Narcotics, kicked off its effort to roll out federal control in 1938 with a series of surveys on arrestees. Bromberg's work, referenced above, was conducted at New York's public Bellevue Hospital and involved individuals experiencing acute intoxication effects. And in the mayor's office in New York, Mayor Fiorello LaGuardia commissioned both a clinical and sociological study to examine cannabis users in the city.

With the notable exception of those featured in the LaGuardia study, the individuals examined in this essay were not given much consideration for their personal views or opinions of cannabis as the studies tended to focus on assessing the risks associated with acute cannabis intoxication, and the violence that was making headlines in the news.[9] Nevertheless, indications of user motive crept into the reports published about cannabis users. Adding in the context of the examined users' similar socioeconomic status and shared anxieties existing on the margins of both consumer society and the public health infrastructure help us more deeply understand their health-based motivations and justifications for use.

"The Results were Most Beneficial:" User Testimony in Newspaper Reports

Newspaper accounts that include healthful articulations from users can be found in arrest and court reports following the flood of local and state-level cannabis regulations that started to appear in the late 1910s. The specific claims of motive from users represents a small portion of the total cannabis

9 "Murder of Child Blamed on Drug," *Helena Daily Independent*, February 21, 1930; "Crazed Mexican Murders Youth," *Big Spring Daily Herald*, February 27, 1931; "Marijuana Weed Blamed for Axe Murder of Five," *Gastonia Daily Gazette*, October 19, 1933; Kenneth Clark, "Murders Due to 'Killer Drug' Marihuana Sweeping United States," *Syracuse American*, February 17, 1935; "Police Blame Marihuana for Majority of Murders and Sex Outrages in Valley," *Alamosa Daily Courier*, August 31, 1936; "Trunk Murder Mystery Solved in New York," *Hammond Times*, August 19, 1937; "Girl Bandits Indicted for Murder in New Jersey," *New York Times*, January 7, 1938; "Former Kern Nurse Held on Murder Charge," *Fresno Bee*, April 19, 1938; "Sensational Irwin Murder Case Trial Opens," *Monessen Daily Independent*, October 26, 1938.

incidents reported during the same period and were reported on largely to illustrate the lack of appreciation of the risks of acute intoxication on the part of arrestees. While these claims certainly could be an effort to elude penalties, some claims were explicitly dismissed as typical of cannabis addicts but, taken with the other examples that follow, display a specific pattern of articulation of both the benefits and risks of cannabis use that strongly suggest intentional health treatment.

In 1928, a Billings, Montana, man named "Gerrero" was questioned in connection to federal Prohibition agents finding a large cache of alcohol intended for Mexican beet farmers who had returned from summer work. Among the contraband was an "apple box full of marijuana," which Gerrero claimed to have cultivated for a friend who brewed a tea to cure stomach pains.[10] In 1931, Gregoria Rangel, mother of nine children in New Braunfels, Texas, claimed to have planted the weed to treat bouts of rheumatism, while later that year in Devine, Texas, Juan Morales told a judge in the 94th District Court, "that he had used marihuana, mixed with olive oil and beef tallow as an ointment for his rheumatism." Philadelphia resident Bartola Morel claimed in 1938 to be "collecting certain plants from which he could brew a tea to ease the rheumatic pains in his legs."[11] The potential of cannabis to manage pain inspired cultivation of the drug for that purpose among these folks. For others, recommendations from friends and acquaintances introduced them to the drug. Al Mann and Edward Martin, two members of a Chicago-based vaudeville troupe claimed in 1937 to have sought out the drug "on advice of a friend who said they were good for colds."[12] Major M. Underwood from Iowa claimed to have purchased eight tins "from a transient in 1930" (eight years prior to his arrest in 1938), and smoked to "make breathing easier when I get the asthma or sinus trouble."[13] Unique among these cases was Brazilian sea-

10 "Mexican Confesses Growing Marijuana," *Helena Daily Independent*, November 20, 1928.

11 "Mexican Woman Held as Officers Find Marihuana," *Abilene Daily Reporter*, August 23, 1931; "Marituana Is Cure, He Says," *San Antonio Light*, November 10, 1931; "Salinas Man Held on Marihuana Charge," *Oakland Tribune*, July 27, 1935; "His Rheumatic Pains Get No Sympathy," *Philadelphia Inquirer*, January 3, 1938; "Flashes of Life Here and There," *Amsterdam Democratic Recorder*, July 19, 1940; "Message to Garcia," *Oshkosh Daily Northwestern*, July 19, 1940; "Foot Bath of Marijuana Places Owner in Prison," *Canton Commercial*, October 1, 1940.

12 "Dancer Warned for Possessing Reefer Cigarets," *Chicago Defender*, July 31, 1937.

13 "Marijuana Used to Ease Asthma, Says Underwood," *Waterloo Daily Courier*, October 27, 1938; James B LaFourche, "Burn $1,000,000 Marihuana Crop,

man Raymundo Santos, arrested in January 1939 at Pier 29 in Brooklyn on a charge of possession, who was actually acquitted by a jury in front of a bemused judge Matthew T. Abruzzo. On a recommendation for cold treatment from a healer in Brazil, he had been preparing "one leaf [of cannabis] in a glassful of hot water, add a little sugar and stir ... and the results were most beneficial."[14]

The drug's ability to comport oneself for the challenges of the day are a much more subtle but more interesting angle on these more overt self-medication claims. There are suggestions throughout the record about the ability of cannabis to induce sleep.[15] It was also used to maintain energy during the day as was the case with Mereciano Vigil, a Mexican beet worker near Las Animas, Colorado, who in 1937 when arrested for the drug claimed that it "kept him from getting tired."[16] But some claims were more sensational than others. In a story that drew press from multiple news outlets, cannabis was touted as a life tonic grown by Chester, Pennsylvania, resident Ludwig Grau, who was eighty-three when arrested for growing cannabis in his back yard. Police found well cared for plants, "systematically planted with stakes and supporting string and wire for the stalks." Twenty years prior, Grau had discovered that a tea brewed from the leaves was a "successful remedy" that had "kept [him] in good health for 20 years." He also mentioned that following his wife's stroke three years prior that he had "experimented ... and discovered that her sufferings were materially aided by daily bathing her in water containing the juices of the weeds."[17]

But thinking about the stakes, balancing their self-declared pursuit of benefits from cannabis against the risks of legal sanction, these responses suggesting self-medication may be more convincing than at first glance. Misrepresenting one's involvement in criminal activity to avoid penalties was common during this time and indeed these comments were more often than not ignored by juries and judges as such. In admitting to a medical motive for use, these users spoke both to the idea that a medical motive legitimized and therefore excused

---

Grown to Cure Asthma," *Atlanta Daily World*, August 9, 1951.

14 "Sailor Convinces Jury Marijuana Is Cure for Cold," *Brooklyn Daily Eagle*, March 10, 1939.

15 And these incidents could often go wrong if a bad reaction caused a user to lash out, as reported in "Houstonian Gets 2 Years in Trial for Stabbing," *Galveston Daily News*, October 16, 1932.

16 "Marijuana Is Found on Mexican Worker," *LasAnimas Leader*, October 13, 1937.

17 "4th Ward Resident, 83, Used Marihuana for Medical Brew," *Chester Times*, September 14, 1938; "Has New Recipe For Longevity – Marijuana," *Charleroi Mail*, September 27, 1938; "'Recipe' for Longevity Revealed as Marijuana," *Nevada State Journal*, December 11, 1938.

their use, as demonstrated by Estofina Diaz who was arrested and pled not-guilty to the misdemeanor charge arguing that "she had been told tea from the leaves was good for the stomach."[18] It is also worth taking seriously their claims to medical use on their own terms, a claim recognized by San Antonio Chief of Police Owen W. Kilday as a motive for targeting Mexicans who, "use the weed for teas, baths and other medicinal purposes."[19]

Benefits Despite Risk: Suicide and Insanity in the Canal Zone and in American Cities

In the summer of 1935, a number of soldier suicides were reported at Fort Clayton in the Panama Canal Zone. Later charged on five counts of libel and acquitted on all but one, Nelson Rounsevell, editor of the bilingual *Panama American* had published a series of editorials alleging that Colonel James V. Heidt and Major General Harold B. Fiske were running a "suicide post" at Fort Clayton, "that the soldiers [had] been driven to the solace of the marijuana drug by the harsh treatment meted out by their officers, and that their use of the drug has led to the suicides."[20]

After the massive canal project was finished in 1914, routine interactions between US soldiers and locals became common. It was through these interactions that soldiers were exposed to cannabis in the canal zone. Primarily cultivated by local farmers and traders for personal use, surplus supplies of cannabis were then sold to soldiers in and around the two army installations in the Canal Zone. Fort Clayton and Fort Davis officials' concerns about the drug's effects on discipline and morale led to the issuing of Army circular No. 5 on January 20, 1923. The circular banned the possession and use of cannabis by army soldiers in the Canal Zone and subjected violators to a court-martial and dishonorable discharge. From 1923 until 1935 a number of inquests, committees, and studies were conducted to determine the effect of cannabis on morale and insubordination, each in various ways rejecting

18 "Officers Object to 'Dream Weed' Crop," *Los Angeles Times*, July 6, 1919.

19 "Officers War on Backyard Marihuana Growers in S.A.," *San Antonio Light*, July 12, 1931.

20 *The Panama American* title is held by two publications, both of which have a gap in holdings for the period when these editorials were published. "Four Suicides Blamed on Doped Cigarettes," *Long Island Press*, July 12, 1935; Gerald Martin, "U.S. Army Begins Probe of 'Suicide Wave' at Fort," *Chicago Daily Tribune*, July 13, 1935; "Too Much Discipline," *Edwardsville Intelligencer*, July 19, 1935.

links between cannabis use and dereliction of duty and recommending relaxation of restrictions on its use off duty, all leading to the summer of 1935.[21]

The suicides in 1935, at least according to Rounsevell's accusations, were due to overwork which drove soldiers to cannabis use which, because it wasn't regulated, caused the psychotic breakdown and subsequent suicides of soldiers at Fort Clayton, and the hospitalizations of several others. There doesn't seem to be much archival information on the suicides or hospitalizations that occurred in the summer of 1935, so it remains difficult to draw definitive conclusions about their specific connection to cannabis use. However, a long history of cannabis use on the base, and several studies that looked at the effects of that cannabis on soldiers who used, can offer evidence that adds credence to self-medication, in this case self-medication to stave off mental health crises brought on by brutal working conditions in the Canal Zone. The 1925 survey, which examined seventeen cannabis-using soldiers, discovered widespread use among soldiers "to relieve headache, spells of the 'blues' and to break the monotony of their lives." The 1931 study, which subjected thirty-five soldiers to exposure to and withdrawal from the drug over several days of hospitalization at Gorgas Hospital, recounted the ways in which users self-reported the drug's action during "mild intoxication." Users were reported to be "brushed up," "high," "happy," "peppy," "rosy," and "dopy" and were "satisfied" that use was a "'pleasant pastime', usually during hours off duty when they had nothing else to do to amuse themselves."[22]

Had it not been for Rounsevell's sensational charges against leadership at Fort Clayton, these observations may not have been particularly remarkable. But due to the libel cases that followed, details of routine brutal working conditions came to light. He was acquitted on one charge and convicted on a second that hinged on a technicality about the liability of Fiske (though not Heidt) for the conditions at Fort Clayton. But the most damaging claims, in which Heidt was labeled as "the Simon Legree of the zone, [relentlessly] driving his men by day and [ignoring] marihuana smoking by night" stuck around after the trial was over.[23] Claiming, on

21 Ernest L. Abel, "Marijuana on Trial: The Panama Canal Zone Report," *International Journal of the Addictions* 17, no. 4 (1982): 667–78; "Marijuana Smoking Is Reported Safe," *New York Times*, November 21, 1926.

22 J. F. Siler et al. to The Governor, The Panama Canal, October 21, 1932, Box 9, File 17, H. J. Anslinger papers, HCLA 1875, Special Collections Library, Pennsylvania State University (hereafter "Anslinger Papers").

23 "Army Accuses Editor in Panama of Libel," *New York Times*, August 3, 1935; Gerald Martin, "Panama Canal Army Heads Jail Editor for Libel," *Chicago Daily Tribune*, August 4, 1935; "Publisher of Panama Paper Under Arrest," *Buffalo Courier*, August 4, 1935; "In Panama," *Hammond Times*, August 8,

the stand, "a desire to alleviate ... unbearable conditions for enlisted men at Fort Clayton," Rounsevell's conviction and $500 fine in the second case was followed by a visit to Washington by Rounsevell's counsel, Louis Waldman, petitioning President Roosevelt to investigate labor conditions on the base.[24] The stress of overwork and isolation on a military base in the tropics had profound effects on the individual soldiers that experienced daily life in the Canal Zone, and many used cannabis as a matter of course to alleviate the boredom, overwork, and perhaps more. While Rounsevell never denied a direct role of acute cannabis intoxication in the suicides, his articles were written to address the conditions of overwork, and not the use of cannabis itself. This relates directly to Walter Bromberg's experience with Case 23 from the beginning of this essay. The experience of risk outcomes and benefit outcomes could often occur simultaneously or at least within the progression of use of the same treatment. What was once palliative could at once become dangerous. In either case, soldiers made the decision to use cannabis, a healthy reactive tendency against the psychological anguish of overwork, until they experienced a tragic adverse reaction. While the adverse effect of cannabis was the likely cause of the suicides, the focus of the editorials and the subsequent investigation was the working conditions.

Reports from the Panama Canal Zone were also followed closely by Harry Anslinger at the Federal Bureau of Narcotics. The Rounsevell incident occurred during a pivotal time in the shaping of federal cannabis policy in the United States.[25] The Marihuana Tax Act of 1937 was a tri-

---

1935; "Try Editor for Libel; Rapped 2 Army Officers," *Chicago Daily Tribune*, September 6, 1935; "U.S. Editor Freed of Libel Charge in Canal Zone," *Chicago Daily Tribune*, September 19, 1935; "Ft. Clayton Insane Called Numerous," *New York Times*, September 26, 1935.

24 "Rounsevell on Stand in Canal Zone Trial," *New York Times*, September 28, 1935; "Canal Zone Inquiry Urged," *New York Times*, October 16, 1935; "Army May Probe Panama Scandal," *New York Evening Post*, November 12, 1935.

25 J. F. Siler et al. to The Governor, The Panama Canal, October 21, 1932, A1 9 Subject Files 1916–1970, Box 108, Folder Drugs – Marihuana – General – 1933, RG 0170 – Drug Enforcement Administration – Department of Justice Bureau of Narcotics and Dangerous Drugs. NARA II (hereafter RG 0170, NARA II); L. W. Robert to Secretary of War, May 19, 1933, A1 9 Subject Files 1916–1970, Box 108, Folder Drugs – Marihuana – General – 1933, RG 0170 NARA II; Secretary of the Treasury to Secretary of War, June 13, 1933, A1 9 Subject Files 1916–1970, Box 108, Folder Drugs – Marihuana – General – 1933, RG 0170 NARA II; Acting Secretary of War to Secretary of the Treasury, June 13, 1933, A1 9 Subject Files 1916–1970, Box 108, Folder Drugs – Marihuana – General – 1933, RG 0170 NARA II; Harry Anslinger to Gertrude Seymour, February 5, 1934, A1 9 Subject Files 1916–1970, Box

umph of bureaucratic maneuvering, public lobbying, and of Commissioner Anslinger's media and public relations savvy.[26] Anslinger's approach to cannabis control involved dominating the media narrative surrounding the drug and repeating accounts of particularly gruesome crimes committed by users in interviews, public speeches, essays, books, and newspaper articles, most famously in his 1937 *America Magazine* article "Assassin of Youth."[27]

The emphasis on potential violence of some cannabis users and the consequences of heroin addiction, prostitution, or even suicide in these articles highlights the risks of acute cannabis intoxication. Some of this indeed was drawn from evidence from cases across the country, but a lot of the rhetoric was rooted in Orientalist myths born in the prior century.[28] Following passage of the Marihuana Tax Act, Anslinger drafted Circular Letter No. 458 referencing "a study ... being made of the extent to which the use of MARIHUANA is responsible for crime." District Supervisors were instructed to cooperate with federal, state and local officials in their districts to submit "detailed reports ... together with the history of offenders involved." Included was a survey, which was revised several times during the

108, Folder Drugs – Marihuana – General – 1934, RG 0170 NARA II; J. P. Wall to Harry J Anslinger, February 6, 1934, A1 9 Subject Files 1916–1970, Box 110, Drugs – Marihuana – By District, RG 0170 NARA II; Jack Golden to Harry Anslinger, June 30, 1937, A1 9 Subject Files 1916–1970, Box 108, Folder Drugs – Marihuana – General – 1937, RG 0170 NARA II; D. H. Huff to Bureau of Narcotics, August 2, 1937, A1 9 Subject Files 1916–1970, Box 108, Folder Drugs – Marihuana – General – 1937B, RG 0170 NARA II; J. Edgar Hoover to Harry Anslinger, August 13, 1937, A1 9 Subject Files 1916–1970, Box 108, Folder Drugs – Marihuana – General – 1937B, RG 0170 NARA II.

26 John C. McWilliams, *The Protectors: Harry J Anslinger and the Federal Bureau of Narcotics, 1930–1962* (University of Delaware Press, 1990).

27 Harry Anslinger and Courtney Ryley Cooper, "Marijuana: Assassin of Youth," *American Magazine*, July 1937; Harry Anslinger, "An Indispensable Weapon Against Narcotic Racketeers," *Kiwanis Magazine*, February 1934; Harry Anslinger, "State Co-Operation Vital in Throttling of Dope Traffic, Says Anslinger," *Syracuse American*, January 20, 1935; Harry Anslinger, "Narcotic Law Enforcement – A Local Problem in Need of Local Action," *American Police Review*, August 1937.

28 Isaac Campos, *Home Grown: Marijuana and the Origins of Mexico's War on Drugs* (University of North Carolina Press, 2012); David A Guba, "Antoine Isaac Silvestre de Sacy and the Myth of the Hachichins: Orientalizing Hashish in Nineteenth-Century France," *The Social History of Alcohol and Drugs* 30 (2016): 25.

1930s, and included questions intended to make this connection.[29] Yet like the Panama study, user perspectives on motive crept in, further illuminating evidence that users were engaging in some form of self-medication.[30]

A man from New Jersey responded that while in Hot Springs, Arkansas, he was introduced to cannabis by a Mexican who recommended it as "treatment for a venereal disease." A mixture of cannabis and Copenhagen snuff was recommended to a Nebraska man by a woman for headache, and another from Pennsylvania, "about 1934 … heard that marihuana smoking would help [his] asthma." An Oklahoma man received a recommendation from a physician in Yuma when he was fifteen after being caught in a surprise snowstorm. The "physician in charge told [him] that the smoking of Indian hemp would help stop pain in [his] legs and lungs."[31]

As with newspaper accounts, several respondents commented on the drug's ability to induce sleep including a Pennsylvania man, who "had been in the hospital for an operation and … heard that marihuana makes one sleep."[32] Willis Green, a dancer, was introduced by a circus performer who said it would give him "pep." A man from New Orleans recalled his first experience arguing that he "knew it was a medicine but did not know in what way it was used." He described it as "scary, believing I was losing my mind, but the next one made me feel satisfied and contented."[33] Arden Chase from Honolulu thought that it would make him feel "happy and light-hearted." He claimed that "at first I looked for an intoxicating effect; now I don't look for more than a relaxing effect."[34] An Ohio man was told: "it would quiet my nerves."[35]

When asked "What effect do you obtain from smoking Marihuana?" Elliot, an eight-year user from San Francisco stated: "I have a sense or feeling of satisfaction and well-being." Meanwhile, a more novice user (of

29 Harry Anslinger, "Circular Letter No. 458 – To District Supervisors and Others Concerned," September 29, 1937, Box 110, Folder Marijuana Questionaire 38–42, RG 0170 NARA II; Harry Anslinger, "Memorandum for District Supervisors," April 1, 1938, Box 110, Folder Marijuana Questionaire 38–42, RG 0170 NARA II; Will S. Wood, "Memorandum to All District Supervisors," May 5, 1939, Box 110, Folder Marijuana Questionaire 38–42, RG 0170 NARA II.

30 See, *Answers to Survey Questions 1* (1938), (Box 9, File 20), Anslinger papers; *Answers to Survey Questions 2* (1938), (Box 9, File 24), Anslinger papers; *Answers to Survey Questions 3* (1938), (Box 9, File 53), Anslinger papers.

31 *Answers to Survey Questions 1.*

32 *Answers to Survey Questions 1.*

33 *Answers to Survey Questions 1.*

34 *Answers to Survey Questions 1.*

35 *Answers to Survey Questions 1.*

seven months) from Massachusetts was more explicit: "enlarged imagination; increased appetite; nerves get steadier; can talk more fluently"; and a New York City teenager offered a cheerier view: "Makes me want to laugh and I am happy. I forget my troubles." A Kansan echoed the "no worries" claim, while an Illinois user said it offered "relaxation from strain of work." Musicians and dancers emphasized that it helped them "keep rhythm" and even gave them "more confidence." But cannabis also kept them at it, as, for one man, it "keeps me awake and alert, and relieves the tension under which I perform as a pianist, if without the weed." Another musician said that "it makes me dizzy and gives me a feeling like I am rich."[36] What's more, the relief from nervous anxiety could turn when deprived of the drug. A Michigan man claimed deprivation "affects my nerves and I seem to be nervous when without the cigarette," while a Tennessee man "gets nervous and craves a smoke like a drinking man would a drink," and a man from Woodilla described "severe headaches and mental torture."[37]

The survey answers are just simply recorded and there is no follow-up. One case did generate some additional reports, that of sixteen-year-old Carl Oliver Walcott of El Paso. Charged with smuggling the drug over the Santa Fe Bridge in October 1938 Walcott was interviewed by District Supervisor Joseph Ball and gave a frank discussion of his use and family history. The youngest of three brothers, his father lost his money drinking, leaving Carl and his brothers to support their mother. One of them introduced him to cannabis when he was eight, and at sixteen years old he boasted that he had "smoked this whole room full of marihuana." He described a young life of intermittent labor, legal trouble, and cannabis use. He discusses his troubled mental state, blaming "trouble after trouble" on his cannabis use, and describing the effects of deprivation in a manner suggesting his self-aware addiction. He also mentioned an incident where his mother threatened to hospitalize him "because I got too crazy." His initial statement to police though, referenced the drug's benefits:

> I am going to tell you something that has never been published before ... in this picture of "Marihuana" [a reference to a 1936 film by that title] ... is just another production ... made to make lots of money. It was good I guess but school girls and boys don't do things like that ... I have smoked Marihuana for eight years – it is just like a kind of narcotic and I can ride anything, write anything or read anything you want me to do. I can do anything. I can work. When I was working I was using a big drilling hammer – I worked 22 hours straight. I don't say marihuana cigarettes gave me the strength to do that, but after you smoke it so long, it steadies your nerves

36 *Answers to Survey Questions 2.*

37 *Answers to Survey Questions 1.*

just like any other cigarette ... I don't bother anybody. It don't make you want to kill –it just makes me awful hungry and makes me sleep good.[38]

Walcott seems to have suffered from a number of adverse effects after a long history of heavy use. Nevertheless, his justifications for his use explicitly tout the benefits of the drug, even as he recognizes the nature and degree of the potential risks, and even as he recognizes his own dependence on the drug's effects. Whether a sixteen-year-old boy could accurately self-diagnose or not, he's still articulating the range of benefits and risks associated with eight years of exposure.

"A Fillip to Existence": Cannabis Users in Depression-Era New York

The Panama investigation and the FBN study took the risks of acute cannabis intoxication as more or less a given. Walter Bromberg and Mayor Fiorello LaGuardia, both based in New York, challenged the extent of those claims with Bromberg's work at Bellevue and via the Mayor's Committee on Marihuana, conducted with the New York Academy of Medicine. In both contexts, subjects had even less motive to misrepresent their relationship with cannabis and therefore shared their experiences openly. As with the prior studies, pursuit of user motive was not explicitly sought, but enough motive can be discerned in their responses to questions.

Bromberg's analysis of his cannabis-using patients during the 1930s, including that of Case 23 which opened this chapter, placed him at the center of psychiatric analysis of cannabis use in the 1930s. He was tapped by Anslinger's Federal Bureau of Narcotics to revise the user survey in 1939, and was invited to advise on the early stages of the clinical portion of the Mayor's Committee (discussed below).[39] In two articles, published in 1934 and 1935, and summarized in a 1939 article in *JAMA*, Bromberg reviews case studies of his patients, a mixture of self-admissions and police admissions during the 1930s. His work sought to reclaim the authority of medical studies in determining the "causation of a psychotic picture" among cannabis

38 C. H. Bowers to Joseph Bell, October 27, 1938, Box 3, File 2, Anslinger Papers.

39 Harry Anslinger to Walter Bromberg, February 8, 1939, Box 110, Folder Marijuana Questionaire 38–42, RG 0170 NARA II; Harry Anslinger to Walter Bromberg, February 20, 1939, Box 110, Folder Marijuana Questionaire 38–42, RG 0170 NARA II; "Minutes of the Subcommittee on the Clinical Study of Marihuana," March 14, 1939, Marijuana 1938–1940, Marijuana, New York Academy of Medicine.

users. Bromberg did not deny the potential for serious adverse effects, but challenged the extent of the risk, countering popular and influential claims made by "police officers, narcotic officers, prosecutors [and] judges."[40]

But more than staking out the boundaries of medical authority in determining risk, Bromberg, perhaps unwittingly, sets out the framework of a self-medication thesis despite having no intention of examining user perspective at all. The only dialogue with patients recounted in his articles were descriptions of how the patient came to Bellevue, and their present state of mind during the examination in response to Bromberg's questions. The only passing reference to motive involved a thirty-four-year-old Cuban man, admitted on March 6, 1938, who had taken cannabis "every day for a year and a half because it took his worries away."[41]

However, most of the patients examined displayed "apathy," "depressive features," and "suicidal impulse," and Bromberg identified racial factors, low intelligence, and homosexual desire as factors contributing to use and susceptibility to adverse effects. These biases do call his conclusions into question, but they also add credence to the claims made in this essay, that the challenges of everyday life, especially for those with socially or medically defined deficiencies potentially led to the use of cannabis and that more of his patients were like Case 23 than he thought.

Like Bromberg, New York Mayor Fiorello LaGuardia also questioned the cannabis consensus during the 1930s. In late 1938, he appointed a committee to study the medical and sociological effects of cannabis in the city.[42] The committee report, published in 1944, stands as a forceful refutation of some of the most extreme reports about the cannabis threat.[43] Several methodological shortcomings limited the value of the results of the survey and Harry Anslinger directly attacked the conclusions drawn. The limited sample size, short duration of the testing, and the controlled setting of the tests certainly bring their conclusions into question. But throughout the study, references to user attitudes demonstrate similar motives for use, and a similar range of risk and benefit assessments as found in the other subjects examined in this essay.[44]

40 Bromberg, "Marihuana Intoxication"; Walter Bromberg, "The Menace of Marihuana," *Medical Record: A National Review of Medicine and Surgery* 142 (1935): 309–11; Bromberg, "Marihuana: A Psychiatric Study."

41 Bromberg, "Marihuana: A Psychiatric Study," 8.

42 George B. Wallace, *Report of the Subcommittee on Marihuana* (City of New York, 1938), 2, Marijuana 1938–1940, Marijuana, New York Academy of Medicine.

43 *The Marihuana Problem in the City of New York: Mayor's Committee on Marihuana, by the New York Academy of Medicine* (City of New York, 1944).

44 *The Marihuana Problem in the City of New York*, 9; Emily Brooks, "Marijuana in La Guardia's New York City: The Mayor's Committee and Federal Policy, 1938–1945," *Journal of Policy History* 28, no. 4 (2016): 568–96.

During the clinical study, a control group of five people was compared to seventy-two subjects (65M, 7F), all of them then supervision of the New York City Department of Corrections. The subjects were given cannabis and then given a series of physiological tests to determine the drug's effect. Of the seventy-two inmates, forty-two men and six women had a prior history of use, and all seventy-two had volunteered to participate in the study. The committee chose subjects from among inmates so they could be kept "under continuous observation throughout the period desired," but also since inmates "constituted an excellent sample of the class … from which the marihuana user comes." Assumptions about "typical" use were extended into selecting the non-using control group as subjects were sought from low socioeconomic backgrounds and with "abnormal" personality traits.[45] Among the conclusions of the clinical study was the finding that the drug produced "feelings of relaxation, disinhibition and self-confidence," but could lead "also [to] feelings of anxiety."[46]

While these self-assessments among users could reasonably stand as an explanation of the explicit healthful benefits, a lack of social setting limited the capacity of the clinical study to reliably ascertain user motive. The sociological portion of the study was explicitly designed to, among other things, determine "the general attitude of the marihuana smoker toward society and toward the use of the drug." To do this, the committee tasked six New York Police cadets with collecting the data for the study by interviewing users in their own environments. They "acted as investigators and social workers and not as police officers" and the committee praised the cadets' supervisors for their "extreme degree" of cooperation in allowing "the marihuana squad" to report directly to the director of the survey. While it is unclear how effective or successful this ruse was, there is some suggestion that users provided a more genuine perspective not filtered through the eyes of the city and its political and medical authorities.

One of the six cadets, Olive J. Cregan's meticulous notes are found with the holdings of the mayor's committee at the New York Academy of Medicine. Primarily tasked with interviewing school principals on the frequency of cannabis use by school children, Cregan's notes included a conversation with Louise, a twenty-four-year-old, "pale skin," and "underweight" woman of German descent, during her travels. Louise was supporting herself as a waitress but never stayed in one job for very long. She smoked "six to twelve [cannabis] cigarettes a day" after learning it from her husband who "smoked it now and then as a fillip to existence." She described her own use (as recounted by Cregan in her notes) "because of her boredom and dissatisfaction with life,

45 *The Marihuana Problem in the City of New York*, 25.
46 *The Marihuana Problem in the City of New York*, 69.

she smokes partly to get out of an emotional apathy into which she falls, but mostly to find solace for her real or imagined woes."[47]

Louise did not appear to have an impending psychosis, nor did she suffer from asthma or rheumatism, but like Bromberg's Case 23, of similar age, status, and situation, an observably malnourished waitress in Manhattan during later part of the Great Depression Louise perhaps could have used a "fillip." Despite her ignorance of her mental/psychological condition or whether cannabis was (or even could) alleviate her "real or imagined woes," and despite the risks of arrest, or the potential effects of acute cannabis intoxication, she still decided to use cannabis deliberately to improve her life.

Conclusion

The conclusions of the mayor's inquiry directly countered the "publicity concerning the catastrophic effects" of cannabis, which the committee described as "unfounded." The conclusions also rejected the direct link between the drug and the "commission of major crime." New York's mayor rejected the draconian approach to cannabis regulation being adopted through state and federal legislation in the 1930s, but the committee did not completely reject the prevailing risk/benefit assessment about cannabis use. While the committee sought potential therapeutic applications for cannabis, their conclusions on that point were not definitive, reinforcing the view from organized medicine that cannabis had no medicinal benefits. In terms of risks, especially to personal and public safety, the mayor's committee merely suggested that reports about the dangerous effects of cannabis were exaggerated, not completely unfounded. The tragedy in the Canal Zone, and the incidents of psychotic episodes at Bellevue add further context to a recognition that while strict enforcement might be counterproductive, some of the dangers of cannabis were very real.

Within this larger critique, the mayor's committee's findings also identified a "consensus among marihuana smokers" that use led to "a definite feeling of adequacy." [48] This assertion is similar to Walter Bromberg's conclusion about Case 23's "healthy reactive tendency," even while his self-designed regiment culminated in an adverse event: a psychotic break due to acute cannabis intoxication. Though it is difficult to assess their claims adequately, users still made individual decisions based on their own health-related circumstances, their exposure to cannabis, and their continued use of

47 Olive J. Cregan, "Notes on Sociological Study," September 1941, Marijuana 1938–1940, Marijuana, New York Academy of Medicine.

48 *The Marihuana Problem in the City of New York*, 21–23.

the drug for specific health benefits, thus directly challenging the consensus risk/benefit assessment. Studies from the Panama Canal Zone, The Mayor's Committee, and surveys and case studies conducted by the Federal Bureau of Narcotics and Walter Bromberg, all have a similar pattern of risk and benefit articulation among users of cannabis. Though much of that articulation was done without the expertise of a physician or even under one's care, there is still plenty to suggest taking those claims seriously.

The evidence from these studies, all initiated through incidents of adverse effects, reveals a previously unrecognized agency among users. A small portion of those users, each likely ignorant of the specific diagnosis and unable to assess the drug's efficacy, expressed their assessments of the drug's risks and benefits in the context of promoting a healthy outcome. They identified as suffering from specific sets of symptoms, occasionally named as an ailment, but not always. These symptoms were described specifically and intentionally, in part to justify use to officials. When directed to describe their experience of use, users identified a range of risks and benefits, but each prioritized description of the benefits of cannabis use, including its alleviation of those symptoms. Users also mentioned experiencing various adverse effects, including increased anxiety, addiction, and even the risk of psychotic break. There is not enough evidence to indicate how individuals might have mitigated those risks, but they clearly figured into users' decision-making. Despite the serious risks, users continued to use cannabis *because* of its benefits.

Indeed, all of the subjects considered for this study were suffering from one of these more serious risks associated with cannabis use during this time, psychotic break and/or arrest. The temporary surveillance and study by officials and other professionals of these specific individuals provide the archival material that this essay relies on. Examiners, interested in those more serious risks to personal and public safety, often ignored or downplayed the "excuses" given for user behavior, but their noting and publication of these assessments give us a glimpse at an explicit risk and benefit assessment on the part of users.

On their own, these anecdotal assessments fall short of providing convincing evidence about user agency during the 1930s and could easily be dismissed as the evasive behavior of individuals trying to avoid potentially serious consequences. The collection of incidents in this essay, considered within the larger context of the user perspectives represented during this period, points to a small portion of cannabis users during this period who used cannabis explicitly for curative and healthful purposes, and articulated a personal assessment of risks and benefits in the pursuit of achieving those healthful outcomes. We cannot adequately assess or evaluate these claims as user voices are limited in the archival record, but we can take those limited perspectives on their own terms to reveal how users made decisions to use cannabis. The decisions challenged the prevailing attitudes of regulators, medical professionals, and the public in general. In each of the cases described in this essay, adverse effects notwithstanding, users determined cannabis to be one option to addressing health concerns during the 1930s.

Chapter Fourteen

When is an Opioid not an Opioid? Loperamide, the Use of Pharmacology, and the Pharmacology of Use[1]

Jeremy A. Greene and Avery Gulino

This chapter uses the case of loperamide, an opioid-receptor agonist developed in the 1970s for the treatment of intractable diarrhea, to rethink pharmacological categories of benefit and risk in terms of the dynamic framing of desired and undesired effects, uses, and users. Loperamide (brand-name Imodium) was first approved by the US Food and Drug Administration (FDA) for marketing as an antidiarrheal agent in 1976 based on claims that it was an opioid-receptor agonist that only functioned on *mu* receptors in the gut. This therapeutic alchemy transformed the known risk of constipation among opiate users into the central benefit of a new class of drugs which could now be recategorized as antidiarrheal agents. Key to the reformation of constipation from undesired to desired effect was the claim that these drugs themselves induced no desire and had no desirable features that would be basis for recreational use. By 1980, as cases of loperamide dependence began to mount (including cases of "loperamide overdose," which were treatable by naloxone), several forms of trial design were deployed to contain this emergent risk by demonstrating that this dependence was strictly a gut phenomenon; that loperamide provided no systemic opioid

1 Thanks to Nils, Joe, and David for the opportunity to consider these questions after a wonderful and stimulating conference in Strasbourg on the eve of the pandemic.

effects, no euphoria, and, in the words of the US "Drug Czar," Jerome Jaffe, "was 'liked' little or not at all." Forms of evidence that emphasized benefit over risk with conventional use sufficed for the DEA to reclassify loperamide from a Schedule V drug to a decontrolled agent in 1982, and to further liberalize its availability as an over-the-counter product in 1988. In the past decade, however, the question of abuse potential of loperamide has re-emerged, leading the FDA to mandate smaller packaging forms in 2019. Like pseudoephedrine (Sudafed), a derivative (decongestant) product whose pharmacological use based on an initial side effect of amphetamines has been revisited in the context of changing patterns of methamphetamine production, the kinship of loperamide to morphine and heroin has also recently been re-evaluated. This chapter explores the framing and reframing of loperamide's desired and undesired effects as a reminder that risk and benefit of any pharmacological compound are highly contingent, not only on biology and chemistry but also on the creative dynamics of use itself.

* * *

Drugs are polymorphously perverse. Since the earliest formulations of Ehrlich's receptor theory, which posited that pharmaceutical agents function like a key in lock by binding to specific sites that cause specific actions to take place in the bodies of living things, pharmacological sciences have sought to differentiate benefit from risk by differentiating the primary, desired effect of a given drug from the secondary "side effects" that hamper their most efficient utilization. Yet, from the point of view of the drug, there is no such distinction. A drug, once ingested, injected, or inhaled, does not work its way through the body according to any teleology of risk and benefit. It interacts or it does not interact, but does not make any distinction between its intended and unintended effects. The distinction between a desired effect and a side effect or an adverse effect can only be made in retrospect by a human agency that declares which outcomes are to be valued (as benefits), which are to be avoided (as risks), and which are merely to be tolerated (as side effects).[2]

This distinction between pharmacological risks and benefits is not arbitrary, but it is not natural either: it is always tethered it is always tethered to a dynamic and contingent set of human values that classifies and reclassifies

2 See, for example, Rein Vos, *Drugs Looking for Diseases* (Springer, 1991); Arthur M. Silverstein, "Paul Ehrlich's Passion: The Origins of His Receptor Immunology," *Cellular Immunology* 194, no. 2 (1999): 213–21; Rod Flower, "Drug Receptors: A Long Engagement" *Nature* 415, no. 6872 (2002): 587; Jeremy A. Greene, *Prescribing by Numbers: Drugs and the Definition of Disease* (Johns Hopkins University Press, 2007); and Nils Kessel's contribution to this volume.

desired and undesired uses and users. These distinctions are informed by the shifting epidemiology and understanding of disease, by the changing nature of medical markets, and by the perception and advocacy of those who would use these agents for medical or non-medical purposes. Above all, in twentieth- and twenty first century medicine the difference between desired and undesired effects has been especially informed by this last step, the delineation of a central *telos* of "legitimate medical need" from the slippery side branches of recreational use and abuse. Nowhere is this distinction clearer than in the career of loperamide – sold in the United States under the brand name Imodium after its approval by the Food and Drug Administration – an antidiarrheal agent whose sole purpose, at least in initial intent, was to produce the double reformation of a "bad" side effect of a "bad" category of narcotics into the "good" principal effect of a new kind of medical "good."[3]

The synthesis of loperamide by celebrated Belgian pharmacologist Paul Janssen in 1969 was a masterclass in pharmaceutical alchemy, an act of spinning dross into gold. Nearly half a century later, that attempt has paid off well for Janssen Pharmaceuticals and its parent company, Johnson & Johnson. Loperamide continues to lead the market for antidiarrheal drugs, a health share of the over-the-counter and prescription drug market with roughly $5 billion in global sales in 2024.[4] Initially treated as a potentially dangerous compound with potential for abuse, loperamide became progressively easier to access in the 1980s, and in the 1990s became available over the counter. Yet the efforts to distance this drug – a synthetic opioid in all but name – from the more dangerous connotations that have tarnished this category have not been entirely successful. It is not merely the case that specters of overdose, withdrawal, dependence, and abuse have haunted this compound since the early years, and risen up anew in the recent re-categorization of twenty-first-century opioid crises. To understand the story of loperamide is also to understand that attempts to control the risks of other forms of opioid use have created conditions for extraordinary creativity and dynamism among loperamide users and usage, which changed in ways that reframed not just the meanings of risk and benefit for this drug, but their biological manifestations in human health as well.

3 David Herzberg, *White Market Drugs: Big Pharma and the Hidden History of Addiction in America* (University of Chicago Press, 2020).

4 "Antidiarrheal Drugs Market Report Up to 2031: Visiongain Research Inc," *New York: NASDAQ OMX Corporate Solutions, Inc.*, 2022.

From Risk to Benefit

New drugs are often made by re-framing an ancillary effect of an older drug and carefully tending the former side-branch as the main trunk. For example, the sulfonylureas – the first successful pills for the treatment of diabetes – owe their origin story to the initial observation that some sulfa-based anti-infective drugs had the inadvertent side effect of lowering the blood sugar of patients being treated for infectious disease. Initially this was seen as an unacceptable risk for an anti-infective, but with some modification and development and repurposing, this side-effect became a highly desirable main effect for manufacturers seeking an oral regimen for diabetes. In the right hands, then, a dangerous risk could become a valuable benefit.

So too with loperamide, whose desired effect began as a reframing of the well-known constipating effect of opioid medications. Opium and its principal alkaloid extract, morphine, were understood by nineteenth-century physicians to be powerful analgesic agents, whose use was associated with profound constipation.[5] In the second half of the twentieth century, a variety of opioid receptors were found to relate to different effects in different parts of the body, including the *mu* receptor whose activity in the human large intestine explained constipation as a physiological response opioids elicited well outside of the central nervous system. How, the industry wondered, might the basic form of the opioid be modified to isolate the risk of constipation as a benefit of a new kind of drug, specifically designed to be an antidiarrheal agent?

Loperamide was first synthesized by in 1969 as part of the frothy outgrowth of synthetic opioid research taking place in the Belgium-based Janssen Pharmaceuticals firm in the 1950s and 1960s. Founder Paul Janssen, who also synthesized the opiates diphenoxylate and fentanyl in 1956 and 1960, respectively, had been working in the field of synthetic opioids for some time. Some of these tweaks, most notable in his development of fentanyl, were focused on amplifying the analgesic potency of opioids on a scale well beyond what morphine was capable of. Loperamide took a different turn.

Janssen and colleagues knew that opium, morphine, and other opioids were effective means of treating severe diarrhea but that this benefit was

5 The constipating effect of opium was well known to early modern physicians, and is captured in the seventeenth-century herbal of Nicolas Culpeper, *The Complete Herbal* (The Project Gutenberg eBook, 1850 edition), 145, https://www.gutenberg.org/files/49513/49513-h/49513-h.htm.

thinly tempered against substantial risks of addiction.[6] Yet some new and extraordinarily potent analgesics produced little constipation. Conversely, Janssen supposed, one might produce a powerful antidiarrhea drug with minimal analgesic or euphoric effects. "It therefore seemed reasonable," he proposed, "to assume that analgesic type compounds devoid of analgesic action but behaving as highly active inhibitors of gastro-intestinal population and defaecation might be synthesized."[7] The challenge for the molecular tinkerer was to synthesize a new opioid that isolated the constipating effect, producing an agent that would be all benefit and no risk.

Janssen and his team tweaked and screened, screened and tweaked, passing hundreds of different versions of synthetic opioids through the bodies of thousands of mice. Two established tests helped them sort through the library of drugs. The first, the "hot plate" test, allowed a standard measurement for pain and its relative degree of abeyance. The second, the "charcoal meal test," allowed a way of quantifying how much food came out the other end of a standard mouse. To peer behind the "hot plate" euphemism for a moment:

> The hot plate was a restring cylinder on a copper bath containing equal parts of boiling (55°–55.5°) acetone and ethyl formate. The reaction time is the interval, measured in intervals of 2 x 10–1 seconds, between the moment the mouse reaches the hot plate and the moment the animal either licks its feet or jumps out of the cylinder. All other signs of discomfort, such as kicking of the hind legs, dancing around the cylinder are disregarded.[8]

Analogously, the "charcoal meal test" was a way to quantify constipation, in which mice were fed "charcoal meals" after receiving a test drug so that, when they were killed an hour later and their intestines stripped from their body, to see how far the charcoal had progressed in the alimentary canal. Successfully antidiarrheal activity was "considered "positive" when the appendix was "white," and "negative" when the appendix was "black" (contained some charcoal).[9]

The first promising result came from R1132, a new series of compounds which had no significant analgesic effects in mice or rats but which were, in Janssen's terms, "more active in reducing the rate of defaecation or

6 Paul A. J. Janssen, Anton H. Jageneau, and Jules Huygens, "Synthesis of Anti-Diarrhoeal Agents – I. Some Pharmacological Properties of R 1132 and Related Compounds," *Journal of Medicinal and Pharmaceutical Chemistry* 1, no. 4 (1959): 299–308.

7 Janssen, Jageneau, and Huygens "Synthesis of Anti-Diarrhoeal Agents," 480.

8 Paul A. J. Janssen and Anton H. Jageneau, "A New Series of Potent Analgesics," *Journal of Pharmacy and Pharmacology* 9, no. 1 (1957): 381.

9 Janssen and Jageneau, "A New Series of Potent Analgesics," 385–86.

gastro-intestinal propulsion in the same species than any other known compounds thus far tested in this laboratory."[10] Subsequent tests in rats counted the number of fecal pellets produced by 150 Wistar rats in fifty cages every six hours for a week, and showed the new drug was demonstrably more effective at constipating rats compared to standard morphine.[11]

R1132 would be marketed in 1960 as Reasec (diphenoxylate), and then as the brand name Lomotil, in combination with atropine. But in therapeutic doses it was found to cause respiratory depression, complicating its utility for people of low body weight, especially children. Later reports by 1970 indicated diphenoxylate also yielded narcotic-seeking behavior and dependency at higher doses.[12] Fortunately by that time another even more specialized agent was emerging from the labs at Janssen.

Loperamide was fourteen times more active at blocking fecal volume than diphenoxylate, and unlike Lomotil it seemed to concentrate all of its activity on the *mu* receptors in the gut. Even though *in vitro* loperamide could bind to opiate receptors in rat brain as well as guinea pig ileum, central nervous effects were not observed *in vivo*.[13] When injected into dogs and rats, loperamide appeared to only bind to peripheral opioid receptors at gastrointestinal sites. In contrast to rats treated with fentanyl, morphine, and methadone, none of the rats who received loperamide would press a lever to get more loperamide.[14] "Studies on morphine, codeine, and diphenoxylate revealed that all of these prominent antidiarrheal agents produce the narcotic cue in a dose-related way," Janssen and coauthors concluded. "In contrast, loperamide at oral doses up to 40 mg/kg was found to be devoid of narcotic stimulus properties."[15] Here, they claimed, was proof of a non-habit-forming antidiarrheal agent shown "not to possess any abuse liability in humans."[16]

Loperamide, marketed as Imodium in Europe in 1975 in advance of its approval by the US FDA, was first designated for extreme cases: patients with ileostomy tubes, or hospitalized children with severe, life-threatening

10 Janssen, Jageneau, and Huygens, "Synthesis of Anti-Diarrhoeal Agents," 300.

11 Janssen, Jageneau, and Huygens, "Synthesis of Anti-Diarrhoeal Agents," 306.

12 Jerome H. Jaffe, "Narcotic Analgesics," in *The Pharmacological Basis of Therapeutics*, ed. L. S. Goodman and A. Gilman (MacMillan, 1970), 237–42.

13 Carl R. Mackerer, George A. Clay, and Esam Z. Dajani, "Loperamide Binding to Opiate Receptor Sites of Brain and Myenteric Plexus," *Journal of Pharmacology and Experimental Therapeutics* 199, no. 1 (1976): 131–40.

14 Francis C. Colpaert et al., "Investigations on Drug Produced and Subjectively Experienced Discriminative Stimuli: 2. Loperamide, an Antidiarrheal Devoid of Narcotic Cue Producing Actions," *Life Sciences* 16, no. 5 (1975): 717–27.

15 Colpaert et al., "Investigations," 723.

16 Colpaert et al., "Investigations," 726.

diarrhea.[17] Larger studies showed it worked well in chronic diarrhea in adults and children as well.[18] Although some early head-to-head trials did not show much difference between Imodium and Lomotil, pharmacologists and practitioners had a sense that the new drug was stronger, safer, and better.[19] Only in doses so high as to be fundamentally implausible – several orders of magnitude higher than a standard dose – could any form of central narcotic effect be seen in nonhuman primates.[20] "Loperamide hydrochloride," one broader review of Imodium's activity in chronic diarrhea claimed, "is of particular interest in that it appears to possess no residual central activity and merely exerts a direct pharmacological effect, inhibiting small bowel motility."[21] Previously incurable chronic diarrhea could be controlled on relatively low doses. Severe cases of uncontrolled fecal leakage were eliminated; chronically anxious and depressed sufferers were so improved they no longer needed psychotherapy. Children, adults, acute, chronic – all patients seemed to respond favorably.[22] Loperamide was hailed as a minor miracle, all benefit and no risk.

Risk in Regulatory Context

The research on loperamide's addictiveness overlapped with a moment of transition in the sciences of addiction in the United States, coalescing around the Nixon administration's War on Drugs. The implementation of the Comprehensive Drug Prevention and Control Act of 1970 put a wave of funding into pharmaceutical research and established government control agencies such as the Special Action Office of Drug Abuse Prevention. These

17 J. P. Buts, B. F. Petit, and R. de Meyer, "Letter: Loperamide in Treatment of Persistent Diarrhoea in Children," *British Medical Journal* 3, no. 5986 (1975): 766–67.

18 P. Mainguet and R. Fiasse, "Double-Blind Placebo-Controlled Study of Loperamide (Imodium) in Chronic Diarrhoea Caused by Ileocolic Disease or Resection," *Gut* 18, no. 7 (1977): 575–79.

19 Gabriel Jaffé, "A Comparison of Lomotil and Imodium in Acute Non-Specific Diarrhoea," *Journal of International Medical Research* 5, no. 3 (1977): 195–98. "Loperamide and Other Antidiarrhoeal Drugs," *Drug and Therapeutics Bulletin* 15, no. 16 (1977): 61.

20 Mackerer, Clay, and Dajani, "Loperamide Binding to Opiate Receptor Sites," 137.

21 I. D. Paterson, "The Use of Loperamide for Treatment of 'Difficult to Manage' Chronic Diarrhoea in Adults," *Journal of International Medical Research* 1, no. 2 (1977): 459–61.

22 R. C. Heel et al., "Loperamide: A Review of Its Pharmacological Properties and Therapeutic Efficacy in Diarrhea," *Drugs* 15 (1978): 33–52.

agencies served to centralize drug enforcement and create one entity to govern how drugs were perceived and how their misuse was punished in the United States. This office was headed by Jerome H Jaffe.

Jaffe, the original White House "Drug Czar," famously set into motion many programs that transformed drug and addiction research in the early 1970s. The domestic drug war ramped up as the Vietnam War was drawing to a close, but the experience of Vietnam veterans linked warfare with pharmacology on multiple levels, as increasing public attention was drawn to the way drugs were utilized to aid soldiers: amphetamines to stay awake, opioids to manage pain, and marijuana and heroin from the Vietnamese countryside for recreation. In 1971, the Department of Defense reported that 10–15% of service members in Vietnam were now using heroin, which increased pressure on the Nixon administration to provide support for treatment programs and rehabilitation efforts.[23] When, in June of that year, Jaffe took his role as the head of White House Special Action Office for Drug Abuse Prevention, his brought with him a research program that focused on multi-modal treatments for drug addiction that utilized not only methadone but also detoxification support and therapy to treat addiction.[24]

When loperamide, an opioid that didn't look like an opioid, appeared before the FDA for approval in 1976, it was silently placed into the lowest-ranked Schedule V drug class. As a subsection of the Comprehensive Drug Control and Prevention Act, the Controlled Substances Act had been signed into effect in 1970. This subsection classified drugs into "schedules" based on their relative risks of abuse potential, and the perceived benefit of their medical use. Schedule I included those with the highest abuse potential and considered unsafe for use, while Schedule V included drugs with little abuse potential and with common uses in a medical setting. The important distinction, though, was that *any* scheduled drug carried some risk of abuse.

Janssen did not publicly object to this classification, but "stated they might in the future raise the issue of whether schedule V controls for loperamide are warranted" after later study. The *Federal Register* recorded that

23 Jerome H. Jaffe, "Conversation with Jerome H. Jaffe," *Addiction* 94 (1999): 13–30; Alvin Shuster, "G.I. Heroin Addiction Epidemic in Vietnam," *New York Times*, May 16, 1971.

24 Jaffe, "Conversation with Jerome H. Jaffe"; Lee Robins, "The Vietnam Drug User Returns: Final Report," *Special Action Office for Drug Abuse Prevention* (1973), https://prhome.defense.gov/Portals/52/Documents/RFM/Readiness/DDRP/docs/35%20Final%20Report.%20The%20Vietnam%20drug%20user%20returns.pdf; Sanjay Gupta, "Vietnam, heroin and the lesson of disrupting any addiction," *CNN*, December 22, 2015, https://www.cnn.com/2015/12/21/health/vietnam-heroin-disrupting-addiction/index.html.

the firm "would not presently oppose control and in fact recognized the need for it regarding substances with a potential for abuse."[25] After all, it was well accepted that loperamide interacted with opioid receptors, most importantly *mu* receptors. Janssen's agenda, then, was clear: to provide convincing proof that loperamide's effects were strictly peripheral, and that there was no potential for abuse. All benefit, no risk.

When Imodium received FDA approval as a Schedule V drug in the US, distributed by Ortho Pharmaceutical and readied for a launch in April 11, 1977, it was already being used in Western Europe, South America, and Asia. Imodium, according to FDA-approved labeling, "is indicated for the control and symptomatic relief of *acute nonspecific* diarrhea and *chronic diarrhea* associated with inflammatory bowel disease. Imodium is also indicated for reducing the volume of discharge from ileostomies." For the FDA, absence of evidence of risk was not evidence of absence of risk.[26] The first US package insert set a normal dose of twelve capsules for acute diarrhea, and carried a boilerplate warnings for "overdosage" deemed relevant to any opioid, including constipation, CNS depression, and gastrointestinal irritation. Ortho proudly marketed Imodium to American physicians as the "first new antidiarrheal in 16 years," and committed a sales force of 300 "detailers" to selling the product, along with an *Antidiarrheal Handbook*.[27]

For the first five years of its existence as a drug in the US market, loperamide remained a Schedule V drug: a drug with modest, if entirely theoretical, "potential for abuse."[28] Repeated studies found no evidence of addiction or central opioid activity for loperamide at low or even moderately elevated doses. In other words, loperamide was a Schedule V drug because it was an opioid, and the entire concept of scheduling "narcotics" was based on the premise that opioids, in particular, were inherently risky drugs that needed to be scheduled.

Yet a drug whose abuse potential was entirely theoretical presented practical problems for those seeking to study addiction. "Since by definition the new drug has not been abused," Jerome Jaffe noted in 1980, "there is no sure way to predict the dose levels at which reinforcing effects (presumably pleasing subjective effects) will occur."[29] Jaffe had for years been authoring

25 "Placement of Loperamide in Schedule V," *Federal Register* 42, no. 96 (1977): 25498–99.

26 Herzberg, *White Market Drugs*.

27 "Imodium Antidiarrheal Clears FDA Dec 28; Ortho Marketing," *FDA Pink Sheet*, January 17, 1977, T&G 6; "Imodium Antidiarrheal Launch Date April 11; Ortho," *FDC Pink Sheet*, April 4, 1977, T&G 2.

28 Heel et al., "Loperamide: A Review of Its Pharmacological Properties," 1.

29 Jerome H. Jaffe, Maureen Kanzler, and Judith Green, "Abuse Potential of Loperamide," *Clinical Pharmacology and Therapeutics* 28, no. 6 (1980): 813.

the opioid chapter of Goodman and Gilman's *Pharmacological Basis of Therapeutics*, the central reference point for clinical pharmacology for the second half of the twentieth century. He had been following the use of narcotics as antidiarrheal agents and was very familiar with the research output of Janssen's laboratory. Now, he presented two studies from his own lab, exploring the appropriate dosage of loperamide and its effects on a group of subjects that had been previously addicted to opioids.

Loperamide helped Jaffe put his finger on a central problem at the heart of addiction research in the Nixon era.[30] Until 1975, US addiction research had come to revolve around the infamous federal "narcotics farm" in Lexington, which he referred to somewhat euphemistically as "the cooperation of federal prisoners with a history of opioid addiction who volunteered to be transferred from various federal prisons to the Addiction Research Center in Lexington." Like Janssen's "precious rats" who had been trained to press levers for fentanyl, and thereby became a screening tool for mass quantities of other potentially habit-forming agents, the prisoner subjects of the Lexington "farm" had provided baseline conditions for "a controlled environment, research designs involving repeated measurements could be undertaken with reasonable assurance that subjects were not simultaneously using nonprescribed drugs, and that the dropout rate would be low."[31] But, in Jaffe's telling, all of this changed in 1973, as a searing critique of the ethics of medical research among prisoners combined with a broader outrage at the growing scandal surrounding the lack of informed consent among the deliberately misinformed subjects of the *Tuskegee Study of Untreated Syphilis in the Negro Male*. In a mounting series of ethical investigations, including the Belmont Report, the federal government suspended the Lexington Farm on the basis that prisoners, by definition, could not give informed consent.[32]

Since the last prisoner left the Lexington program on the last day of 1976, Jaffe observed, "the evaluation of the abuse potential of loperamide has, of necessity, required the cooperation of nonprisoners." [33] Nonprisoners would now need to be evaluated using the new structure of Institutional Review Board (IRB) approval; and since "many who become dependent on opioids outside of a medical context often exhibit a degree of unreliability exceeding

30 See Caroline Jean Acker, *Creating the American Junkie: Addiction Research in the Classic Era of Narcotic Control* (Johns Hopkins University Press, 2006); Nancy D. Campbell, *Discovering Addiction: The Science and Politics of Substance Abuse Research* (University of Michigan Press, 2007); and Nancy D. Campbell, *OD: Naloxone and the Politics of Overdose* (MIT Press, 2020).

31 Jaffe, Kanzler, and Green, "Abuse Potential of Loperamide," 812.

32 On the closing of the ARC at Lexington, see Campbell, *Discovering Addiction*.

33 Jaffe, Kanzler, and Green, "Abuse Potential of Loperamide," 812.

that of the general population,"[34] it would be very hard to guarantee reliable follow up in test subjects that weren't reliably incarcerated.

Loperamide presented a unique opportunity for the study of narcotic risk and benefit in this new regime. As a drug with evidently low adverse effects and minimal abuse potential to date, "loperamide presented an opportunity to explore in practice all the above problems that might arise in testing opioid abuse potential in nonprisoner subjects with histories of opioid dependence." [35] Jaffe paid nine subjects, "all male, who were not opiate addicts but had prior experience with other drugs, such as alcohol and marihuana," willing to take loperamide orally along with a placebo and an active control (codeine). All subjects had their vitals, pupils, and perceptions of the drug monitored to determine its likability and the dosage range at which participants felt any "drug effects," whether good, bad, or neutral.[36] While Jaffee admitted that "the frame of reference for recognition of 'dope' in these presumably opioid-naïve subjects is unclear," and a few subjects "liked" the sensation of low-dose loperamide, none of the majority of subjects who reported a "drug effect" at high dose of loperamide found the experience pleasurable.

Jaffee then moved on to nine new subjects that had previously been addicted to opioids. These men took loperamide in low, medium, and high doses to specifically determine if they felt any opiate-like effects from the drug. Only one said the feeling was similar to that of "dope". Overall, loperamide was more similar to the placebo and subjects only felt minimal opiate-like effects, with one participant commenting, "an addict in search of a mood-altering drug would prefer cough medicine with codeine over the loperamide preparation."[37]

In February, 1980, Ortho and Janssen presented data showing that after two and a half years and some 80,000,000 doses prescribed to more than 3,000,000 patients, there had been no overdose deaths and only a single report of possible abuse sent in to Jaffe's new Drug Abuse Warning Network (DAWN) epidemiological surveillance system.[38] In retrospect, the data suggested it was possible that loperamide had never truly ever been a narcotic. Jaffe was inclined to agree, suggesting the 1977 decision to place loperamide as a Schedule V drug came simply from its classification as an opioid, and that the sum total of epidemiological and clinical trials data

34 Jaffe, Kanzler, and Green, "Abuse Potential of Loperamide," 813.
35 Jaffe, Kanzler, and Green, "Abuse Potential of Loperamide," 813.
36 Jaffe, Kanzler, and Green, "Abuse Potential of Loperamide," 814.
37 Jaffe, Kanzler, and Green, "Abuse Potential of Loperamide," 818.
38 Jaffe, Kanzler, and Green, "Abuse Potential of Loperamide," 819.

since then suggested the drug could be moved towards "complete decontrol," or descheduling.[39]

This was a highly unusual recommendation at a time when the federal government was mostly preoccupied with "upscheduling" drugs to make them less accessible for casual use.[40] Loperamide was moving in the other direction: an opioid that no longer needed to be considered a narcotic. When the Secretary of Health and Human Services formally proposed the removal of loperamide from Schedule V in 1982, no objections were raised. That fall, the DEA and HHS jointly declared that loperamide "does not have sufficient potential for abuse to justify its continued control in any schedule of the Controlled Substances Act."[41] Opioid no more.

Opioid No More: Imodium as an Everyday Consumer Good

As risks reduced, potential benefits multiplied. No longer a potentially "bad" drug whose consumption needed to be controlled, loperamide was now free to be perceived simply as a consumer good: an antidiarrheal with no other effects that warranted concern. Marketers at Ortho and Janssen immediately sought larger markets for the drug. As a potentially dangerous agent its use had been demonstrated in pediatric cases of potentially fatal diarrhea – and even cholera. Now its use could be expanded to those forms of diarrhea that might merely be inconvenient.[42] In the early 1980s, Imodium was increasingly marketed as a traveler's medication: an everyday object like a birth control pill or a diaphragm that one might obtain from one's physician, not as a treatment but as a form of prevention.[43]

39 Jaffe, Kanzler, and Green, "Abuse Potential of Loperamide," 819. A 1981 study of the mechanism of action of loperamide pointed out that even though the anti-overdose drug naloxone reversed the antidiarrheal action of loperamide: "the action of naloxone suggests, but does not prove, that loperamide exerts its effects *via* opiate receptors." B. K. Sandhu et al., "Loperamide: Studies on Its Mechanism of Action," *Gut* 22, no. 8 (1981): 658–62.

40 See, for example, the case of Talwin, "another non-opioid opioid," which met a very different fate from Imodium in the late twentieth century, accumulating more and more restrictions at the same time that Imodium was descheduled. This is discussed in greater detail in David Herzberg, *White Market Drugs*.

41 "Schedules of Controlled Substances: Removal of Loperamide From Control," *Federal Register* 47, no. 213 (1982): 49840–41.

42 Sandhu et al., "Loperamide: Studies on Its Mechanism of Action."

43 B. Wade, "How to cut the risk of diarrhea when traveling abroad," *Orlando Sentinel*, August 7, 1988; J. Morris, "Panel tackles an old ailment for travelers," *Boston Globe*, February 24, 1985.

In January of 1985, some 250 epidemiologists, GI specialists, and representatives from the travel industry gathered en masse for a National Institutes of Health Consensus Conference for Traveler's Diarrhea, a messy category that contained a wide variety of infectious agents united by geographical concern and transmission through contaminated food and waste. "Although it is rarely life threatening," the *NIH Record* reported, "travelers' diarrhea can cause considerable discomfort, days in bed, and restricted activity." The economic cost alone merited expert attention and innovative pharmacology.[44] The conference explicitly shifted the focus of prevention away from prophylactic antibiotics towards a pocketful of Imodium. Treating diarrhea with Imodium, the *Washington Post* reported, is "a more sensible approach that can shorten the disease to 30 hours or less in most people."[45] Imodium was now the first-line treatment.[46]

As Imodium became primarily regarded as a travelers' medication over the course of the 1980s, something a patient could use when needed, based on their own symptoms, it increasingly fit the category of an over-the-counter (OTC) medication.[47] Many manufacturers of other formerly prescription-only medications had discovered the benefits of the "OTC switch" over the course of the 1980s; consonant with the anti-regulatory transformations of the Reagan administration. The category of "OTC" had been created much earlier as a by-product of the laws generating prescription-only drugs and described a set of products which were both effective and safe for self-treatment, specifically for the symptomatic treatment of self-limiting conditions.[48] In the 1980s, the project of deregulating access to symptomatic drugs so that prescribing decisions could devolve to everyday consumers became a new focus of activity for the FDA. These drugs could still be dangerous, however: OTC Tylenol became a leading cause of liver failure through unintentional overdose, and played a new pharmacological role as an agent of suicide.[49]

44 Judy Murphy, "Avoid Drugs to Prevent Travelers' Diarrhea; Prompt Treatment Is Best and Safer Method," *The NIH Record* 36, no. 5 (1985).

45 Sandy Rovner, "Diarrhea-Prevention Tactic Criticized," *Washington Post*, January 31, 1985, A12.

46 "Diphenoxylate, loperamide and bismuth subsalicylate are first line drug treatment for mild travelers' diarrhea, NIH conference finds; fluids first," *The Pink Sheet*, February 4, 1985.

47 Wade, "Cut the risk of diarrhea"; "Diphenoxylate, loperamide and bismuth subsalicylate"; Morris, "Panel tackles an old ailment for travelers."

48 Jeremy A. Greene and Elizabeth Siegel Watkins, eds., *Prescribed: Writing, Filling, Using, and Abusing the Prescription in Modern America* (University of Chicago Press, 2012).

49 W. C. Myers, T. A. Otto, E. Harris, D. Diaco, and A. Moreno, "Acetaminophen overdose as a suicidal gesture: a survey of adolescents'

In 1986, Johnson & Johnson sought a New Drug Application to promote loperamide as an OTC option. The consumer landscape was confusing, as pharmacologist G. E. Dukes lamented: more than a hundred antidiarrheal remedies were available over the counter, many of them (like charcoal, pectin, and rhubarb extract) grandfathered in from before 1938 and often not even "drugs" but instead marketed under the laxer regulations for "dietary supplements." Earlier that year, the FDA had declared that only two of these agents were found safe and effective: polycarbophil (Fibercon) and attapulgite (Kaopectate).[50] Loperamide, believed to be between three to twenty times more effective than any other antidiarrheal agent on the market, stood to make a killing. "The most significant development in the category of antidiarrheal products," the industry weekly *Pink Sheet* reported in 1991, "was the recent Rx-to-OTC switch of Imodium A-D." [51] Sales had grown in double digits each year since its release. "It's been the No. 1 brand in antidiarrheal products since it went OTC in June 1988," Imodium A-D product director David Goldsmith told *The Pink Sheet*, and the sky was the limit.[52]

Misuse, Abuse, and the Return of the Repressed

As Johnson & Johnson was celebrating the OTC release of Imodium as an inherently safe agent whose responsible use could easily be placed in the hands of American consumers, the chair of pediatrics at Nishtar Hospital publicly appealed to Johnson & Johnson to withdraw Imodium from the market in Pakistan entirely. Dr. Tariq Bhutta wrote in *The Lancet*, in the immediate aftermath of a crisis in which ten babies, all less than seven months of age, died after being admitted to his hospital for abdominal distension and paralytic ileus after being given Imodium for diarrhea. Consumers in Pakistan, Bhutta argued, were unable to benefit from consumer protections designed for middle-class Americans. Although "the package states that the drug should not be used in children less than one year of age," Bhutta reported, "in practice this warning is useless in a country where drugs are freely available over the counter, where 99% of patients can't read, and

---

knowledge of its potential for toxicity," *Journal of the American Academy of Child and Adolescent Psychiatry* 31, no. 4 (1992): 686–90.

50 "Antidiarrheal Drug Products for Over-the Counter Human Use: Tentative Final Monograph," *Federal Register* 51, no. 83 (1986): 16138–49.

51 Iris Rosendahl, "Antacids/Antidiarrheals Churn Up Sales Gains," *Drug Topics* 135, no. 14 (1991): 55.

52 Rosendahl, "Antacids/Antidiarrheals Churn Up Sales Gains," 55.

where unqualified people (quacks and *Hakim*) use drugs without knowing the side-effects."[53]

Bhutta saw a double standard between the West and the rest, or more precisely between global North and South, especially in the domain of pharmaceutical safety. Medications banned for sale in the US and Europe were flooding into unregulated markets in states with lax regulatory schemes and used for symptomatic control without prescriptions. The same year that Imodium was approved as an OTC drug in the United States, the WHO had explicitly recommended against drugs like Imodium for children, pushing oral rehydration therapy as a more appropriate response to diarrhea.[54] An earlier scandal involving a different antidiarrheal in Kenya had already inflamed the subject. After the Pakistan incident, the WHO produced a larger review on the appropriate use of drugs for diarrhea in children found that more than 450 different products were being marketed in the developing world for diarrhea, nearly three-quarters of them specifically marketed for use in children.[55]

In the WHO's framework, there was rational use of drugs, there was misuse, and then there was abuse. In this framework, "loperamide abuse" now became an index case of "irrational use" of drugs, in which the relative risks and benefits of a given drug depended on the differential regulation of drug markets between North and South, or in his formulation, East and West. "If such a thing happened in the West," he told *The Lancet*, "and even one child had died as a result of poisoning due to this drug, there would have been such an uproar that the firm would have withdrawn the drug and banned it from the whole world."[56] And yet, it did not – though Janssen and Johnson & Johnson did agree to withdraw the pediatric syrup version in all developing countries in which WHO maintained a diarrheal disease control program. Between 1989 and 1993, sixteen countries passed regulations limiting the use of loperamide in children.

53 T. I. Bhutta and K. I. Tahir, "Loperamide Poisoning in Children," *The Lancet* 335, no. 8685 (1990): 363.

54 "Drugs in the Management of Acute Diarrhea in Infants and Young Children," *Bulletin of the World Health Organization* 67, no. 1 (1989): 94–95; Hilbrand Haak and Mariam E. Claeson, "Regulatory Actions to Enhance Appropriate Drug Use: The Case of Antidiarrhoeal Drugs," *Social Science & Medicine* 42, no. 7 (1996): 1011–19; *A Manual for the Treatment of Acute Diarrhoea: WHO/CDD/SER/80.2* (World Health Organization, 1980); Andrew Chetley, "Antidiarrhoeals: dying for lack of a drink," in *Problem Drugs* (Health Action International, 1993), 1–3.

55 "The Rational Use of Drugs in the Management of Acute Diarrhea in Children" (World Health Organization, 1990).

56 Bhutta and Tahir, "Loperamide Poisoning in Children," 394.

This is not to say that the drug was not abused in sites both north and west of Pakistan. France restricted the sale of loperamide for use in children in 1991, and Norway reclassified loperamide as a prescription-only drug in 1993. Yet while the WHO mailed its critical review directly to the US FDA in 1990, a public hearing was not held until 1993, after consumer watchdog group Public Citizen sent a petition to the FDA to ban or relabel both Imodium and Lomotil. In that year, two physicians at the Mount Sinai School of Medicine in New York described a case of loperamide abuse in a thirty-five-year-old male physician who presented to their emergency department with appendicitis after excessive use of the drug. Their use of the term "abuse" was not meant to suggest he sought hedonic effects from the narcotic agent, but that he used it outside of the rational drug use policies supported by the WHO, the CDC, and the FDA.

Having taken the medicine for a week, "he exceeded the eight teaspoons per day maximum recommended dosage during all of the 7 days he used the medication." The authors could have called it "overdose" had they so chosen: the high doses were enough to cause ileus, fecal stasis, and appendicitis. They reminded the readers that loperamide, though available over the counter, was still a narcotic, even if only peripherally active. Contrary to Bhutta's suggestion that health-literate consumers were more protected, they pointed out that the patient in question was a physician: "Despite package insert information, medical training, and the knowledge of possible adverse effects, the patient continued to use loperamide exceeding the daily recommended dosage and beyond the recommended number of days."[57]

Other examples of "loperamide abuse" trickled in as case reports in medical journals throughout the 1990s, the inverted cousins of a much larger literature on "laxative abuse," – though the effects of the latter were universally mild and non-life-threatening.[58] People abused laxatives for a number of reasons, ranging from secondary gain in forms of anorexia and bulimia (using laxatives to attain weight loss) to simple dependence (i.e., developing a new physiology in which the ability to have regular bowel movements now depended on increasing doses of laxatives). Either way, physicians considered laxative abuse and loperamide abuse to have a strong overlay with

57 Jeffrey P. Katz and Kai M. Sturmann, "Appendicitis Associated with Loperamide Hydrochloride Abuse," *The Annals of Pharmacotherapy* 27, no. 3 (1993): 369–70.

58 "Loperamide Abuse: Dependence Case Report," *Reactions Weekly* 438, no. 1 (1993): 10; "Loperamide Abuse: Constipation and Tolerance: 3 Case Reports," *Reactions Weekly*, no. 661 (1997): 8; T. Litovitz, C. Clancy, B. Korberly, A. R. Temple, K. V. Mann, "Surveillance of loperamide ingestions: an analysis of 216 poison center reports," *Journal of Toxicology: Clinical Toxicology* 35 no. 1 (1997): 11–19

mental illness, especially anxiety disorders. As one series of cases reported in 1997 emphasized:

> Two of the patients, a 25-year-old man and a 16-year-old boy, were anxious about the availability of toilet facilities outside their homes and took loperamide to prevent defaecation when they were on outings. The third patient, a 14-year-old boy, had "an obsession about moving his bowels" and was given loperamide by his mother to prevent frequent bathroom stops when they were away from home. The first patient took loperamide for over 2 years and experienced several episodes of severe constipation during this time. The second patient developed tolerance after taking 1–2 loperamide tablets per situation and started taking 3–6 tablets 1–2 times/week. In all 3 patients, appropriate psychiatric diagnosis and treatment resulted in the cessation of loperamide.[59]

Abuse, tolerance: these were not just incidental words, and they continued to re-emerge in descriptions of nonstandard administration of Imodium through the early 2000s. Yet although their language overlapped with the language of addiction research, they were not the same concerns as Jaffe's regarding the "abuse potential" of the drug. Tolerance, a key element of the understanding of narcotic addiction, in which a dependent body comes to need more and more narcotic in order to maintain the same drug effect obtained on first use, had since become a more generalized element of pharmacology.

This changed in 2013, when *Clinical Toxicology* reported two different patients who presented with syncope (fainting) and a potentially fatal ventricular arrhythmia after "loperamide abuse."[60] One of the patients was a twenty-eight-year-old man with Crohn's disease, whose dangerous heart rhythm was only explained after he admitted to taking up to 400 tablets of loperamide daily – a situation that could perhaps be understandable, if unorthodox, self-treatment by a patient with a chronic inflammatory bowel disease. The other case, however, was directly to opiates. The patient in question, a forty-three-year-old woman, had clearly been taking loperamide to help mediate the effects of opiate withdrawal. She admitted to taking 140 tablets of loperamide daily as a form of DIY detox when methadone was not available.

How did this happen? A clue came from a group of "substance abuse researchers" at the University of Ohio who were developing new forms of

59 "Loperamide Abuse: Dependence Case Report"; See also N. Langlitz, K. Schotte, and T. Bschor, "Loperamide abuse in anxiety disorder," *Nervenarzt* 72, no. 7 (2001): 562.

60 J. M. Marraffa et al., "Syncope and recurrent polymorphic ventricular tachycardia following loperamide misuse," *Clinical Toxicology* 51, no. 7 (2013): 653; "Loperamide Abuse: Syncope and Recurrent Polymorphic Ventricular Tachycardia: 2 Case Reports," *Reactions Weekly*, no. 1478 (2013): 24.

internet-based epidemiology to learn about evolving substance abuse patterns through new social media. "The World Wide web has been identified as one of the 'leading edge' data sources for detecting patterns and changes in drug trends," they explained, "and as a useful tool for reaching hidden populations."[61] While looking for user-generated content, they stumbled over a cache of new information on the extra-medical use of loperamide. Although loperamide was believed to have no abuse potential, their content analysis of a random sample of 1290 posts on an opioid use website between 2005 and 2011 now indicated otherwise.

They were surprised to discover an online community itself actively in the process of discovering the use of loperamide to self-treat withdrawal symptoms in real time when methadone could not be located. "Back in the day when I would run out of pills early, I would take 8–10 loperamide tabs and get some pretty good relief from withdrawal," one of the earlier posters noted. "If you take a shitload of lope [loperamide] like 10–20 pills at once in withdrawal, you'll get relief from some of the physical symptoms," another poster added; "I'm not sure exactly how it works, but it's definitely more than just relieving the GI [gastro-intestinal] symptoms. I'm guessing if you just bombard your blood with it, some of it has to make it through? Not sure." [62] Different users valued risks and benefits differently.[63]

The key to success was a new dosing strategy that online posters dubbed the "megadose." "I just wanted to tell you that loperamide WILL WORK," another poster added: "I take 105 mg of methadone per day, and recently have been running out early due to a renewed interest in IVing [intravenous use] that shit. 200 mg of lope (100 pills) will make me almost 100[%] again. It brings the sickness down to the level of, say, a minor flu. Sleep returns, restlessness dissipates. Sometimes a mild 'opiation' is felt."[64] With one pill: no euphoria; with eight to ten pills: no euphoria; but with 100 pills: maybe? As an online networked community of innovative users and innovator-users continued to experiment with very, very high doses, a few even reported that there might be ways, at a large enough quantity, to find some kind of high from Imodium.

New risks of potentially fatal cardiac side effects from a drug previously believed to be safe were the direct result of new patterns of consumption: the increasing popularity of Imodium megadoses for both self-treatment

61 Raminta Daniulaityte et al., "'I Just Wanted to Tell You That Loperamide WILL WORK': A Web-Based Study of Extra-Medical Use of Loperamide," *Drug and Alcohol Dependence* 130, nos. 1–3 (2013): 241–44.

62 Daniulaityte et al., "Loperamide WILL WORK," 242.

63 Campbell, *OD*.

64 Daniulaityte et al., "Loperamide WILL WORK," 242.

and euphoric use as "the desperate junky's methadone."[65] To date, these side effects had been cause for concern, even hospitalization. But when the first death attributed to "loperamide abuse" was reported two years later, in 2015, the *British Medical Journal* moved to list loperamide dependence as a new disease.

The index case was a twenty-six-year-old man who checked into an emergency department in Tacoma, Washington, requesting detox. By the time he presented, he had already developed an 800mg per day loperamide habit – consuming 400 2mg pills of Imodium per day. He related a life history that started with recreational use of prescription opiates at age seventeen, then shifted to alternate sources of opiates to manage withdrawal and also seek pleasure, at one point ingesting home-batch extracts of poppy seeds bought in bulk from a supermarket. After he learned about the loperamide hack through social media, and found it gave him an "opiate-like effect," his habit grew into its present state. Several times, concerned with the sheer volume of his dependence, he tried to quit, but found any attempt to quit on his own led to severe withdrawal symptoms, including tremor, vomiting, and diarrhea. After being denied access to detox services because loperamide dependence was not an acceptable diagnosis, he reported obtaining prescription opiates in order to get a positive urine tox and be admitted for narcotic detox. By that time, he had experienced severe cardiac complications, having been diagnosed with Brugada syndrome and fitted with an implantable cardiac defibrillator. After a second failed detox, he was found in cardiac arrest.

The authors of the *BMJ* report imply that his death could have – should have – been prevented: that this patient who had sought care for loperamide abuse had been unable to receive it within a world of detox centers that maintained that such a condition could not exist. Thus the urgency of recognizing loperamide addiction as a "new disease" – the "first of a patient with significant loperamide dependence on its euphoric effects" to achieve public recognition for other patients who might be suffering similarly in the future.[66] A few months later, a nineteen-year-old man was found dead in his Houston home after hosting a party the previous night, next to a pill-crusher, with a combination of minor tranquilizers and high-dose loperamide in his blood. The reporting pathologists likewise suggested that "loperamide toxicity may be at a higher incidence in the United States than currently reported due to its easy availability as an OTC medication … and lack of awareness of loperamide's potential for abuse."[67]

65 Daniulaityte et al., "Loperamide WILL WORK," 242.

66 Ryan MacDonald et al., "Loperamide Dependence and Abuse," *BMJ Case Reports* (2015): bcr2015209705.

67 Jennifer Dierksen, Morna Gonsoulin, and Jeffrey P. Walterscheid, "Poor Man's Methadone: A Case Report of Loperamide Toxicity," *American Journal of Forensic Medicine & Pathology* 36, no. 4 (2015): 268–70.

More reports followed, along with a realization that the toxicity profile of loperamide itself was changing rapidly in response to rapid changes in patterns of use. Earlier studies suggested that poison control centers only received a handful of calls about loperamide, and all were benign. But between 2009 and 2015, the number of loperamide-related calls doubled, mostly among teens and young adults, with 18% of cases involving serious cardiotoxic effect. Google Search analytics showed a sharp increase during this period in Google searches for both "loperamide high" and "loperamide withdrawal."[68]

Media attention complicated matters. The *New York Times* published its first report on "loperamide abuse" after two deaths in New York in 2016. On the one hand, this increased the visibility of the problem to physicians and pharmacists and poison control centers; on the other hand, it made the possibility of the practice still more visible and net-searchable for other would-be users. A retrospective analysis of the National Poison Data System found that where there had been almost no cases of loperamide abuse before 2008, between 2010 and 2015 the rate of "intentional misuse and abuse" of loperamide effectively doubled. "Misuse" in their terms denoted the use of high-dose loperamide as an agent to manage opioid withdrawal; "abuse" now referred explicitly to the use of even higher doses to achieve euphoric effect.[69] Though the numbers were still small, the rate of increase looked potentially exponential, as did the spread of loperamide-using knowledge on internet chatboards, which included strategies to increase potency of effect through grapefruit juice and other modalities.[70]

The timing of all of these shifts appeared closely related to crackdowns on other opioids.[71] In 2010, as a response to the increasing visibility of deaths due to overdose of prescription opioids, the US FDA had approved changes in the formulation of oxycodone to make them less amenable to misuse; in 2014 the DEA had bumped codeine up from Schedule III to Schedule II

68 Stephen W. Borron et al., "Intentional Misuse and Abuse of Loperamide: A New Look at a Drug with 'Low Abuse Potential,'" *The Journal of Emergency Medicine* 53, no. 1 (2017): 73–84.

69 J. Priyanka Vakkalanka, Nathan P. Charlton, and Christopher P. Holstege, "Epidemiologic Trends in Loperamide Abuse and Misuse," *Annals of Emergency Medicine* 69, no. 1 (2017): 73–78.

70 Cornel N. Stanciu and Samantha A. Gnanasegaram, "Loperamide, the 'Poor Man's Methadone': Brief Review," *Journal of Psychoactive Drugs* 49, no. 1 (2017): 18–21.

71 W. Eggleston, J. M. Marraffa, C. M. Stork et al., "Notes from the field: cardiac dysrhythmias after loperamide abuse New York, 2008-2016." *CDC Morbidity and Mortality Weekly Report* 65, no. 45 (2016): 1276e1277.

to achieve a similar goal.[72] It is not a surprise, pharmacoepidemiologists argued, that innovative users would find ways to shift their usage to adapt another opiate still available for purchase, much as methamphetamine users had shifted to bulk orders of over-the-counter pseuedphedrine (Sudafed) a decade or so earlier as a reliable way to produce an amphetamine effect after the crackdown on meth markets. In response, pharmacists called for a greater control of Imodium – to put the drug "behind the counter," like Sudafed, to limit purchases of the large scale of pills this required.[73]

Others called for the drug to be removed from the market.[74] In 2016, the FDA changed the package label of Imodium to warn against the cardiac risks of high doses, but this did little to blunt overdoses.[75] In turn, in January of 2018 the FDA changed the packaging of Imodium to "use blister packs or other single-dose packaging and to limit the number of doses in a package."[76] Yet, five years later the FDA admitted that "we continue to receive reports of serious heart problems and deaths with much higher than the recommended doses of loperamide, primarily among people who are intentionally misusing or abusing the product, despite the addition of a warning to the medicine label and a previous communication."[77]

72 "FDA approves new formulation for OxyContin," US Food and Drug Administration, http://www.fda.gov/NewsEvents/Newsroom/PressAnnouncements/ucm207480.html; "DEA to publish final rule rescheduling hydrocodone combination products," United States Drug Enforcement Agency, https:// www.dea.gov/divisions/hq/2014/hq082114.shtml; both cited in Heather Miller et al., "Loperamide Misuse and Abuse," *Journal of the American Pharmacists Association* 57, no. 2 (2017): S45–50.

73 Miller et al., "Loperamide Misuse and Abuse," S49.

74 Amr Idris, Danielle C. Mihora, and Kenji Kaye, "Loperamide Abuse Cardiotoxicity. Should Loperamide Still Be an over the Counter Medication?," *The American Journal of Emergency Medicine* 36, no. 9 (2018): 1716.e1-1716.e3.

75 Laurie McGinley, "FDA Wants to Curb Abuse of Imodium, 'the Poor Man's Methadone,'" *Washington Post*, October 26, 2021.

76 "FDA Limits Packaging for Anti-Diarrhea Medicine Loperamide (Imodium) to Encourage Safe Use," FDA Center for Drug Evaluation and Research, September 20, 2019, https://www.fda.gov/drugs/drug-safety-and-availability/fda-limits-packaging-anti-diarrhea-medicine-loperamide-imodium-encourage-safe-use.

77 "FDA Drug Safety Podcast: FDA Limits Packaging for Anti-Diarrhea Medicine Loperamide (Imodium) to Encourage Safe Use," FDA Center for Drug Evaluation and Research, January 12, 2022, https://www.fda.gov/drugs/fda-drug-safety-podcasts/fda-drug-safety-podcast-fda-limits-packaging-anti-diarrhea-medicine-loperamide-imodium-encourage.

News of "loperamide abuse" spread outward from user discussion boards and poison control centers. As the Missouri Poison Center put out in a public dispatch:

> Does anything surprise us anymore? – Yes, even the over-the-counter **antidiarrheal drug, loperamide (Imodium), can be abused**. It is a legal, inexpensive, and accessible alternative for someone with opioid use disorder, or merely curious about the pleasurable effects of opioids. It is also used for self-treatment of opioid withdrawal symptoms, giving it the moniker "poor man's methadone." The high doses needed to produce CNS effects carry an unanticipated **risk of significant cardiotoxicity resulting in life-threatening arrhythmias**. Between 2010 and 2015 the National Poison Data System showed a 91% increase in intentional loperamide exposures with 11 related deaths, and 13 deaths in a one-year period in 2016–2017.[78]

As before, the added media attention had the risk of inflaming, rather than resolving the issue. As pharmacologist William Eggleston, who studied the cyber-epidemiology of loperamide use, told *The Washington Post*, the FDA's actions on blister packs only really affected those who bought their drugs at the pharmacy. The online purchasing of drugs still offered easy means to massively accumulate the megadoses required: "Even if you limit the quantities available in any individual package, if you can buy a lot of packages online, that doesn't fix the issue that the drug is easily accessible."[79]

Conclusion

The story of loperamide confounds our categories of risk and benefit, of effects desired an undesired. This chapter provides a light sketch of the traces left by loperamide in the scientific, clinical, and regulatory literatures. Even within the relatively sanitized archive of medical publications and regulatory actions, the trajectory of loperamide offers a complex bio-social narrative. This narrative is constrained on the one end by the physical manifestations of 4-[4-(4-chlorophenyl)-4-hydroxypiperidin-1-yl]-*N*,*N*-dimethyl-2,2-diphenylbutanamide, and the location and function of the *mu* receptors that it agonistically activates more generally in the walls of the intestine than in the brain. Yet it remains open on the other end to the shifting historical context of regulatory systems, marketing classifications, broader constellations of narcotic and

78 Julie Weber, "Loperamide – An Unexpected Drug of Abuse," Missouri Poison Center, January 17, 2019, https://missouripoisoncenter.org/loperamide-an-unexpected-drug-of-abuse/.

79 McGinley, "FDA Wants to Curb Abuse of Imodium."

amphetamine crackdowns, and the informatic media and body-hacking genius of "abusers" who can just as easily be understood as highly innovative users – social, technological, and biomedical innovators in their own right.

To gather together the strands of this story again at the end: opium, for hundreds of years before the advent of synthetic opiates, was always understood to be a polyfunctional drug. As Nicholas Culpeper described in his widely read seventeenth-century pharmacological treatise, *The English Physician*:

> The garden Poppy heads with seeds made into a syrup, is frequently, and to good effect used to procure rest, and sleep, in the sick and weak, and to stay catarrhs and defluxions of thin rheums from the head into the stomach and lungs, causing a continual cough, the fore-runner of a consumption; it helps also hoarseness of the throat, and when one have lost their voice, which the oil of the seed doth likewise. The black seed boiled in wine, and drank, is said also to dry the flux of the belly, and women's courses.[80]

Without making too gross of a reduction of Culpeper's categories into biomedical ontologies, it is still safe to say that opium was understood as a narcotic, an analgesic, an effective agent against cough and sore throat, which also helped with menstrual cramps as well as the treatment of excessive diarrhea. By the early nineteenth century, all of the above properties could be attributed directly to morphine, once this alkaloid was derived from opium as the first chemically defined opiate.

Imodium begins its life as an opioid with more gut action than brain; it enters commercial life, at least in the United States, as a closely monitored entity all the same, coming into existence as a consumer good in the dual-edged moment of the deployment of the Nixon Administration's Controlled Substances Act, on the one hand, and the dissolution of the Lexington narcotic farm on the other. It becomes the posterchild of a transnational attempt to use postmarketing surveillance to document the consumer safety and non-abusability of a potentially addictive substance, subject to the scrutiny and laboratory work of none other than Jerome Jaffe, Nixon's first Drug Czar. And it receives these blessings in time to not only be the first drug ever to be de-scheduled as a narcotic, in 1982, but then teed up for the wave of "Rx to OTC Switch" projects of the Reagan administration. Subject to the greatest scrutiny, on the largest stage, this safe consumer product seemed as far away from a dangerous drug as anything could be, even if technically some pharmacology textbooks referred to it by its seemingly arcane description as a synthetic opioid.

When the insulatory fabric of Imodium's non-abusability came undone in the first decades of the twenty-first century, then, it was not for lack of effort or surveillance on the part of pharmaceutical chemists, drug enforcement

80 Culpeper, *The Complete Herbal*, 145.

agencies, regulatory laboratories, pharmacists, and other epidemiologists of drug use. It was not because of a sudden transformation in the physical structure of the drug or the physiology of the human organism. It was because the benefits and risks of a drug are never fixed, but are always responsive to a dynamic ecology of uses and users that extends well beyond categories we might seek to use to name and bind them. Loperamide never was merely an antidiarrheal agent, as much as we might wish to think that we might make any pharmacological agent act as a "good" and not a "bad" simply by calling it by the name whose effects we desire.

Chapter Fifteen

Containing a Gray Market Drug: The Rise and Regulation of the US Poppers Industry (1969–1991)[1]

Joseph Jay Sosa

In the early twenty-first century, there are a few things gay men know they can and can't say about poppers, a product popular with gay men to facilitate anal sex. The commercial and vernacular name for alkyl nitrite inhalants, poppers are a class of vasodilators that elevate the heart rate, reduce blood pressure, increase tactile sensations, and relax smooth muscle. Starting in the 1970s, the poppers industry has operated upon one simple dictate: don't call them poppers! Manufacturers could compound butyl nitrite and consumers could buy it without facing criminal charges for inhaling it. But manufacturers could not tell consumers to inhale it nor advertise the effects of inhalation. This incentivized the gay men who manufactured butyl nitrite products and the gay men who consumed them to use coded vocabulary around what nitrites did, down to avoiding the very name "poppers." Advertisements in gay media labelled butyl nitrite products as odorizers, VHS cleaners, or nail polish removers to avoid regulatory scrutiny, and they simultaneously

1 An enormous thanks to David Herzberg for his interest in this project and to David, Joseph M. Gabriel, and Nils Kessel for inviting me to join this volume at a late stage and working with me to bring this chapter in conversation with the book. Additional thanks to Shenila Khoja-Moolji for reframing feedback and Beth Hoppe for archival strategies. This research has been supported by the Leather Archives and Museum in Chicago and by the Knowledge of AIDS Network (NSF #2240822; #2240637; #2240673).

communicated the benefits of inhaling using the masculine, eroticized vocabulary of "power" and "potency." A specialized language of risk and benefit circulated among gay men, developing creatively within the limits of what those men knew they could and could not say about poppers.

The distinctive features of poppers markets resulted from their complex pathway through US consumer protection regulations. The physiological effects of alkyl nitrites were first being investigated in the late 19th century, as the pharmaceutial industry was consolidating. The category of pharmaceutical emerged slowly through a series of state and market interventions in the industrial production of chemicals. The modern regulatory state of the early twentieth century saw a need to help citizens distinguish between "good" chemicals and "bad" ones.[2] Alkyl nitrites have fallen on one side or another of this divide at various moments. One alkyl nitrite compound, amyl nitrite, was in wide medical use as a treatment for angina before the Food and Drug Administration (FDA) restricted it to prescription-only status in 1969. In the 1970s, gay men seeking alternatives to amyl nitrite started producing butyl nitrite, a compound with similar pharmacological properties that was not covered by FDA restrictions. The FDA refrained from evaluating butyl nitrite for medical use, and other potential oversight agencies such as the Drug Enforcement Agency (DEA) and Consumer Product Safety Commission (CPSC) were slow to address butyl nitrite. As a result, butyl nitrite sat in an ambiguous position, neither normalized nor criminalized. Without explicit FDA guidance, major manufacturers were reluctant to make butyl nitrite, giving rise to a "chemical cottage industry," the term Jason Pine uses to describe the decentralized, community-protected, small-scale production of (in Pine's case) methamphetamine labs.[3] In this cottage industry, gay entrepreneurs and consumers developed their own methods of evaluating the risks and benefits of nitrite products, and they communicated those evaluations through coded advertising and community grapevines. Ironically, the claims around risks and benefits communicated in advertisements were in some ways aspirationally modeled on the regulatory apparatus that had excluded poppers, yet the advertisements themselves were seen as evidence of malpractice by those same hands-off regulators.

This chapter recounts how a pharmaceutical third space for poppers emerged between regulated medicines and controlled substances. I consider this third space as a gray market with its own standards of risk and benefit

2 David L. Herzberg, *White Market Drugs: Big Pharma and the Hidden History of Addiction in America* (University of Chicago Press, 2020); James Harvey Young, *The Medical Messiahs: A Social History of Health Quackery in 20th Century America* (Princeton University Press, 1992).

3 Jason Pine, *The Alchemy of Meth: A Decomposition* (University of Minnesota Press, 2019), xvi.

that trouble the licit/illicit divide while also operating as a buffer zone that stabilizes that same divide by quarantining unapproved, but not prohibited, behavior.[4] The gray market is, crucially, informal, defined in part by the absence of regulation. It falls between prohibition-market drugs (controlled substances), whose consumers are criminalized, and white market drugs (pharmaceuticals), whose consumers are protected by formal regulation. Within this gray market, poppers operated as a boundary object – one that is part of many social worlds and invites (sometimes contentiously) interactions between them.[5] They appeared differently to consumers, manufacturers, physicians, regulators, and journalists who were each attuned to different potential risks of butyl nitrite. These different perspectives are not the result of poppers' position between licit and illicit substances; rather, disputes between these actors over the risks and benefits of poppers produced the malleable demarcation between the licit and illicit.

Queer Containment

Counter to expectations, poppers' gray market status emerged not from regulatory scrutiny but through targeted state neglect. Federal regulators maintained poppers sales in a gray market by rejecting potentially viable paths for product approval sought by some butyl nitrite manufacturers while simultaneously being reluctant to fully enforce ways in which butyl nitrite production could be shut down. Regulators repeatedly upheld the status quo of the poppers market – what all parties saw as an unresolved status – by carefully managing claims around potential risks and benefits around nitrite inhalation. This is in line with how the FDA traditionally determines the claims around safety and effectiveness that can make a pharmaceutical approvable; but it is the inverse of how this power over safety and effectiveness normally operates.[6]

This regulatory strategy is similar to what Damon Scott labels "queer containment" – where the state cordons off certain sectors of the economy as a place for non-normative use to avoid exposing the majority population to

4 On pharmaceutic "gray markets," see Herzberg, *White Market Drugs.*

5 Susan Leigh Star,and James R. Griesemer, "Institutional Ecology, 'Translations' and Boundary Objects: Amateurs and Professionals in Berkeley's Museum of Vertebrate Zoology, 1907–39," *Social Studies of Science* 19, no. 3 (1989): 387–420.

6 Daniel P. Carpenter, *Reputation and Power: Organizational Image and Pharmaceutical Regulation at the FDA* (Princeton University Press, 2010), 16.

vice.[7] As Scott documents with zoning and alcohol laws, containment practices unintentionally incentivized bar owners to employ extralegal tactics to stay in business and hastened the consolidation of bars serving homosexuals to identify as "gay bars" in the 1950s and 1960s. Queer containment offers a useful perspective to characterize the sometimes erratic shifts in regulation regarding how nitrite inhalants were regulated and the corresponding strategies with which manufacturers marketed them. Amyl nitrite had many off-label applications from the 1870s through the 1960s. When regulators restricted amyl nitrite in response to consumer advocates' concern about the risk of teenage inhalant usage, however, the butyl nitrite industry that took its place solidified poppers' status as a drug oriented to providing benefits towards sexual enjoyment.

Poppers' gray market status was sustained primarily through the careful management of which claims could be made regarding nitrite inhalants' potential risks, and especially regarding their potential benefits. Political actors outside of the gay community such as public officials, consumer advocates, and mainstream journalists discounted the knowledge about the benefits and harms around poppers usage that developed within gay male communities. Butyl nitrite manufacturers and vendors, mostly gay men, endeavored to communicate community knowledge about poppers' benefits without running afoul of prohibitions on making specific pharmaceutical claims. Coded language in advertisements didn't fool public officials, but it did make it difficult for many state and federal agencies to justify restricting poppers based on product claims alone. Instead, anti-poppers consumer advocates and allied public officials characterized advertisements and other public statements of the poppers industry as misleading, i.e., creating consumer risks.

The attention to manufacturers' claims as the basis of whether poppers were a licit or illicit substance (or somewhere in-between) demonstrates the performative character of drug claims. As mentioned, the FDA enforces pharmaceutical standards primarily by controlling what statements manufacturers can make regarding drug safety (what are the risks of use) and efficacy (what benefits a drug may have). In linguistics, performative statements are not judged according to whether they are truthful (i.e., reflecting reality) but whether they are successful (i.e., enacting the reality they describe). Further, performatives are buttressed by all kinds of other statements and social relations that determine the rules of whether a statement can be successfully uttered.[8] The FDA exercises the performative power to make some

7 Damon Scott, *The City Aroused: Queer Places and Urban Redevelopment in Postwar San Francisco* (University of Texas Press, 2023).

8 J. L. Austin, *How to Do Things with Words: The William James Lectures Delivered at Harvard University in 1955*, 2nd ed. (Harvard University Press, 2009).

statements successful and others unsuccessful through the authority that the agency's reputation lends them.[9]

Federal authority over pharmaceutic statements, however, accrued over time. And the period when the poppers industry emerged and consolidated, from 1969 (the restriction of pharmaceutical amyl nitrite) to 1991 (the federal ban of butyl nitrite for purposes of human consumption), witnessed significant changes that would impact how manufacturers could make claims about benefits. Loosening restrictions on obscenity in media in the 1950s enabled a rapid expansion of gay and lesbian print publications by the 1970s, providing a space where butyl nitrite could be advertised to a national public.[10] In the same period, however, Congress strengthened classifications between prescription vs. over-the-counter (OTC) medications and introduced drug effectiveness requirements that restricted drug markets. A generation earlier, poppers advertisements would most likely have been seized by the US Postal Service on moral grounds. By the early 1980s, they were used as evidence in state and local boards of health on public safety grounds.

Business records for the poppers industry are hard to obtain. Instead, this chapter documents the poppers industry through an archive of claims made about the benefits and risks of amyl nitrite and butyl nitrite. In advertising, journalism, and state records, a coterie of actors made claims about what nitrite inhalants could do for, or to, consumers. These claims, in turn, provided the justification for the queer containment practices maintaining a gray market status for poppers. This chapter also considers the many unuttered and unutterable claims around poppers, keeping in mind queer theory's observation that the unsaid is not the mere absence of speech but the manifestation of power imbalances making only certain speech possible and facilitating the weaponization of ignorance.[11] This allows for rereading the silences and coded language of poppers advertisements, not as evidence of malfeasance (as regulators did), but as a counterpublic means of communicating the risks and benefits of nitrite products.

9 Carpenter, *Reputation and Power*, 15.

10 The rapid expansion of pharmaceuticals and curtailment of obscenity policing are key factors in development of "pharmacopornographic" politics in the mid-twentieth century. See Paul Preciado, "Pharmaco-pornographic Politics: Towards a New Gender Ecology," *Parallax* 14, no. 1 (2008): 105–17.

11 Judith Butler, *Excitable Speech: A Politics of the Performative* (Routledge, 1997); Michel Foucault, *The History of Sexuality* (Vintage Books, 1990); Eve Kosofsky Sedgwick, *Epistemology of the Closet* (University of California Press, 2008).

Pharmaceuticalization and Prescription Controls of Amyl Nitrite

First compounded in 1844, amyl nitrite was a wonder product of nineteenth-century synthetic chemistry and was proposed in the popular press as a remedy to conditions as diverse as feinting, chloroform overdose, angina, sea sickness, and the hiccups.[12] By 1910, British manufacturers Burroughs Wellcome had started selling amyl nitrite under the product name Vaperole. Amyl nitrite would have been a common, well-known treatment to middle-class consumers in the US and Great Britain. The influential long-term editor of the *Journal of the American Medical Association*, Morris Fishbein, instructed readers to give amyl nitrite to individuals experiencing chest tightness.[13] *The Complete Book of First Aid*, published in 1955 by John Henderson, the medical director of Johnson & Johnson, also recommends amyl nitrite for acute coronary thrombosis and cyanide poisoning.[14] When US president Dwight Eisenhower had a heart attack in Denver in 1957, amyl nitrite was widely reported as the first drug administered to him.[15] Beyond its therapeutic uses, however, amyl nitrite had a reputation for pleasurable effects, leading to off-label usage. Poppers manufacturer W. Jay Freezer described this hidden history of amyl nitrite off-label usage, asserting that "once in a generation, a medical student would write a paper about their discovery of amyl nitrite and its amorous effects."[16] Warning and titillating its audience about fashionable "amyl and cocktail parties," the *Brooklyn Eagle* wrote in 1931: "amyl nitrite, which can be bought without any embarrassing questions ... when inhaled causes intense exhilaration."[17] Journalists' reports of

12 "The Coming Method of Warfare," *The Weekly Calistogian*, August 1, 1888; Theodore Van Dellen, "Hiccups Easy to Control If You Know How," *New York Daily News*, October 24, 1947; "Inquisition as to the Death of Mrs. Minnie Ninnis," *Grass Valley Daily Union*, January 14, 1882; Andrew Currier, "How to Keep Well: Angina Pectoris," *The Standard Union*, March 5, 1926.

13 Morris Fishbein, "Angina Victim Must Not Take Hard Exercise," *Spokane Chronicle*, May 19, 1937.

14 John Henderson, *The Complete Book of First Aid* (Bantam Books, 1955).

15 "Detailed Account Given of Eisenhower Heart Attack," *The Tampa Tribune*, December 25, 1955.

16 "Interview with W. Jay Freezer," *The Gay Life with Randy Alfred*, Aired December 27, 1981, on KSAN, GLBT History Archives, Randy Alfred Subject Files and Sound Recordings, Reel 116, Box 161991-24.

17 "London Smart Set Is Finding Thrill in Amyl," *The Brooklyn Daily Eagle*, December 13, 1931.

vendors like "Poppers Bill" in New York or "Tugboat Annie" in Miami in the 1950s and 1960s offers a glimpse into its non-pharmaceutic sales.[18]

Although amyl nitrite had been included on the list of drugs that required a prescription according to the 1951 Durham-Humphrey Amendment, in 1960, the FDA removed prescription requirements for amyl nitrite at the request of manufacturer Burroughs Wellcome. For the next decade, amyl nitrite was available for OTC sales in pharmacies. Adult customers could now walk into a pharmacy and purchase amyl nitrite, but its widespread availability spilled into street sales. Outreach workers in San Francisco's Tenderloin district in 1967 noted the ubiquity of amyls (labelled in the report as "sniff" and listed alongside marijuana, the only two substances included without a street price).[19] Often characterized as a "cheap high" in journalistic accounts, amyl nitrite's availability to adolescents soon alarmed the public. Exacerbating the situation, the legal status of amyl nitrite was not always clear. Local authorities in Rochester, New York, for instance, found that some amyl nitrite packaging continued to list the product as by prescription only while other amyl nitrite was readily sold at pharmacies without prescription.[20] It was a precipitous moment to expand sales, as middle-class consumer norms were also becoming more amenable to the recreational and mind-altering capabilities of a variety of chemical products.[21] Over the 1960s, amyl nitrite usage also entered the pharmacopeia of the 1960s counterculture.

By the mid-1960s, the FDA began reversing course. In June 1964, public officials in Buffalo, New York, complained to the FDA about the recreational use of amyl nitrite. Determining that at least four(!) teenagers had obtained

18 On Poppers Bill, see John Lauritsen and Hank Wilson, *Death Rush: Poppers and AIDS* (Inland Book Co., 1986). On Tugboat Annie, see Herb Rau, "They Get Their Kicks Sniffing Amyl Nitrite," *Miami News*, March 30, 1966.

19 Outreach workers in the Tenderloin District of San Francisco reported that amyl nitrite was one of cheapest substances available to homeless youth, who purchased it in conjunction with marijuana. See "The Tenderloin Project" (Unpublished manuscript, 1967). Source: Tenderloin Project, Homophile Organizations. February 1–August 16, 1966, n.d. MS Phyllis Lyon, Del Martin and the Daughters of Bilitis Box 19, Folder 15: Gay, Lesbian, Bisexual, and Transgender Historical Society, Archives of Sexuality and Gender.

20 John van Buren, "New Teen-Age 'Kicks' Can Be Fatal," *Democrat and Chronicle*, June 5, 1964.

21 David Farber, "The Intoxicated State/Illegal Nation: Drugs in the Sixties Counterculture," in *Imagine Nation: The American Counterculture of the 1960s and '70s*, ed. Peter Braunstein and Michael William Doyle (Routledge, 2002), 17–40.

amyl, the FDA officials vowed to revisit the question of amyl nitrite.[22] The FDA issued a directive to over 200,000 recipients including pharmaceutical companies, physicians, and pharmacists that prohibited marketing nitrite- and nitrate-based products of claiming effectiveness in treating anything other than angina pectoris.[23] Even Burroughs Wellcome communicated to the FDA their concern that teenagers had too much access to OTC amyl nitrite.[24] The FDA maintained that existing approved nitrite medications were "safe and widely regarded as useful under medical supervision."[25] Writing in 1967, the FDA reiterated that "amyl nitrite inhalant in units no more than .3 cc been available over the counter for self-medication for a number of years without evidence of harm to the users," but decreed that it not be sold commercially in units above twelve dosages.[26] In 1968, the FDA went further, citing numerous reports of abuse, and described amyl nitrite as "a drug with a potentiality for harmful effect and that it should be removed from over-the-counter status and restricted to sale on the prescription of a practitioner licensed by law to administer such drug."[27] In 1969, the FDA renewed its prescription requirement for amyl nitrite sales.[28]

Gay journalists chronicling the origins of the poppers industry speculated on the political motivations for loosening and then tightening prescription requirements for amyl nitrite in such a short time. Some accounts emphasized a profit motive. Either they saw the diminishing use of amyl nitrite in cardiology with the prevalence of nitroglycerin tablets, or they saw the

22 Van Buren, "New Teen-Age 'Kicks' Can Be Fatal."

23 "U.S. Moves Against Drug Firms," *Boston Globe*, April 20, 1966.

24 The public health psychologist Ronald Wood, who documented the regulation of amyl and butyl nitrite, noted repeated correspondence between the Wellcome Burroughs and the US FDA during this period around what both parties saw as a concerning increase in amyl nitrite uses among teens. See Ronald Wood's unpublished 1987 report "A chronology of the regulation of volatile nitrites," in Randy Shilts Papers, LGBTQIA Center, San Francisco Public Library, Series 5b, Box 128.

25 "U.S. Moves Against Drug Firms."

26 "Nitroglycerin and Amyl Nitrite as Over-The-Counter Drugs for Humans: Proposed Statement of Policy," *Federal Register* 32, no. 165 (1967): 12404.

27 "Statements of General Policy or Interpretation: Amyl Nitrite Inhalant as Prescription Drug for Human Use," *Federal Register* 33, no. 232 (1968): 17751.

28 "Statements of General Policy or Interpretation: Amyl Nitrite Inhalant a Prescription Drug for Human Use; Change in Effective Date," *Federal Register* 34, no. 50 (1969): 5254–55.

growing sales for off-label use, or both.[29] Some proposed that Burroughs Wellcome had advocated for restriction because of either homophobia or fear of lawsuits.[30] But the mechanics of queer containment were more haphazard and lacked a singular trajectory. Amyl nitrite was being reclassified at a moment when pharmaceutical approval procedures were being transformed. The Durham-Humphrey Amendment had only solidified the distinction between prescription and OTC drugs in 1951, and the Kefauver-Harris Act of 1962 redefined standards for drug approval, introducing the requirement for drug effectiveness. Although poppers were not considered addictive, the Drug Abuse Control Act of 1965, which created new oversight requirements for the registration, record-keeping, and labelling of nonprescription drugs deemed habit forming, further reflected state attitudes towards off-label drug use. Changing prescription status may have reflected these still-consolidating standards as much as a clear decision to limit authorized circulation of amyl nitrite. It is helpful here to think of prescriptions as Jeremy A. Greene and Elizabeth Seigel Watkins do, as "a shorthand reference for the complex relations among producers, providers and consumers of medicine."[31] The FDA used prescription status to respond to varied interests of local police departments, pharmacologists, and concerned parents, but in the morally-removed language of dosages, efficacies, and misuse. Yet its effort to contain amyl nitrite misuse from certain groups would transform the entire culture around poppers.

The Rise of the Butyl Nitrite Gray Market

The renewed restriction of amyl nitrite posed a challenge for gay consumers, for whom I use pseudonyms to protect their privacy. T. M., who lived in San Francisco in the late 1960s, explained: "I can remember buying those boxes of Vaperole and you didn't need a prescription, things were a lot easier those days about getting chemicals. ... We all went in [the drugstore] on Friday afternoons, picking up our bottles [*sic*] of poppers." In the wake of a sharp restriction, demand for amyl nitrite poppers outpaced supply in the early 1970s. "It was still the preferred [poppers]," T. M. recalled, "[y]ou would look for someone who made bathtub amyl. It was hard to find doctors who

29 The first explanation was put forth by journalist David Reed in "The Multi-Million-Dollar Mystery High," *Christopher Street* 2 (1979): 21–27.

30 Reed, "The Multi-Million-Dollar Mystery High."

31 Jeremy A. Greene and Elizabeth Siegel Watkins, "Introduction: The Prescription in Perspective," in *Prescribed*, ed. Greene and Watkins, 2–3.

would write you scripts for amyls."[32] T. M. was not alone. Gay men tried to procure amyl nitrite from hospital stockpiles, friendly druggists, obliging doctors, and certain jurisdictions like Puerto Rico and British Columbia where amyl nitrite was still unrestricted. In 1976, a reported 330,000 boxes of amyl nitrite were sold annually far outpacing the only 5000 prescriptions written for it, while the street price for amyl nitrite reportedly skyrocketed from $2.50 to $15.[33] Low supplies and highs costs encouraged gay consumers to find creative alternatives alternative to amyl nitrite.

The most obvious solution was making poppers from butyl nitrite, which was molecularly similar but not regulated by the FDA. Butyl nitrite wasn't difficult to make. The compounding and titrating techniques required to make alkyl nitrites require only basic mixing equipment and perhaps an undergraduate-level knowledge of chemistry.[34] And through the experimental ethos that prompted off-label uses of amyl nitrite since the nineteenth century, users eventually trusted the similar effects of butyl nitrite inhalation. Over the 1970s, butyl nitrite production operations started in Chicago, Houston, Indianapolis, Los Angeles, Miami, New York, San Diego, San Francisco, and possibly more places.[35] These companies often tapped into or sprang from local economies in gay urban enclaves. The different origin stories of each company present a tapestry of queer practices. Often credited as the first successful brand of butyl nitrite poppers, Locker Room was manufactured by LA-based medical student Clifford Hassing. Jac Aroma, another early brand, was a product from the sex toy manufacturer Jac Masters. The brand Super Bullet was made by entertainment entrepreneur Jim Flock, who owned the Houston gay bar Silver Bullet Saloon. Brands like Locker Poppers and Crypt Tonight emerged as the in-house poppers brands of New York gay bookstore The Studio and San Diego erotic store the Crypt, respectively. And there was Liquid Hardware, produced in Indianapolis, curiously close to the Eli Lilly production headquarters, which remained a major producer of amyl nitrite for anti-poisoning kits.

32 Zoom Interview with T. M., poppers consumer, Toronto, conducted April 28, 2022.

33 See Dick Brass, "Sex and the Aching Heart: Angina Drug Sells Big to Lovers," *Daily News*, May 6, 1976; and Roger Watson, "Butyl Poppers the Other Juice That Puts More Hum in Your Cum!," *Queen's Quarterly: The Magazine for Gay Guys Who Have No Hangups*, December 1977.

34 This was the estimate of an entrepreneur making poppers in a major US city at the time of publication. In-person interview with M. P., butyl nitrite maker, conducted July 14, 2022.

35 This list was compiled by reviewing advertisements for poppers in *Drummer Magazine*, *Blueboy Magazine*, and *The Advocate* from 1974 to 1981.

Advertising butyl nitrite carried more legal risk than making them or selling them. Its oversight fell to the CPSC as a hazardous substance. But butyl nitrite did have some uses in industrial production; CPSC therefore limited its concern over whether manufacturers were telling consumers to inhale the product. In the 1970s and 1980s, federal regulatory agencies largely accepted this impasse. As one regulator stated in 1977: "The Commission [CPSC] has two options. We can require stronger labeling or we can ban it outright. Right now we don't have the data to back banning butyl nitrite products. What disturbs us is these manufacturers advertising it as a room deodorizer or incense when it is clearly sold for inhalation purposes."[36] Local law enforcement might respond in any number of ways. In 1978, the sheriff's office in Broward County, Florida, tried to shut down a local bookstore selling poppers. But they ran into an obstacle when they discovered the products being sold were butyl nitrite. As one sheriff anonymously told the *Fort Lauderdale News*: "We tried to get the adult book stores on a rap of operating as a pharmacy without a license by selling the stuff. ... But what it boiled down to was that their chemists were smarter than ours." Yet even if the sheriff couldn't do anything regarding butyl nitrite, they noted that the store stopped selling butyl nitrite after their visit.[37] Alternatively, one Chicago-based lawyer who represented local bathhouses and countless gay and trans clients targeted by vice squads, couldn't recall a single case he worked where police included possession of butyl nitrite in their charge. When police raided a now-defunct erotic bookstore, the lawyer remembered the police thumbed through magazines looking for obscene material but left the poppers alone. Two vendors of nitrites in different cities told me similar stories of local raids (although neither kept records nor could remember dates). In each case, a small group of federal officers went around to local stores and confiscated all their nitrite products, and local vendors collaborated hurriedly to move one another's product in advance of agents. These stories, some I have chosen to leave anonymized, reflect the haphazard regime of enforcement that periodically broke the general regulatory détente around nitrites.

Despite the risk of (albeit) uneven enforcement, many gay men persisted in poppers' gray market economy. "I was always concerned," said J. R., who co-operated a gay bathhouse from the 1970s to the 1990s, "but never enough to stop selling them." Although he paid attention to national regulatory battles, "particularly in California ... I thought in my mind, they know

36 From Wood, "A chronology of the regulation of volatile nitrites," 2.

37 Karen Snead, "FDA Allows OTC Sales of Drug, Butyl Nitrite," *Fort Lauderdale News*, April 24, 1978, 33.

how difficult it will be for the police [to stop poppers sales]."[38] The burgeoning number of gay bars, bathhouses, sex stores, and erotic bookstores offered an alternative point of sale than the pharmacies that had controlled amyl nitrite circulation until 1969. Many of these businesses had themselves been targets of criminalization or continued to operate semi-informally. The poppers gray market blended into the informal economies of other community institutions. Many of the informal economy practices continued intergenerationally through gay men's social networks. One key rule for was to never ask for or offer to sell poppers, and instead to refer to a particular brand name or a popular euphemism for the product. Many stores kept their poppers out of eyesight of walk-in customers, and some maintained valued customer lists specifically for selling. L. T. told me about a system he encountered in San Francisco's Castro district in the 1990s: "If you went in looking for poppers you were highly screened. They asked, 'How did you know about us?' and [they] ask people what bars they went to. If you passed their questions, you were given a card after your first purchase in the store. On return visits you could present the card and buy poppers."[39] Such tactics were reminiscent of underground gay bars of the 1950s and 1960s and show how knowledge around evading enforcement was applied to poppers sales.

In addition to increasing points-of-sale for poppers in gay urban enclaves, direct-to-consumer sales made poppers a national product. Print advertising shaped the discursive field through which butyl nitrite was elaborated as a gray market product. Like other parts of queer economies, the publication of these ads in the 1970s had only recently become legal, made possible by a wave of thirteen Supreme Court decisions beginning in the mid-1950s that challenged federal definitions and enforcement of obscenity.[40] Most consequentially, the court severely restricted the power of the US post office to limit sexually explicit material sent between consenting adults.[41] Today, these decisions are interpreted as the first Supreme Court cases promoting LGBTQ civil rights, and they paved the way for an immediate explosion in the national gay and lesbian press in the 1970s.[42]

38 In-person interview with L. T., San Francisco, conducted January 10, 2023.

39 In-person interview with J. R., former bathhouse operator, Chicago, conducted July 13, 2022.

40 Rodney A. Grunes, "Obscenity Law and the Justices: Reversing Policy on the Supreme Court," *Seton Hall Law Review* 9, no. 3 (1978): 403.

41 Jason M. Shepard, "The First Amendment and the Roots of LGBT Rights Law: Censorship in the Early Homophile Era, 1958–1962," *William & Mary Journal of Race, Gender, and Social Justice* 26, no. 3 (2019): 599.

42 Carlos A. Ball, "Obscenity, Morality, and the First Amendment: The First LGBT Rights Cases before the Supreme Court," *Columbia Journal of Gender & Law* 28, no. 2 (2014): 229; Gregory Briker, "The Right to Be Heard: ONE

Advertisements operated as a key semiotic technology where competing containment practices exercised control and through which the performative politics of the gray market emerged. Butyl nitrite manufacturers advertised in major gay publications of all stripes – from the BDSM-directed *Drummer* to the elite lifestyle magazine *Blueboy* to the mainstream *Advocate* and in gay city newspapers across the country. In addition to reaching consumers directly, manufacturers also advertised that they encouraged distributors to contact them to also sell their product.[43] By the early 1980s, some distributors themselves would advertise multiple brands and even sell sampler packs. Free from obscenity control, advertisements often portrayed white, shirtless, physically fit men (reflecting normative beauty standards) and used unsubtle references to sex to sell their product. Yet they were circumspect around the intended use and claimed physiological effects of their product. Advertisers implicitly communicated intended aphrodisiac properties of butyl nitrites as benefits while not letting regulators catch them explicitly directing consumers to inhale them. A thin line separated what could and couldn't be communicated. The euphemistic reference to their products as odorizers or liquid incense and some brand names like Locker Room and Dirty Feet communicated that these products were meant to somehow get up one's nose. And product branding like Locker Room's claim to be known for its "Power, Purity, and Potency" telegraphed the efficacy and quality control of their product properties. Finally, the most popular brand of poppers, Rush, made no apologies in its name about being a recreational substance.

Butyl nitrite manufacturers adapted to the realities of the gray market, even as some of them aspired to make the product legitimate in the eyes of the public and the state. The two most prominent producers of the 1970s, Clifford Hassing and W. Jay Freezer, both gave interviews to major news outlets while revealing few details about their businesses. Speaking to the *Wall Street Journal* in 1978, Freezer stated his hope that butyl nitrite would go mainstream enough to be sold in supermarkets.[44] Freezer wanted to convey scientific legitimacy and consumer safety to the product. To that end, Freezer founded a clinical research lab, Pharmex, which employed four university-credentialed researchers in the fields of pharmacology, cardiology, pulmonology, and sociology to research the effects of inhaling butyl nitrite. The group's single ninety-five-page publication, *Isobutyl Nitrites and Related Compounds* (1979), presented data on nitrite inhalants with an

---

Magazine, Obscenity Law, and the Battle Over Homosexual Speech," *Yale Journal of Law and the Humanities* 31 (2020): 64.

43 Joseph Jay Sosa, "Decoding Poppers Ads," *Queer Pasts* (forthcoming).

44 Stephen J. Sansweet, "A New Way to Glow And Giggle, and Get A Headache Besides," *Wall Street Journal*, October 10, 1977.

emphasis on butyl nitrite's vasodilatory properties, toxicology, and behavioral effects. The empirical evidence drew largely on emergency room survey data and a workplace toxicology study of people who worked at an isobutyl nitrite bottling facility.

Freezer's media statements and publications offer a glimpse into his vision of what a licit butyl nitrite industry might have looked like – one with standardized product testing, expert verification, brand reputation, regulatory cooperation, and consumer confidence. But regulatory oversight went in almost the exact opposite direction that Freezer envisioned. From 1976 to 1988 municipal, state, and federal government bodies made it harder, not easier, to sell butyl nitrite. As a result, poppers did not jump from queer enclaves to mainstream vendors. But neither were poppers sales extinguished by outright criminalization and police crackdowns. Far from resolving contradictions of the gray market, attempts at regulation only solidified the poppers industry's position between licit and illicit economies.

Regulating the Gray Market

At the 1981 meeting of the Society of Forensic Toxicologists, pharmacology professor Roger Maickel voiced his concerns over butyl nitrite: "My feeling is, some federal agency ought to take a stand and say 'These things are illegal,' before there is a spate of deaths that such action could have avoided or even impeded."[45] Despite Maickel's concern, he acknowledged that there were no reported deaths from inhaling butyl nitrite and two deaths from drinking butyl nitrite (which popper ads would have expressly dissuaded consumers from doing). Yet, Maickel insisted, "[r]ight now, if you get enough of this stuff in your body, medically, the chances of saving you are zero."[46] Maikel wasn't alone in his call for federal regulation. Beginning in 1977, municipal and state governments opened hearings on the safety of butyl nitrite – and many acknowledged their lack of jurisdiction over the classification of chemical products.

The concern over butyl nitrite was fueled by several factors. Poppers were increasing in prominence in advertisements, mainstream news articles, and popular media, and they were gaining the attention of the general public.[47] By the late 1970s, the consumer power movement in the United States was growing, marked by new regulatory agencies, consumer

45 "Disco Frenzy Drug Could Be Deadly, Professor Warns," *The Tampa Tribune*, November 6, 1981.

46 "Disco Frenzy Drug Could Be Deadly, Professor Warns."

47 Reed, "The Multi-Million-Dollar Mystery High," 22

watchdog groups, and landmark legislation, that focused on increased product safety and consumers' access to information.[48] Additionally, the Controlled Substances Act of 1970 introduced automated monitoring of controlled substances in hospitals, pharmacies, and other points of sale/service. New agencies like the Drug Abuse Warning Network (DAWN) and the National Institute on Drug Abuse (NIDA) began creating new epidemiological accounts of butyl nitrite, such as ER-visit counts, that provided an evidence-based justification for further containing the industry. To many of these new organizations, poppers appeared most similar to inhalants and were easily applied to concerns over teenager and adolescent misuse of everyday chemicals.

The first major test of the poppers industry was in Connecticut. In May 1977, after reportedly receiving complaints from several local police departments, Consumer Protection Commissioner Mary Heslin announced her intention to open hearings on the status of butyl nitrite.[49] Hartford, CT, police officer Lt. John Burns described butyl nitrite as "hav[ing] the same effect as glue."[50] For her part, Heslin commented: "The use of butyl nitrite to produce or remove household odors or for young people to obtain a high is extremely dangerous and cannot be permitted. The hazard of butyl nitrite vapors presents such a hazard to the public health and safety that the sale of such products should not be allowed to continue."[51] The hearings that took place in July elicited testimony from numerous actors. Former medical advertisement salesman Robert Kleinman testified that the product was being misused. Pharmacologist Alex Cardoni from the Connecticut Poison Information Center reported that he had received two calls for information about butyl nitrite but no complaints. Cardiologist John Parker and lawyer Alan Kaplan, both representing the San Francisco-based Pharmex, emphasized the lack of evidence towards butyl nitrite's toxicity. And Richard Ferjanec, identified by the Bridgeport *Post* as a church organist, testified to his personal consumption and insisted that he knew of no one who reported dangerous side effects.[52] The eventual ruling against butyl nitrite was the

48 For a background on the consumer regulation movement, see Michael Pertschuk, *Revolt against Regulation: The Rise and Pause of the Consumer Movement* (University of California Press, 1982).

49 Nancy Pappas, "Heslin Asks Butyl Nitrite Ban," *Hartford Courant*, May 17, 1977, 22.

50 Pappas, "Heslin Asks Butyl Nitrite Ban," 22.

51 "Ban Proposed on Sale of Butyl Nitrite," *Naugatuck Daily News*, May 17, 1977, 12.

52 "Butyl Nitrite Sales Ban Urged by Consumer Chief," *The Bridgeport Post*, July 21, 1977, 14.

first of a wave of state decisions from 1978 until 1986, when Congress would begin legislating butyl nitrite.

As debates over regulating butyl nitrite continued, the onset of the AIDS epidemic beginning in 1981 dramatically shifted the discussions on the risks of poppers. In the 1970s, questions about butyl nitrite toxicity dealt primarily with acute effects of overdosing and the risks of methoglobemia (poor oxygenation of the blood) or maculopathy (intense pressure on the eyes). At the outset of AIDS cases, poppers were suspected as a possible cause of the syndrome, and speculation about poppers-AIDS connections lasted long after the HIV virus was proven as the definitive cause of AIDS. Beyond discredited theories about poppers causing AIDS, the epidemic prompted additional studies on the chronic effects of poppers usage, including studies on carcinogenic and immunosuppressant effects.[53] These studies yielded no conclusive correlations, but the general risk-aversion prompted during the AIDS epidemic allowed for regulators to presume the risk of poppers as sound policy.

An early example of the new discourse on the risks of poppers took place in 1983, when the Board of Supervisors Public Health Committee held hearings on butyl nitrite. The city's public health commissioner Mervyn Silverman opened testimony at the hearings, explaining to the supervisors present: "I think we are dealing here with something here that is a little bit unique," highlighting misleading advertisements marketing poppers as "odorizers." Like the Connecticut police officer, Silverman also compared butyl nitrites to sniffing glue. Yet, unlike glue, Silverman contended, butyl nitrite had no constructive purpose. While refraining from making a direct link between poppers and AIDS, Silverman brought up the current health crisis in the gay community as another factor for which more epidemiological research was needed. Curiously, in their questions and statements, the Supervisors focused less on potential health hazards of butyl nitrite and more on what public officials could and could not do on the municipal level. Silverman lamented that only the state or federal government could prohibit the sale of butyl nitrite, and that the FDA had issued no rulings on butyl nitrite. Silverman proposed and the Supervisors concurred with a point-of-sale warning on all butyl nitrite sales in the city.

By 1987, the sale of butyl nitrite had been banned outright in nine states and prohibited for use as an intoxicant in another nine states.[54] Later campaigns to restrict poppers faced less opposition than earlier ones, as butyl nitrite manufacturers were most likely neither organized nor resourced

53 Anti-poppers consumer advocates Hank Wilson and John Lauritsen compiled these studies in their book *Death Drive: Poppers and AIDS.* 1986. Pagan Press.

54 National Association of State Controlled Substance Authorities, 1987 Survey. Source: Hank Wilson Papers, Box 7, Folder: Haverkos Laws 1988, GLBT Historical Society, San Francisco.

enough to defend their product amidst the increasing number of hearings. W. Jay Freezer, whose research company Pharmex had been a key figure in defending the industry, died in 1985. Ads for poppers also dropped precipitously. Whereas the number of butyl nitrite ads in *Drummer* magazine averaged 7.6 per issue between 1976 and 1979, that average dropped to 2.7 between 1980 and 1983. Other advertisements show how some manufacturers and distributors sought to maintain compliance even as new regulations and public health information were coming out. For instance, one distributor selling a six-pack sample of different nitrite products continually changed advertising warnings in their ads placed in *Drummer*. In Issue 57 (1980), distributors warned consumers that their product was not legal in Connecticut or Georgia, reflecting contemporary bans on butyl nitrite. By Issue 63 (1983), their warning label had been updated: "The health effects of nitrites/nitrates [*sic*] are currently under investigation. Offer void in CT and GA." These small changes to advertisements reflect nitrite manufacturers' and distributors' attempts to adapt to a changing regulatory field. Keeping this in mind, it is helpful to understand how butyl nitrite manufacturers responded when they did respond directly. Rather than arguing for the legitimacy of their product, manufacturers emphasized their adherence to the contradictory rules of the gray market.

Butyl nitrite manufacturers were largely absent in the debates over poppers regulation at the federal level that began in the 1980s. By the beginning of the decade, pharmacologists and consumer advocacy activists began petitioning the Environmental Protection Agency, the Food and Drug Administration, the Consumer Product Safety Commission, and the Federal Trade Commission in attempts to determine which agency might be able to pursue regulatory oversight over poppers.[55] These initial petitions were unsuccessful, but Congress eventually took up the question of butyl nitrite's unclear status in two omnibus drug bills. The Anti-Drug Abuse Act of 1986 mandated a review of alkyl nitrites to be conducted jointly by the FDA and the National Institute on Drug Abuse (NIDA). The FDA and NIDA were tasked with addressing four questions: (1) "the extent and nature" of alkyl nitrite use; (2) whether the use of products conformed to advertisements; (3) health risks to the product; and (4) a recommendation as to whether alkyl nitrites should be regulated by the Food, Drug, and Cosmetic Act of 1938. The two agencies responded to the questions in a way that reenforced the gray market status of poppers and also demonstrated the logics of queer containment. First, they maintained a strong distinction between amyl nitrite, which they described as "pleasant smelling, five carbon molecule," and butyl nitrite, which they described as "four carbon molecules" and "unpleasant,

55 For a partial list of these actions, see Wood, "A chronology of the regulation of volatile nitrites."

like a locker room or dirty socks."[56] Further, they argued: "butyl nitrite is much more volatile than amyl nitrite, and has never been marketed to treat any medical condition."[57] There was a certain circularity to their reasoning: butyl nitrite was never marketed as a medicine; therefore it had no ostensible medicinal properties. The report once again found butyl nitrite advertising misleading, but believed that the FDA should not regulate the substance. Essentially, the report maintained the status quo.

By the time of the Anti-Drug Abuse Act of 1988, sentiment against butyl nitrite had increased. Congressmen Mel Levine (D-CA) and John Conyers (D-MI) who wrote the butyl nitrite amendment to the 1988 bill were supported by major LGBT organizations like the National Gay and Lesbian Taskforce and Act Up Golden Gate.[58] The 1988 bill banned the sale of butyl nitrite for personal consumption, and instructed the CPSC to restrict sales of the substance except for "legitimate purposes." In the Anti-Drug Abuse Act of 1988, Congress followed up on the FDA/NIDA report by classifying butyl nitrite as a "banned hazardous product," except for "any commercial purpose other than for the production of consumer products containing butyl nitrite that may be used for inhaling or otherwise introducing butyl nitrite into the human body for euphoric or physical effects."[59] While ensuring oversight by the CPSC, the 1988 bill did little to change the de facto situation of butyl nitrite sales. Manufacturers could continue to use coded language to sell their products, or they might move to ethyl nitrite (which a few manufacturers did briefly). The 1988 bill failed, at least according to Hank Wilson. The San Francisco AIDS activist had been a strong supporter of 1983 municipal hearings to put safety warnings at butyl points-of-sale.

By 1994, Wilson busily wrote to media and politicians to warn that "poppers were back!" as a new generation of gay men coming of age after the first generation of the AIDS crisis were wholly unaware of their dangers.[60] "It's

56 "Study on Alkyl Nitrites (poppers), Section 4015 of Public Law 99–570, by the Department of Health and Human Services Food and Drug Administration, National Institute on Drug Abuse," 1986–1987. GLBT History Archives. Steve Morin Papers. 1994–02. Box 11, Folder 1. p 3

57 "Study on Alkyl Nitrites (poppers), Section 4015 of Public Law 99–570, by the Department of Health and Human Services Food and Drug Administration, National Institute on Drug Abuse," p. 3

58 Series II. Field Files: AIDS Project: Alphabetical Files: Poppers, 1986. MS The National Gay and Lesbian Taskforce Records, 1973–2000: Series II: Field Files Box 125, Folder 8. Cornell University Libraries, Archives of Sexuality & Gender, http://tinyurl.galegroup.com/tinyurl/BSK6w5.

59 Anti-Drug Abuse Act of 1988, Pub. L. No. 100-690, 102 Stat. 4181 (1988), Sec 2404.

60 Letter from Hank Wilson to Michael Elkins (Editor at *The Advocate*), March 23, 1994, GLBT Historical Society, Hank Wilson Papers (1996–02), Box 7, File: Media 94.

reasonable to sound the alarm," Wilson told *Out News* in 1990, "[i]t's fueling the epidemic."[61] Wilson's was an example of the continued consumer advocacy that sought to limit the butyl nitrite industry in the 1990s and 2000s. By lodging complaints or finding sympathizers in the federal government, Wilson and his small organization, called the Committee to Monitor Poppers, successfully prompted sporadic enforcement by the CPSC, especially when butyl nitrite crossed state lines. But the poppers industry continued relatively unabated well after the issue was settled by Congress. One possible rationale for continuing this gray market might be read in a 1994 memo from the United Kingdom Department of Trade and Industry to the CPSC. In the memo, the Department of Trade and Industry informed the CPSC that they did not intend on banning poppers, as this might "drive supply underground, most likely into the hands of suppliers of hard drugs, where the problems associated with misuse would, we believe, escalate with more serious consequences." While this by no means the represented the policies of the US government, it provides some insight as to a possible reason US regulators might ultimately be okay with the gray market economy.

Conclusion: Queering Pharmaceutics

In March 2025, in a coordinated national action, federal agents seized the inventory of three major butyl nitrite manufacturers and sex shops in several cities.[62] As no involved parties have spoken publicly at the time of writing, many details remain unclear. In the confusion, however, queer businesses and consumers quickly reverted to gray market tactics to contend with the uncertainty brought by federal actions. Vendors who weren't affected moved their poppers under the counter, and customers inquired after "leather cleaner" or other traditional euphemisms for poppers. Whole websites simply erased their online presence.[63] By June, however, poppers business seemed to return to usual, minus a few major manufacturers. These events are a reminder that the poppers industry was born out of imposed scarcity and adapted to a pharmaceutical market that could never quite determine its

61 Randy Dotinga, "San Francisco Wants Poppers Regulated," PlanetOut.com, October 31, 2004. Printout accessed GLBT Historical Society, Hank Wilson Papers (1996–02), Box 7, File: SF 2004.

62 Sonja Sharp, "FDA Crackdown on Poppers Prompts Rush on Popular Gay Party Drug," *Los Angeles Times*, March 21, 2025.

63 On vendors changing sales practices in Los Angeles, see Sharp, "FDA Crackdown on Poppers." I also witnessed altered sales practices when visiting three stores in Chicago on March 15, 2025. After first reporting via Instagram that they had been raided by federal agents, Double Scorpio, a company based in Austin, TX, removed all online content, a move followed by other vendors.

licit or illicit status. Scarcity is cyclical in the poppers market. A major manufacturer folds, or a regulation changes, or an epidemic causes panic. Yet the fundamentals of its gray market status remain unchanged.

The queer containment of the poppers industry has worked for so long because risk and benefit are calculated differently in distinct spheres of drug regulation, leading to a performative imbalance in the way such claims can be made and assessed. In pharmaceutic markets, claims of effectiveness can be crafted through credentialed experts, clinical trials, and frameworks of benefits that emphasize therapeutic value rather than say pleasure or sexual health.[64] No such apparatus exists in prohibition markets or gray markets, where benefits can only be referenced in code. Claims of risk don't need to be authoritative in the same way to be successful. When discussing prohibition, evidence is needed to refute risk, but not to sustain its consideration. US federal regulators maximized this uneven performative field to maintain the indeterminate status of poppers at every opportunity. Their continued scrutiny of advertisements, the site where contradictions became unavoidable, shows how these impasses were managed rather than resolved. Trying to keep adolescents away from amyl nitrite laid the groundwork for butyl nitrite as a queer chemical commodity. Further restriction ran the risk of pushing this industry ever more underground.

But the status quo relies on not saying the obvious, at least with respect to poppers' benefits. One cannot claim that vasodilation causes pleasure, at least not in the sphincter. (Meanwhile, the vasodilator sildenafil has become a blockbuster pharmaceutical for erectile disfunction.) At the same time, poppers' risks, such as FDA warnings about butyl nitrite fatalities if drunken (2021), or confusing poppers with five-hour energy drink bottles (2023), ignore the fact gay men's communal knowledge that would find such practices absurd.[65] These FDA warnings effectively shield the wider public from knowledge about poppers as much as they contain poppers use itself. This shows that gray market drugs like poppers are not exceptions to the logic of pharmaceutic governance; they are central to it.

64 For more on prioritizing therapeutic value over pleasure see Kane Race, *Pleasure Consuming Medicine: The Queer Politics of Drugs* (Duke University Press, 2009).

65 Adam Mack, "This Man Does Not Make Poppers," *BuzzFeed News*, July 27, 2021, https://www.buzzfeednews.com/article/davidmack/poppers-factory; Nick Logan, "The FDA Says People Are Confusing Poppers with Energy Shots, and Dying. Experts Want Proof," *CBC News*, June 4, 2023, https://www.cbc.ca/news/health/fda-poppers-energy-shots-warning-1.6863960.

Contributors

Beat Bächi, University of Zurich

Beat Bächi is a historian who undertakes research at the University of Zurich (Institute of Biomedical Ethics and History of Medicine, Chair for the History of Medicine). He is the author of *LSD auf dem Land. Produktion und kollektive Wirkung psychotroper Stoffe* (Konstanz: University Press, 2nd edition 2024) and co-authored together with Magaly Tornay *Drogen. Zur Einführung* (Hamburg: Junius 2025). He is currently working on a social history of pigs in Switzerland.

Bob Beach, University at Albany, SUNY

Bob Beach is an adjunct instructor at Mohawk Valley Community College. His dissertation examines user perspectives on cannabis in the United States during the 1920s and 1930s, and he is a former contributor to "Points," the blog of the Alcohol and Drug History Society. He lives in Rome, NY with his wife and one-year old daughter. When not teaching or parenting, Bob performs standup comedy.

Christian Bonah, Université de Strasbourg

Christian Bonah is Professor for the History of Health and Life Sciences at the University of Strasbourg. He has worked on comparative history of medical education, medicaments, human experimentation, and drug scandals. Recently he was principal investigator of the ERC-funded "BodyCapital" project on twentieth-century health history through audiovisual sources and of the ARCHIMED project "Mining medical archives and pathological collections in the digital age."

Nancy D. Campbell, Rensselaer Polytechnic Institute

Nancy D. Campbell is Professor of Science and Technology Studies at Rensselaer Polytechnic Institute and author of *OD: Naloxone and the Politics of Overdose Prevention* (MIT Press, 2020); *Discovering Addiction: The Science and Politics of Substance Abuse Research* (University of Michigan Press, 2007); *Gendering Addiction: The Politics of Drug Treatment in a Neurochemical World* (co-authored with Elizabeth Ettorre; Palgrave, 2011); *The Narcotic Farm: The Rise and Fall of America's First Prison for Drug Addicts* (co authored with J. P. Olsen and Luke Walden; Abrams, 2008); and *Using Women: Gender, Drug Policy, and Social Justice* (Routledge, 2000).

Joséphine Eberhart, Laboratoire IRISSO, Université Paris Dauphine, and Cermes3, Université Paris Cité

Joséphine Eberhart holds a PhD in sociology. She is affiliated with the IRISSO laboratory (CNRS, INRAE, Paris Dauphine University) and is an associate researcher at the Cermes3 laboratory (CNRS, Inserm, EHESS, Université Paris Cité). Her research in the social sciences of health focuses on studying healthcare professions through the lens of medicines. Sited at the intersection of science and technology studies and the sociology of health, her work explores why certain drugs become particularly successful among specific categories of prescribers, such as general practitioners or veterinarians.

Joseph M. Gabriel, Florida State University

Joseph M. Gabriel is Associate Professor in the Department of Behavioral Sciences and Social Medicine at Florida State University. He writes about the history of pharmaceuticals, intellectual property, ethics, and related topics. He lives in Tallahassee.

Jeremy A. Greene, Johns Hopkins School of Medicine

Jeremy A. Greene, MD, PhD is William H. Welch Professor of Medicine and History of Medicine at Johns Hopkins School of Medicine. Dr. Greene's published books and articles explore the ways in which medical technologies influence our understandings of what it means to be sick or healthy, normal or abnormal, on personal, regional, and global scales. His newest project, *Syringe Tide: Disposable Technologies and the Making of Medical Waste*, focuses on the shift towards disposable technologies in hospitals and clinics, with inevitable environmental consequences.

Avery Gulino, University at Massachusetts

Avery Gulino, MD, is a first-year Internal Medicine resident at the University of Massachusetts. Dr. Gulino earned her Bachelor's degree in the History of Science, Medicine, and Technology from Johns Hopkins University before attending Cooper Medical School at Rowan University in Camden, New Jersey. Throughout her medical training, Avery has maintained a deep appreciation for history and strives to understand the broader context in which she meets her patients, integrating their experiences, environments, and stories into compassionate, informed care.

David Herzberg, University at Buffalo, State University of New York

David Herzberg is Professor of History and Director of the Drugs, Health, and Society program at the University at Buffalo (SUNY). His research explores the nature and trajectory of drug commerce, drug use, and drug policy in America, with a primary focus on psychoactive pharmaceuticals.

He is author, among other books and articles, of *White Market Drugs: Big Pharma and the Hidden History of Addiction in America.*

Nils Kessel, Université de Strasbourg
Nils Kessel is Associate Professor (maître de conférences) at Université de Strasbourg. He holds a PhD in history and his research focuses on the history of drugs and medicines, particularly user practices, medical markets, and the pharmaceutical industry. Nils is also interested in the history of emergency medicine and currently works on sustainable disaster risk reduction.

Solène Lellinger, Laboratoire SPHERE (UMR 7219) – Université Paris Cité
Solène Lellinger is Associate Professor in History and Philosophy of Health in medicine faculty at Université Paris Cité. Her research focuses on the socio-history of therapeutic agents, which she studies through their production, regulation, monitoring, and use in care relationships. She leads the research project VIGICAMENT "Monitoring drugs: changes in the actors and practices involved in surveillance of therapeutic agents since 1970" funded by the French National Research Agency.

Dan Malleck, Brock University
Dan Malleck, Professor of Health Sciences, is a medical historian specializing in drug and alcohol policy. His books include *Try to Control Yourself: The Regulation of Public Drinking in Post-Prohibition Ontario* (2012); *When Good Drugs Go Bad: Opium, Medicine, and the Origins of Canada's Drug Laws* (2015); and *Liquor in the Liberal State: Drink and Order Before Prohibition* (2022), as well as three edited collections.

Alex Mold, London School of Hygiene & Tropical Medicine
Alex Mold is Professor of Public Health History at the London School of Hygiene & Tropical Medicine. Her research focuses on the history of public health in Britain since 1945. Alex is especially interested in the history of substance use, including illegal drugs and alcohol. She is a Co-Investigator on a Wellcome Trust Discovery Award project entitled "Kicking the habit," which examines the history of "addictive" sports sponsorship in Britain since 1965.

Samuel K. Roberts Jr., Columbia University
Dr. Samuel Kelton Roberts Jr., PhD, is Associate Professor of History (Columbia University School of the Arts and Sciences) and Sociomedical Sciences (Columbia University's Mailman School of Public Health), and is also a former Director of Columbia University's Institute for Research in African American Studies (IRAAS). Dr. Roberts writes, teaches, and lectures

widely on African American urban history, especially medicine, public health, and science and technology. Roberts is currently researching and writing a book-length project on the United States's troubled history of race and recovery, examining the social and political history of heroin addiction treatment from the 1950s to the early 1990s.

Caroline Rusterholz, Graduate Institute, Geneva and Fribourg University
Caroline Rusterholz is assistant professor at the Graduate Institute, Geneva, and professor at Fribourg University. She has published widely on the transnational history of sexual and reproductive health, population, and family in the twentieth century. She leads the research project "RE:SHARE. Race and Ethnicity: Sexual Health and Reproductive Experiences in postwar Britain," which explores the racialization of sexual and reproductive health (SRH) charities and the ways that minoritized communities advocated for their SRH needs.

Joseph Jay Sosa, Bowdoin College
Joseph Jay Sosa is Associate Professor of Gender, Sexuality, and Women's Studies at Bowdoin College in Brunswick, ME. A political anthropologist and queer theorist, his work focuses on sexual governmentality, ideology, citizenship, and political affect. He is the author of *Brazil's Sex Wars: The Aesthetics of Queer Activism in São Paulo.*

Index

Printed and bound by CPI Group (UK) Ltd, Croydon, CR0 4YY

15/09/2026

14962416-0003